Getting
the Sex
You Want

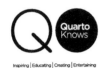

Inspiring | Educating | Creating | Entertaining

Brimming with creative inspiration, how-to projects, and useful information to enrich your everyday life, Quarto Knows is a favorite destination for those pursuing their interests and passions. Visit our site and dig deeper with our books into your area of interest: Quarto Creates, Quarto Cooks, Quarto Homes, Quarto Lives, Quarto Drives, Quarto Explores, Quarto Gifts, or Quarto Kids.

This book is dedicated to Bruce,
who has shown me true passion and love.

Text © 2008 Tammy Nelson
Paperback edition published 2013

First published in 2008 by Quiver,
an imprint of The Quarto Group,
100 Cummings Center, Suite 265-D,
Beverly, MA 01915, USA.
T (978) 282-9590 F (978) 283-2742
www.QuartoKnows.com

Quiver titles are also available at discount for retail, wholesale, promotional, and bulk purchase. For details, contact the Special Sales Manager by email at specialsales@quarto.com or by mail at The Quarto Group, Attn: Special Sales Manager, 100 Cummings Center, Suite 265-D, Beverly, MA 01915, USA.

ISBN: 978-1-59233-526-8

Library of Congress Cataloging-in-Publication Data
Nelson, Tammy.
    Getting the sex you want : shed your inhibitions and reach
new heights of passion together / Tammy Nelson.
        p.   cm.
    ISBN 1-59233-301-X
    1. Imago relationship therapy. 2. Marital psychotherapy.
3. Communication in sex. I. Title.
RC488.5.N45 2008
616.89'1562--dc22
                                    2007051459

Book design and layout: Rachel Fitzgibbon

Printed in USA

Getting
the Sex
You Want

Shed Your Inhibitions
and Reach New Heights
of Passion Together

Tammy Nelson, Ph.D.

QUIVER

CONTENTS

INTRODUCTION

In my clinical work as a psychotherapist over the past twenty-five years, I have discovered that couples have a greater likelihood of staying together, and for longer periods of time, when they improve their sexual communication skills.

Unfortunately, the therapeutic world has had little training in helping couples explore their sexuality and communicate their erotic needs. If therapists are inexperienced when it comes to talking about sex, how can they help their clients work on these issues in their relationships?

Using a communication method called the "Imago dialogue," I have developed specific techniques that have helped men and women recharge their relationships, and bring passion back into their lives. It's not unusual for couples to be relieved after learning how to talk about their fantasies and fears and discovering what can happen just from doing the exercises in these chapters. Anyone who hopes to be in a satisfying relationship can benefit from this work (and play!).

Learning ways to communicate about sex can help you become a better lover; you will bring more skills to your relationship. The intensity and eroticism will deepen, and the passion between you and your partner can connect the two of you for life.

Using the Imago dialogue is a new way of exploring your sexuality together that can bring you to new places. It provides you with a structure in which to explore your deepest fantasies and desires. It will give you the safety to talk to each other and finally experience being seen and heard. You will find a new way to ask for the sex you have always wanted. Perhaps there are parts of your sex life that you currently enjoy. There might also be some new things you would like to try. Maybe you have sexual desires that you have been afraid to talk about. Now you will have a language in which to express these desires.

Imago therapy was developed by Harville Hendrix, the author of the best-selling book, *Getting the Love You Want*. His book has helped thousands of couples around the world ask for what they want and express their love for each other. Now you can use these time-tested techniques to expand your love-making and experience the intimacy and connection that will give you the passion you want and create a truly long-lasting partnership.

When you learn how to talk openly about sex, you will experience a greater level of intimacy and safety in your relationship. Loving feelings will then naturally increase toward your partner. A vital and healthy interest in sex along with a passionate curiosity for life are the ways to keep your relationship alive for a very long time.

Long-Term Passion Starts with Early Communication

"Imago: An idealized mental image of another person or the self."
—*The Merriam-Webster Dictionary*

"Normal wife" closes her book and lies back on her pillows, exhausted. She listens for the kids, wondering whether they will get up for water or to use the bathroom. The night before, both children had climbed into bed with her and her husband and she wonders whether they are both coming down with colds.

She remembers that she has forgotten to check the dryer and let the cat in for the night. She thinks about getting up, but her feet are cold and she snuggles down deeper into the bed. Every muscle aches from her day—running to the grocery store, cleaning out her son's closet, picking up her husband's shirts at the dry cleaners, and painting the hall bathroom. She scratches her head for a moment, running her fingers through her hair and tries to remember whether she took a shower that day. Her flannel shirt and boxer shorts are warm and she closes her eyes for just a moment.

Another thought suddenly occurs to her. She wonders whether her husband will want to have sex tonight. She rolls over and pretends to sleep.

"Average husband" sits in bed with his laptop balanced on his knees. He peruses the long list of e-mails he has still not opened from work that day. He glances over at his wife as she snuggles down lower in the bed. He sees she is wearing her flannel shirt. He wonders whether this is the signal that there will be no sex again tonight.

Sighing, he turns back to his computer and flips down through his e-mails until he comes to one unfamiliar e-mail address. Unsure whether it is spam, he hesitates for a moment, and then clicks on it. It is a poorly disguised invitation to visit a porn site. He sneaks another glance at his wife, and she rolls over onto her side away from him. He clicks on the link. His computer screen immediately flashes onto a catalog of young, busty, half-clad girls promising to fulfill all of his erotic dreams. He moves his cursor over one particular girl, who looks him in the eye, and he clicks on her image. A larger shot of her, with her legs spread open, invites him to charge $9.99 to his credit card for another peak, to go deeper into the site.

He sighs, and taking his glasses off of his face, rubs his tired eyes. What he really wants is to have sex with his wife, to feel connected to her. But he wonders where the passion and energy have gone.

Getting over the Fear of Talking about Sex

Marriage and long-term cohabitation breed familiarity, which can lead to a mundane erotic life. Marital familiarity can be comforting, but it doesn't lend itself to intense passion and sexual connection.

Learning to communicate sexual needs and desires early in a relationship can help contribute to an easier and smoother erotic connection later on. Sometimes it's scary to talk about sex, especially in the beginning phases of a relationship. And yet, an early pattern of relating to each other in an open and honest way can make sex more rewarding later on. Consider the following example:

Girlfriend "A" lies under Boyfriend "B." It is a Saturday night, and they are having sex. Missionary style.

This feels good, she thinks, but she wonders whether she should try and tell him that she would like to make love in a different way, using a new position. They have had sex in the missionary position every Saturday night for weeks now. How can she talk to him about what she would really like?

He seems to try so hard, she thinks. Her thoughts jump around as she lies under him: "I don't want to make him think I don't appreciate how hard he

He wonders whether his girlfriend will still want to have sex with him if he can't perform like the porn stars. His performance is a large part of what makes him feel like a man.

is trying to please me. But I wonder what else there is? And I wonder if he would mind if I used my own hand to give myself an orgasm? I don't think I could ever ask him that. I wonder if I should just fake an orgasm and make him feel good?"

As Boyfriend "B" pumps into his girlfriend he worries that he might lose his erection. It has never happened before, but he has heard stories from his buddies that sometimes they have a tough time staying hard. He wonders whether she will still want to have sex with him if he can't perform like the porn stars. His performance is a large part of what makes him feel like a man. What happens if he can't always please her?

"What if I can't last?" he thinks. "What if I come too soon?"

He keeps pushing inside her, trying not to focus on how good it feels. He begins to feel more anxious. He wonders whether he can hold out until she climaxes. He wonders whether he will he know when she comes.

"How long does it take her to come?" he thinks to himself.

He has never asked her, nor has she told him. He would like to know because he wants desperately to please her. He begins to feel the buildup and knows he is getting closer to ejaculating.

"Oh, boy, please let me last," he thinks. "I need to try harder not to think about what feels so good. This can't be the way it's supposed to be. Aren't I supposed to be gazing into her eyes or something? Maybe I should think about baseball."

Getting the Erotic Connection

Like the couples above, many people are not having the sex they really want and they aren't talking about it. Most couples want more sex, or better sex, and they don't know how to ask for it. How do we get the sex we really want? And how do we tell our partner what our fantasies are?

By using a technique called the Imago dialogue, this book will teach you and your partner ways to resexualize your partnership and have the erotic connection you truly desire. Exercises will teach you how to increase passion and connection with your partner. Writing exercises will help you clarify what you need in your erotic life—you will discover what your fantasies are and what your sexual needs are all about. You'll learn better ways to communicate with one another and talk about your deepest desires.

If you practice these skills, you *will* get the sex you want!

Introducing Imago

Imago relationship therapy was created by Harville Hendrix and Helen Hunt, authors of the book *Getting the Love You Want*, a national best-seller describing a revolutionary new way to love. The development of Imago relationship therapy is based on the theory that we choose a partner, many times unconsciously, who is perfectly suited to us, based on our image, or *imago* in Latin, that we have created from all of our experiences from childhood.

These partners have the unique ability to heal our childhood wounds. They have qualities that are similar to the positive and negative qualities of our original caretakers, and cleverly, we have chosen them because they hold the special characteristics that, when combined with our own personality traits, will help us to finish all of our unfinished business from childhood. We will get the love we always wanted! It is no coincidence that we choose the mates we do based on their similarities to and differences from our childhood experiences.

Because of this amazing and uncanny ability we all have to pick our partner, we end up with someone who can also bring up all of our issues! Although our partners can heal us from our pain like no one else, they can also hurt us in some of the same places where we have leftover wounds from childhood.

This is why relationships seem like such hard work sometimes—and why they feel so painful.

We continue to be wounded again and again in the same places that have hurt since we were young. Our partners have an almost magical way of poking us in those vulnerable places like no one else can. And yet we seem determined to continue our old behaviors, hoping against hope that if we keep repeating the same thing over and over, we will somehow get our partner to stop wounding us and give us the love we really want.

On the other hand, the partner we choose often fills our needs from childhood that were left out of our parenting. Even in the best of childhoods, we sometimes don't get our needs met. Mom doesn't always hear us when we cry; Dad doesn't always come running when we are hungry. And that's okay. Having "good enough" parents enables us to grow up and take care of ourselves as independent, functioning adults.

We then fall in love with people because we love who we are when we are with them. We feel they fulfill us in ways we cannot feel fulfilled alone. We feel safe, connected, and relaxed.

However, when they no longer complete us, or fulfill all of our needs, we no longer love ourselves when we are with them. We then withdraw from them or attack them. We are no longer quite sure how to get our needs met. We enter a power struggle or conflict stage. We either run away or settle in. If we decide to stay, we put on the old sweatpants and prepare for the long haul. This is the point where the sexual needs in the relationship begin to get split off. The sex slows down. The passion wanes. We no longer feel "in love." Some of us split off from our sexual needs; others compartmentalize their need for sex into a box deep inside themselves.

Sometimes we have a fantasy that if we trade in our partners for someone new, we might be happier. And sometimes we do. And for a while that new relationship feels better because we get to experience the romantic phase again, and all is well. However, slowly we slide back into conflict and out come the sweatpants, and we find ourselves back in that power struggle place where sex becomes maintenance sex and sometimes even part of the power struggle.

To avoid this scenario and to stay connected and experience romance and passion over the long term, communicating is the first step. But communicating is not the only step. Having a safe way to talk will increase the passion in your partnership, and many times that passion will improve your communication. Taking the first step toward communicating means sitting down together and starting with exercises like the one described below, exchanging appreciation the Imago way.

The Difference between Dialogue and Conversation

Often when we are talking with our partners—particularly when it's over a conflict—we don't really listen. We have a tendency to prepare our "rebuttal" before they even finish their sentence. We respond and cut them off before they say what they wanted to say. They then don't feel heard. And they don't feel seen for who they are.

Using the Imago dialogue, couples can practice really listening to each other and asking for what they need in the relationship. This way of communicating can go a long way toward healing our unmet needs. It can also bring us the love we truly want.

Participating in a conversation is different than being in a dialogue. Being in a dialogue means you are each totally present and in the moment, that is, you are focused solely on what your partner is saying, and not on what your response is going to be. When we listen intensely to what our partners are saying, we are more available to hear what they are trying to tell us. They experience us differently in those moments. They feel our presence, and not our distraction.

We can use the Imago process to reconnect sexually and improve our intimacy. The beginning steps of creating long-term, passionate partnerships involve working on the erotic connection as well as the companionship piece of our relationships. This includes learning to talk about sexual needs. The way to do this is to feel safe enough to share our desires and fantasies with our partner. Using the structure of the Imago dialogue, this sometimes difficult conversation becomes an experience of being deeply held and listened to by our partner.

Participating in a conversation is different than being in a dialogue. Being in a dialogue means you are focused solely on what your partner is saying, and not on what your response is going to be.

Beginning the Imago Dialogue

The Imago dialogue process involves two people—the person doing the talking—the **sender**—and the other person who is listening—the **receiver**.

For our partners to hear us, or "receive" the information we want to "send" them, we have to somehow pave the way. In other words, we have to make it safe. Most of us get defensive right away when our partners are trying to have a "serious" conversation with us. We are afraid of being criticized or that we will have to defend ourselves from something we may have done wrong. We also want to make sure they are able to hear what we are saying.

The best way to create safety for them is to start off all of our dialogues with an **appreciation.** Most of us respond well when we hear positive feedback about ourselves. So, we always start a dialogue with something we appreciate about our partner. An appreciation is something that we like about our partner. Perhaps it is an action that he has taken, or something he has done that has meaning for you. Perhaps it is a part of her personality that you love.

For instance, telling your partner that you appreciate him can mean recognizing something he does. Perhaps you normally wouldn't take the time to mention it. These can be simple things, such as "How nice he remembered that I like my coffee with sugar instead of cream." Or "I really appreciate that she came to therapy with me." Or "I am so appreciative that he mowed the lawn."

Appreciations are a way of getting more of what we want, and also a way of softening our relationship with our partner. Often our partners do things in our daily life that we appreciate but neglect to mention, when a few words from us could mean so much to them. Our relationship becomes softer when there is less tension and criticism and more positive feedback.

Try this exercise with your partner. Remember there is no right or wrong way to do this. This is the beginning of practicing a new way of talking and relating to your partner. It may feel awkward at first. That's fine. Try it anyway! Fumbling around is one way we learn how to do something that we haven't mastered yet.

EXERCISE
Exchanging Appreciations the Imago Way

For this first exercise, you will need at least fifteen minutes of uninterrupted private time together. Find a quiet place where you can sit comfortably facing each other in chairs, on the floor, or on a bed, and maintain eye contact for the entire exercise.

You are beginning the process of a new form of communication, the Imago dialogue. You will build on this format throughout the book, creating a safe structure to talk about your relationship, and later your erotic needs and fantasies. Let's start by sharing some appreciations, and learning how to **mirror** each other. This is a basic dialogue skill, explained below, and one we will use for many of the more advanced exercises to come.

This exercise will feel awkward and even a little corny in the beginning. The words may feel stilted and forced at first. Don't worry about that yet. Let the exercise feel awkward for now. Later it will feel more comfortable and you will use the technique effortlessly while talking about more erotic topics.

You may find yourself giggling or breaking eye contact. That's fine. You may feel the urge to get up and look in the refrigerator or make a phone call or check your e-mail. Try to stay focused on the exercise for the duration of both sending and receiving. The sender is the first one to talk, and the receiver is the first one to listen.

Step One
First, choose who will be the sender and who will be the receiver. The sender will talk, and the receiver's only job is to listen and mirror exactly what the sender says. **Mirroring means saying back what the sender has said with no other comments.**

Step Two

Senders will say or "send" over three things they appreciate about their partner. An example might be the following:

Sender: "I appreciate that you are having a dialogue with me tonight."

Step Three

After each appreciation, receivers will simply repeat, or mirror, what the sender has said. Continuing the example above, the receiver will simply say back while maintaining eye contact, "You appreciate that I am having a dialogue with you tonight."

In all Imago dialogues, there are only two responses a receiver might have:

1. "Please send that again" if they didn't understand or remember what they heard. Then the sender would simply repeat it and the receiver would try mirroring again.

2. Receivers mirror back what the sender says and then ask, "Is there more?"

The sender can say "yes" and send more or "no" and stop there. After three appreciations, the sender switches and becomes the receiver.

Exploring Sexual Curiosity with Empathy

The possibility of waking up a partnership and experiencing that erotic charge again sometimes feels impossible. And yet, throughout our life cycle, we continue to have erotic needs and crave intimacy through sex.

The way to increasing the erotic connection in a relationship is to begin talking to each other and empathizing with your partner. Mirroring is the first step in using these exercises, where you will practice sharing and listening.

You will, through this book, come to understand normal erotic curiosity. Erotic curiosity is simply a way to define our thoughts, fantasies, and sexual desires. We all have curiosity about things that are sexual, and we explore erotic thoughts and fantasies in our minds all the time, even if we don't

(continued on page 18)

Exploring Sexual Curiosity (continued)

share these thoughts with our partner. Understanding our partners' erotic fantasy life will help us understand what will make them happy and give us clues about what will give them a passionate, loving partnership.

In our relationship, sexual empathy needs to be present to make exploring fantasies safe. Sexual empathy means feeling connected to your partner so that you can share your fantasies. If you know that you will not be judged or dismissed by your lover for having erotic curiosity, then you will be more likely to share those thoughts.

Sexual empathy does not mean your partner will agree with your thoughts and fantasies or want to act them out with you. Sexual empathy instead means that you understand that these are your partner's erotic thoughts, and not your own. Empathy also includes being happy that your partner feels safe enough to share them with you. Feeling safe enough in a relationship to share your fantasies is a big step toward finding passion and connection.

However, we can only share our fantasies when we feel safe and respected. If we know that our partner will listen and mirror back what we are saying without judgment, then we will be more likely to share our thoughts and desires.

The Imago dialogue process is a great way to make this happen. If we can share our erotic thoughts and fantasies in a dialogue, our partner simply mirrors back what we are saying and doesn't have to respond. We then feel listened to and heard. We can talk without fear that there will be any response at all, either positive or negative. This creates a space for the fantasy to be expressed.

Sexual empathy means your partner will listen to your erotic thoughts and hold that space. We will talk more about how to be a more sexually empathetic partner later on in this book.

The Risk of Revealing Yourself

Talking about sex can be hard, even with a partner you have known for years. We think that the longer we are in a relationship with a partner, the easier it will be to communicate what we really want in bed. It's not. It actually becomes more difficult, because in the beginning of a relationship there is less to lose.

We take different risks in our sexuality. In the beginning of a relationship, we are able to share parts of ourselves in ways that we later repress. As we begin to feel safe with our partner, our sex becomes "safer," and we shut down the more wild parts of us for fear of hurting our partner or hurting the safety of our connection. If our relationship is to remain safe, we strive to keep the sex safe.

One of the ways that couples can begin to share their fantasies is through this next exercise, in which we will build and expand upon the first exercise. Using the appreciation dialogue outlined above, we will add to what we've learned, creating a safe space to begin to talk about sex. This is a great way for couples to create an opening in which an erotic conversation can happen. Remember, appreciation is the way to create that opening. If you want to get your needs met, appreciation is the doorway in.

EXERCISE
Starting to Talk about Sex

For this exercise, you will need at least twenty-five minutes of uninterrupted private time together. Find a quiet place where you can sit comfortably facing each other in chairs, on the floor, or on a bed to maintain eye contact for the entire exercise.

You may want to turn down the lights, put on soft music, light some candles, and put on comfortable and sexy clothes. Setting the right mood is a great way to get started, and can help lead to more passion later on.

First, we'll start by again sharing appreciations and mirroring each other. This is a basic dialogue skill, and one we will use for many of the more advanced exercises to come. This may still feel awkward, but you may have now felt some of the nice feelings that come with the experience of being mirrored. The words may still feel

(continued on page 20)

(continued)

stilted and forced. Don't worry. How fast you get this is not a reflection of how much you care about each other. Let the exercise feel awkward for now. Giggle, squirm, blush, and feel silly... it's all normal.

Try to stay focused on the exercise for the duration of both sending and receiving.

Step One

First, choose who will be the sender and who will be the receiver. Senders will "send" over one thing they appreciate about their partner. Receivers will mirror back what the sender says.

Step Two

Senders will send over one thing they appreciate about their partner sexually. Receivers will mirror this back as well.

Step Three

Finally, senders will say one thing they really like sexually and would like more of. Receivers should try not to comment on what their partner is saying, but just mirror back exactly. This is important. The receiver does not need to agree, make promises, refuse, make excuses, or answer in any way. There does not need to be any response whatsoever. This exercise is only about mirroring.

Again, there are only two responses a receiver might make—"please send that again," or the receiver can mirror back what the sender says and then ask, "Is there more?" The sender then can say "yes" and send more or "no" and stop there.

Now that you have shared your appreciations for each other, how do you feel? Can you tell your partner what it was like to hear those things? Try not to judge what you heard, or disagree, or argue. You do not have to agree, compromise, or commit. Just sit with what you heard. You can ask questions, but try to soak up the appreciation for now.

The History of Love

Men and women have different emotional needs, and physically respond differently during sex. But we have one thing in common—we are all looking for love.

"Eros," or the creative urge to love, is also the drive to stay alive and to live passionately. Eros is what makes us feel desire in our relationships, giving us that wonderful, energized feeling that we all long for. This is the energy we call passion.

Love is natural; it is the instinct for passion, or the Eros urge. Eros was a figure from Greek mythology; the son of Aphrodite, the Greek goddess of love. As the representation of all that was passionate, romantic, and sexual, Eros was worshipped as a god of fertility—he was the *life* urge. Ancient Greeks felt Eros represented unbridled sexual passion. Yet he was also famous, like Cupid, for being deceitful, overly playful, and unfaithful to his lovers. In English, "Eros" is the root of the word *erotic*.

The Romans had their own interpretation of Eros; they called him Cupid, the god of love. Cupid tortured his lovers with arrows that put them under his spell and left them powerless. The name *Cupid* is a variation of Cupido, from Ancient Rome, meaning "desire," and this god was also known by the name Amor, or "love." It was thought that Cupid was the son of Venus, the Roman goddess of love.

Eros is at the root of our archetype of erotic love and gives us our concepts of the lover overcome with passion, undone by need, and slain in the heart by love. Our understanding of love in relationships is that it is a passionate, intense emotional bond, solidified by intimacy and connected most deeply by desire.

Is it any wonder that we want to stay in this stage of a relationship? We want that passionate, intense energy. It feeds us and makes us feel alive. This is how we identify love. When that energy fades, we fear that we have fallen out of love.

(continued on page 22)

The History of Love (continued)

Yet much of the early stage of love is about brain chemistry. Our bodies release hormones and brain chemicals that actually make us feel high, and these chemicals promote attachment to each other. Unfortunately, our brains cannot maintain that level of chemical production indefinitely. So, over time, the hormones naturally decrease and our brain chemistry returns to normal. We lose that intense state of desire we call "love." This is when we begin to long for more intensity again.

This is also the phase of our relationship when we have to start working at love. To create passion, we have to make a decision to commit to a deeper connection. The way we do that is through our intimate, erotic connection with our partner.

Better sex often requires more connection, and more intensity.

When you crave more passion in your relationship, you really crave more depth or intimacy. You want a deeper connection to your partner. There is a desire within you to know your partner at a deeper level and to be known at a deeper place. To be connected to another person is a need that both men and women share equally. We fulfill this need through sex. And the more erotic our connection, the more connected we feel with our partner. When our erotic fantasies are fulfilled, we feel a connection with our partner that adds depth and dimension to our partnership.

The Six Stages
of a Relationship

Falling in love is easy to recognize. There are signs and symptoms. For example, we long for our lovers. We feel excited to see them. We think about them often. We desire them sexually. And sometimes we feel like we can't get enough.

Then, when the ardor and thrill of this phase of relationship moves into the more settled stages, we wonder whether we are still "in love." When the signs are different, the highs are not as high, and the attraction is not the same, does this mean that we are no longer in love? And does this mean that the passion is gone?

No. Long-term relationships are not necessarily a death sentence for passion. These phases of partnership are normal and common to everyone. Sexual excitement and eroticism can be part of the life cycle of a relationship if both people are willing to recognize the stages and work on having a long-term, passionate partnership.

Below are the identifiable stages of a relationship.

Romantic love stage. In this stage, we feel alive and awake, and the sex is great. We feel hope and connection. Romantic love generally lasts anywhere from three to twenty-seven months. This is a time of passion and it gives us the bond we need to stay connected during the later stages of love.

The "sweatpants" or comfort stage. At this phase, we feel comfortable in our relationship with our partner and we start to relax. The more familiar we are with each other, the safer we feel, and more of our real selves come to the surface. We also begin to relax the need to focus on our appearance. After the first year, we sometimes start to put on weight and not shave as often, becoming careless about our looks. We also stop worrying about things we might have been concerned about initially and generally settle into the partnership.

The conflict or power struggle stage. In the power struggle phase of a relationship we begin to feel the conflict inherent in every long-term partnership. We become reactive and defensive, trying to protect the love we felt in the beginning of the relationship.

Conflicts happen because we see our partners differently now. After the haze of romantic love has passed, we begin to see our partners without the blur of our projections that we initially saw them through. In the beginning, we see our partners as the people who complete us and make us feel whole. This is because they have personality traits that we ourselves have, but have repressed. We repress those parts of ourselves for lots of reasons, including the feeling that they really aren't effective ways to get love and attention.

For example, if you are a man and you are taught as a child that "big boys don't cry"—a common phrase told to young boys—it is entirely possible that by the time you reach adulthood you will be totally shut off from your capacity to cry when you feel sad. This means that you have repressed the part of yourself that cries.

When you meet a woman and take her to a movie on a date and she cries at the commercials, you might feel overwhelming attraction for her. This is because she has the personality trait that you have repressed. And with her, you can feel whole and complete.

Unfortunately, if you fall in love and marry that woman, eventually her crying will make you crazy! It will feel irritating and annoying, and it will create conflict in your relationship. You will no longer feel attracted to that part of her, but instead will see her crying as distasteful and a way to keep you at a distance instead of attracting your love.

Other reasons that everyday conflicts occur have to do with how we keep score. Men and women are different in the way they relate to the world. Men generally solve problems by retreating and taking time to mull over the problem, coming out of their cave when they have a solution. Women generally talk about their problems until they feel less anxious about them. Men may perceive this as a way to discount their offer of a solution. Women may experience men as "shutting them down" when they don't want to hear about their issues repeatedly.

When we feel conflict in our relationship, our anxiety and stress levels increase and we respond in an almost primitive way. Our brains sense danger and we respond by preparing for a fight, where our systems tense and become ready for physical attack. We might feel we have to defend ourselves or intensify an argument when we feel this response, and unknowingly we heighten the tension for our partner. In many relationships, this stage leads to a withdrawal phase.

Withdrawal stage. Our primitive brain responds to the conflict by going into our defensive behaviors. This is called the fight-or-flight response. We may fight more with our partner when we are scared and feel conflict, or we may withdraw. Our partners react to our defenses by feeling anxious, stressed, and scared. They then respond with their own defenses.

One way people respond to a perceived threat is by going into "flight" mode. This could look like withdrawal. Sometimes your partner may withdraw, to create a sense of safety around him- or herself, to have some space, or to regroup.

Or you or your partner may respond to a power struggle by "freezing." This is the "deer-in-the-headlights" response. This response can look several ways. Your partner may look frozen, be uncommunicative, or freeze, with his mouth open, drool coming out of the corner of his mouth, staring blankly at you while you demand a verbal explanation. You may remain frozen in your pattern, repeating the same things over and over, trying to be heard.

You might forget what you wanted to say, or you might feel foggy or confused during a conflict. This leads to the feeling of "if I don't move, maybe they won't notice me"—camouflage behavior. People who use this defense might try to blend into the background, hoping they won't get hurt, and they will wait out the conflict until the other partner appears to be "done." Then they will breathe a big sigh of relief and "unfreeze."

When conflict goes on for too long, and there is a lot of defensive behavior in both partners, we have a natural tendency to withdraw from each other. We pull back slightly from the relationship, trying to protect ourselves from harm.

We might accept the situation and decide that it's worth staying in for a variety of reasons, including the fact that we still remember the romantic love stage and hope that someday we can get back to that initial feeling. We make a choice, instead of ending the relationship, to go to sleep, sinking into the inevitability of the unhappiness, and focus on outside interests to keep us feeling energized. This begins the "sleep" phase of the relationship.

Sleep stage. In the "sleep" stage of the partnership we may feel at home and comfortable with our partner, but the sexual relationship begins to wane.

Couples at this stage of their relationship may begin to complain about lack of interest in sex, sexual dysfunction, noninitiation, feelings of rejection, abandonment, and resentment toward their partner. (Note: Many physical reasons exist for sexual dysfunction, including blood pressure medications, heart medications, cholesterol medications, menopause, hormonal imbalances, thyroid medication, birth control pills, and antidepressants. See your doctor for physical symptoms of sexual dysfunction, including erectile dysfunction and lack of interest in sex.)

Sex at this point in a relationship may turn into maintenance sex, where you are able to please each other but do so more out of physical need and habit than out of a desire to experience the intensity of your romantic interest in each other. Couples begin to live parallel lives at this stage, creating enough of an individual existence to keep them happy, but not putting the energy into the partnership.

At this point the passion and the eroticism of the relationship begin to get split off. We no longer view our partners as erotic, but as someone to feel safe with. Now we are safe, but we are not fully awake and erotic. We are, essentially, asleep.

Waking up stage. The good news is that there is another stage of a relationship—the "waking up" stage. Sometimes one or both partners recognize that the partnership needs help to return to or begin a new stage of passion and connection. This is the time that many couples come to therapy. One partner recognizes the problem and doesn't want to stay asleep. Both partners remember the "alive" feeling of sexual connection and of being in love. They want to feel energized and passionate again. The process of learning to talk to each other begins.

Learning to explore and share erotic fantasies can create new ways to connect. Connecting can keep a partnership awake and alive for the long term. Before the "waking up" stage of the relationship can begin, we have to take a look at what has happened to our erotic needs along the way.

Love Is in the Longing

New relationships often come with an erotic charge between partners. We don't necessarily feel safe and secure yet, but we may experience an intense sexual feeling, a longing for the other person that happens when we are separated.

We think about our new partners when we are apart from them, and begin to fantasize, guessing about their body parts, which we might not have seen yet, and wondering what sexual positions might feel good with this new person in our lives. Our sexual attraction is created in the longing. It is in the distance between us that we feel desire for the other.

Our experience of romantic love includes a feeling of longing, of missing our loved one. We romanticize the missing of our loved one. Most poetry and love song lyrics are about longing and the intensity of separation. For most of us, this is how we experience falling in love.

As the newness of a relationship wears off, desire for each other seems to decrease and we settle into a nice, safe form of loving that can feel secure, but not always passionate. With familiarity, the longing decreases. We no longer have distance between us. We have found someone to whom we can feel close and connected. This stage of the relationship feels wonderful, safe, warm, and loving. And yet we don't necessarily stay in that same state of bliss we experienced when we were falling in love and longing for connection.

How to Bring Back the Sex You Want— The Next Steps

Margaret Mead, the famous anthropologist, said we have three marriages in our lifetime. The first is for children, the second is for sex, and the third is for companionship. And we can experience all three of those "marriages" in one relationship, or several. Furthermore, we can have a lasting sexual relationship through our child-rearing years, and later through our companionship times.

Sex is a way to feel connected and loving toward our partner. Eroticism can be a physical language in which we express intimacy. It is the closest we can get to our partner on a physical level. It shows trust and openness and can express attraction and affection. Throughout the life span of a relationship, sex can repair hurt, heal grief, bond us after arguments, provide tenderness, comfort us, and help with self-esteem and self-confidence.

Most of all, sex is an expression of love.

We are all looking for love. Love has two components—companionship and erotic connection. Companionship, or "hang-out ability," is what we feel when we enjoy spending time together. Companionship becomes more and more important over time.

The other component of a relationship is eroticism. Eroticism is what keeps the relationship vital and awake and makes us feel sexually connected. Without it, a long-term partner can feel more like a roommate. Working on the eroticism in a relationship is a key element to keeping it vital and alive.

Some couples are willing to give up the sexual part of the relationship because it seems too hard to work at keeping it alive. Communicating about sex, working on the erotic needs of the relationship, and focusing on a healthy partnership where sex is a priority can be a challenge and a commitment.

When there are other priorities like children and work, couples can take their relationship for granted. Being companions can feel easier than working on a sexual connection.

The Need for Honesty

The beginning of this journey to increased erotic connection starts with learning how to talk to each other about sex, as you are learning to do in these exercises. Most of us aren't really honest with our partners about sex.

For example, more than 70 percent of women fake orgasms, according to studies. More and more men are faking it, too. (Men can fake orgasm easily, particularly if they ejaculate inside a woman's vagina. Women take it for granted that if a man says he orgasms that he has indeed ejaculated, regardless of appearance of ejaculate. This can happen more and more as men get older.)

It is sometimes difficult to talk to our partners about our deepest fantasies because erotic needs are many times a part of us that we keep hidden, especially from those we are closest to. Sharing a need or desire that is different than what we have been practicing in our intimate lives can feel threatening to our relationship.

Long-term partnership and intimacy can be reinforced by honest and direct communication about sexual needs. This can happen when we feel free and open enough to share our fantasies with our partner.

Establishing Trust through the Imago Dialogue

We've all heard that an important part of relationships is communication, but why then can't we do it? It seems like most people don't have any problem telling each other what is bothering them or what is lacking in their relationship. It is fairly easy to point out in our partners all of their shortcomings. And many times we repeat this list of complaints, hoping to get our needs met.

In the beginning romantic phase of our relationships we use "appreciation" to get the love we want, and yet later on in the "conflict" phase of a relationship we think we can demand love by telling our partners all the ways in which they are doing it "wrong."

Forcing our partners to give us what we need doesn't work. We have to create a new way of relating to each other. The Imago method of communication does this by providing a safe, structured way to communicate concerns and appreciations. This way of increasing connection allows us to find the passion from the beginning romantic phase of our relationship. It is normal and healthy to crave that erotic connection. But to feel this connection, we need to do the work of communicating intimately, which can help us have that connection and begin to have the sex we really want.

This process is not for the faint of heart. We don't talk about sex easily in our culture. And, interestingly, we talk about sex the least often with the person we are having sex with. Learning the language of intimacy is sometimes, for many couples, a whole new language of love. The language of sex and erotic need is sometimes a difficult and new language to learn.

Talking to each other using words that have been forbidden, dangerous, and illicit can be guilt provoking and feel "bad." Yet this new language can also be a way to add spice and erotic electricity to the relationship, all without even a physical touch.

In this next exercise, you will try to create a safe space to talk about sex, and later explore your fantasies, using words and language that you will grow more comfortable with.

Try this exercise without touching and notice what happens between you and your partner. Can you feel the erotic energy increase? Do you feel yourself blush? Can you feel the pull of the words? Notice what you feel in your body and what you respond to. Try to discuss these feelings and responses with your partner after the exercise.

EXERCISE
Talk Dirty to Me

In this exercise, we will expand on the previous exercise, and take our erotic language skills to a whole new level. This is another great way for couples to create an erotic conversation. You may feel silly, embarrassed, and guilty. All of this is normal and healthy. Do the exercise anyway. You may be pleasantly surprised at how connected you feel to your partner, and how turned on you are when you are through.

(continued on page 32)

(continued)

You will need at least thirty minutes of uninterrupted private time together. Make sure the kids are taken care of, and you have total privacy, so that you will have no fear of being overheard or disrupted. This will help you feel comfortable and safe using whatever language you need to with your partner. Find a quiet place where you can sit comfortably facing each other, close enough so that you can whisper in each other's ear.

In this exercise you will write and share what you write with each other. Make sure you have paper and something to write with and that you can see in the low light of the room. Dark markers or pens work well. Make sure you have a surface to write on that is comfortable for you. A small clock or timer may work if you want to limit the time you both take for the writing portion of this exercise.

You might want to turn down the lights, put on soft music, light some candles, and put on comfortable and sexy clothes. Setting the right mood is a great way to get started, and can help lead to increased passion. Turning down the lights so that there is slightly more darkness in the room can make this exercise easier, but make sure the room is not totally dark. You do not need to be ashamed and hide to do this work. Everything you do here is between loving and safe partners.

Try to stay focused on the exercise for the duration of both sending and receiving.

Step One

Choose who will be the sender and who will be the receiver. The sender is the first one to talk, and the receiver is the first one to listen. The sender will talk and the receiver's only job is to listen and mirror exactly what the sender says. Remember, mirroring means to say back what the sender has said with no other comments.

Step Two

After deciding who will be the sender, both of you should write down ten sexual words. They can be words that describe your or your partner's body parts or they can be words that describe sexual acts. Take five minutes to do this portion of the exercise. If you want to set a timer to remind you both when the time is up, you can do this, or just give each other time to write down the words.

Step Three

After you've done this, senders should say the words quietly to their partners, slowly whispering them in the receiver's ear.

Step Four

Now lean back, make eye contact, and say the words out loud while facing your partner. Remember, giggling is okay.

Step Five

Now say them one more time, and let the receiver mirror each word back, maintaining eye contact.

Step Six

While maintaining eye contact, add an adjective or descriptive word before each word on your list and say them out loud to your partner, who should mirror back after each one.

Examples might be "beautiful vagina" or "hard penis."

Step Seven

Switch roles.

When you are finished with the exercise, discuss with your partner how it felt to do the exercise. How did it feel to say the words? How did it feel to hear the words? How do you feel now?

Talking about sex is not easy, but it is worth it. This type of dialogue can help a partnership that has turned stale become the exciting relationship you crave. It can also take a good relationship and make it hot.

Mirroring, Validating, and Empathizing

Let's review the Imago dialogue, and add more depth to the parts we already know.

Mirroring is simply listening, but in an active way, without inserting our opinion. Mirroring is a way of responding by only repeating what we have heard and "sending" the information back. Giving our partners a chance to say what's on their mind and then mirroring it back allows them to hear what they have said and gives them a chance to change what they meant to say, clarify it, and get to the heart of the matter.

Example:

Sender: "I really appreciate you taking the time to massage my back this morning when we made love."

Receiver: "So what I hear you saying is you really appreciate me taking the time to massage your back this morning when we made love."

Sender: "Well, I really meant that I loved that you made time to touch me in that caring way, since I know we usually are so rushed in the morning."

Receiver: "So, you really loved that I made time to touch you in that caring way, since we are usually so rushed in the morning. Did I get that?"

Sender: "Yes, that's what I meant."

Validating is the second step in the Imago dialogue. This is an important step for both the sender and the receiver. It helps the sender to feel understood, like what they said made sense. The receiver does not have to agree with what the sender has said, but being validated means the receiver has tried to make sense of the sender's experience. The receiver tries to understand the sender's point of view.

Example:

Receiver: "That makes sense to me; I know you really love it when I massage you."

Sender: "Yes, it really helped me to relax and get into the sex today."

Validation is an important part of a dialogue. Many times in a conversation with our partner we feel misunderstood and are not sure our partner really understands us. Sometimes it can feel like we are speaking different languages or that we come from different planets altogether.

The third part of the Imago dialogue is empathy. Receivers imagine what the senders might be experiencing, and try to step into their shoes and understand what the senders are feeling. Understanding our partner's feelings is what creates empathy. This is important when we talk about each other's sexual feelings as well. To be sexually empathic, we have to begin to understand how our partners feel sexually. What might feel good to them, what they might desire, and what might turn them on could be different for them than for us.

If we empathize with their feelings, it doesn't mean we have the same experience as them. It just means we understand what they might be feeling. When we empathize with our partners, we try to imagine feelings and emotions they might be having.

Example:

Receiver: "So I imagine you feel happy and turned on when I massage you first."

Sender: "I do! I get really happy and I feel hot and then I can't wait to make love to you!"

Receiver: "So you get really happy and you feel hot and can't wait to make love to me!"

The Right Time

You can use this dialogue process to go to the next step and talk about your sexual fantasies, as in the following exercise. Again, using this process may feel stilted, goofy, or silly at first, but it will make your partner feel safe and validated. They will feel listened to and understood. And when your partner feels like this, they will be more likely to give you the connection you want. Your communication will feel safer and more comfortable, and ultimately, become easier. In time you will both feel like your needs are finally being met.

As the receiver for your partner, all you need to do is listen and mirror. The only response needed is empathy and validation. You don't need to react to hearing your partner's fantasies by promising to take them into action. All you need to do is hold the space by having the dialogue. Three important things to remember about the dialogue are

- Remember to always ask your partner "Is now a good time to have a dialogue?" Sometimes we set ourselves up for disappointment if our timing is off.

- If the time isn't right, make an appointment. An appointment to have a dialogue about sex is a great idea, because a longer wait time often leads to a greater erotic charge. Also, our partner might need a safer time or space to talk about erotic needs. Make sure your partner can commit to a later date or time.

- And finally, always start your dialogue with an appreciation!

Exchanging Fantasies

In this exercise, we will take the appreciation exercise and add *validation* and *empathy*. We will create a safe space to talk more specifically about sex. Remember, appreciation is the doorway into a more connected and intimate sex life with your partner.

For this exercise, you will need at least thirty-five minutes of uninterrupted private time together. Find a quiet place where you can sit comfortably facing each other in chairs, on the floor, or on a bed and maintain eye contact for the entire exercise.

You might want to turn down the lights, put on soft music, light some candles, and put on comfortable and sexy clothes. Setting the right mood is a great way to get started, and can help lead to increased passion later on.

Make sure you have nowhere to go after this exercise. Many times it can lead to lovemaking, but do not put pressure on each other to make that happen.

Step One

Start by again sharing appreciations and continuing to mirror each other. This is a basic dialogue skill, and one we will continue to use. This may still feel awkward and a little goofy, but you may now feel safer with this structure. Giggle, squirm, blush, and feel silly—it's all okay.

Try to stay focused on the exercise for the duration of both sending and receiving.

First, choose who will be the sender and who will be the receiver. The sender is the first one to talk and the receiver is the first one to listen.

This exercise may be more difficult than previous exercises. Now you are talking about your sex life, and being very specific. If you are courageous, trust the process, and follow the dialogue structure, you will find that you can stay in the dialogue with your partner without difficulty. You may feel anxious or embarrassed. Don't be afraid to share those feelings with your partner before or after your dialogue.

Senders will "send" over one thing they appreciate about their partner. The receiver will simply mirror back what the sender says. For example:

Sender: "One thing I appreciate about you is how kind you are."

Receiver: "One thing you appreciate about me is how kind I am."

Step Two

Senders will send over one specific thing about your sex life that they like. The receiver will mirror back what the sender says. For example:

Sender: "One thing I appreciate about being in a sexual relationship with you is how open you are to trying new things."

Receiver: "So one thing you appreciate about being in a sexual relationship with me is how open I am to trying new things."

Step Three

Finally, senders will say one thing they may have fantasized about. The receiver will simply mirror back exactly what the sender sends over. For example:

Sender: "One thing I have fantasized about but possibly not shared before is having sex on an airplane with you."

Receiver: "One thing you have fantasized about but possibly not shared before is having sex on an airplane with me."

Step Four

After the senders have sent over all three steps, receivers will validate what they've just heard. Validation means that you share with your partner how it makes sense to you that he or she might be feeling or fantasizing these things. You don't have to agree with those thoughts and fantasies, and you don't have to do them. Hold all those thoughts and ideas for now. Instead, let your partner know you understand where he or she is coming from.

In response to the first three steps in this exercise, validation might sound like this:

Receiver: "So, knowing you the way I know you, it makes sense that you would appreciate my kindness because I know it means a lot to you when people are thoughtful."

Receiver: "It also makes sense that you like how open I am to trying new things because I know you love to experiment."

Receiver: "It also makes sense that you would fantasize about having sex on an airplane because you like to try risky things."

Step Five

After validation, the sender empathizes with the receiver. Showing empathy for our partners goes a long way to helping them feel understood. Empathy does not

(continued on page 38)

mean that you agree with what they are saying or that you are promising to participate in anything. Instead, it shows that you understand their emotional state. Sharing with your partner how you think he or she might feel could sound like this:

Receiver: "I can imagine that if you were to act out your fantasy you would feel excited and turned on. Did I get that feeling?"

Sender: "Yes, and I would also feel loved and appreciated by you."

Receiver: "So you would also feel loved and appreciated by me."

Sender: "You got me."

Now that you have done this exercise, how do you feel? Can you tell your partner what it was like for you? You do not have to disagree, agree, argue, compromise, or commit. Just sit with what you heard. You can ask questions, but try to soak up the appreciation for now, and read on.

A Sample Dialogue

This is a sample of how to use the Imago dialogue. Try following these steps to make it easier to practice the Imago form of communication.

A specific example of the above dialogue might look like this:

Sender: "One thing I appreciate about being partners with you is that you are committed to improving our relationship."

Receiver (mirrors): "So one thing you appreciate about being partners with me is that I am committed to improving our relationship."

Sender: "One thing I appreciate about being in a sexual relationship with you is how attentive you are to making sure I always have an orgasm."

Receiver (mirrors): "So one thing you appreciate about being in a sexual relationship with me is how attentive I am to making sure you always have an orgasm."

Sender: "Yes, and one specific thing you do while we are having sex that I really like is that you squeeze my breasts when you are kissing me."

Receiver (mirrors): "So one specific thing I do while we are having sex that you really like is when I squeeze your breasts when I am kissing you."

Sender: "Yes. And one thing I have fantasized about but never really shared is that you would squeeze my nipples really hard, maybe pinch them, while we are making love."

Receiver (mirrors): "So one thing you have fantasized about that you have never really shared is that you would like it if I would squeeze your nipples really hard, maybe pinch them, while we are making love. Did I get that?"

Sender: "Yes, you got that!"

Receiver (validates): "So, knowing you the way I know you, it makes sense that you would appreciate the way I always make sure you have an orgasm. I know you appreciate my thoughtfulness, and I know you love to have orgasms! Did I get that?"

Sender: "Yes, you got me!"

Receiver (validates): "It also makes sense to me that you would like it when I squeeze your breasts when I kiss you because I know how sensitive your breasts are."

Sender: "Yes."

Receiver (validates): "And it sure makes sense to me that you might have fantasies about me pinching and squeezing your nipples harder because I know when I have played with them in the past it has really felt great to you. Is that right?"

Sender: "Yes! You got me."

If you are having trouble validating, think about your partner and what you know about her. What do you know about her that would make it seem reasonable that she would feel these things? You don't have to understand, but does it make sense to you that your partner would feel these things, knowing her the way you do? How can you relate to these feelings that she has?

(continued on page 40)

A Sample Dialogue (continued)

If your partner is bringing things up that seem totally out of character, or sharing thoughts and fantasies that are shocking to you, it might be hard to validate what she is saying in this exercise. If you are trying to stay in a dialogue with her and really want to make this exercise work for you, it can be a challenge to stay with it. Mirroring what your partner says can help her feel safe to tell you what's really on her mind. She will feel like you are not judging her, and will be more likely to be honest with you in the future about her desires and fantasies.

After mirroring your partner as well as you can, try validating what she said. Can you find something in what she said that makes sense to you?

After validating your partner, try empathizing with her.

Receiver (empathizes): "I can imagine that when you receive those things in bed you feel—*loved, appreciated, safe, cared for, desired, attractive, alive, young, and excited*. Did I get that?"

Receiver (empathizes): "And I can imagine that having those things makes you feel excited and that if you could fulfill that fantasy you would feel really turned on and alive!"

What are some emotions that you imagine your partner might feel now, and that she might feel if she had her fantasy come true? If you were to put yourself in her shoes, what do you think makes sense about the way she might feel? Now check it out with her.

Receiver: "Did I get that?"

Sender: "Yes, I feel that, and I would feel that, and I would also feel sexually fulfilled if I had that fantasy come true."

Receiver: "So I got your feelings, and you would also feel sexually fulfilled if you had that fantasy come true."

Sender: "You got me."

Real-Life Experiences

Let's take a look at a couple who came into a therapy session and used these techniques to improve their sex life. Notice how they use the dialogue and see whether there are ways that you can use their experiences to help you and your partner improve your communication skills.

Alma and Don came into my office to talk about their issues around sexuality and the blocks in their relationship. For many years they had been sexless. They came to therapy to begin the conversation they both wanted to have about sex.

Don's fears about telling Alma his fantasies were deeply rooted in his past. He had always been afraid to talk about sex because in his childhood he had heard from his church and his family that talking about sex was wrong and that anything outside of sex for procreation was a sin.

Don and Alma built up to the following Imago dialogue, which is a good example of a successful exchange. Using the Imago dialogue, Don asked Alma whether she was ready to hear his fantasies.

Don: "Is now a good time to tell you about one of my fantasies?"

Alma: "Yes, now is fine."

Don: "I am nervous to tell you about this, but have always wanted to share this fantasy with you."

Alma: "So you are nervous to tell me about this, but have always wanted to share this fantasy with me. Is that right?"

Don: "Yes. Well, okay, um, please don't judge me, but … "

Alma: "Oh, so you are asking if I would please not judge you."

Don: "Yes. One of my secret erotic fantasies is actually to masturbate in front of you."

Alma did not respond for a moment. Instead of reacting in any way, positively or negatively, she continued to mirror him.

Alma: "So one of your secret erotic fantasies is to masturbate in front of me. Did I get that?"

Don: "Yes, you got it. I guess I have had that fantasy for a long time."

Alma mirrored his words.

Alma: "So what I hear you saying is that one of your fantasies is that you have thought about masturbating in front of me. Is there more?"

Don described in detail what his deepest and most hidden fantasies were about masturbating for her.

Slowly, as the process continued, Alma was able to hear what Don described, and why he felt the feelings he did. He described his fears about sharing these thoughts with her. He talked about feeling ashamed of his thoughts.

Don: "I don't think it's wrong, but part of me feels like that should be private. I want you to know that I love you and want to share this with you."

Alma: "Oh, so part of you thinks that masturbation should be private, but you don't really think it's wrong. You also want me to know that you love me and want to share this with me."

Don talked about his fears and his childhood prohibition against masturbation. He wondered if he was going to break their marital bond. Alma listened and simply mirrored back, always asking:

Alma: "Is there more?"

Don: "Yes. I was thinking that if we took this fantasy into action, I would want you to do it too, in front of me. Maybe we could do it together, at the same time. That would really be exciting for me, and I would see what you like."

Alma mirrored Don's fantasy, without agreeing or disagreeing. She encouraged Don, simply by staying in the process, to talk through all of his fears and insecurities. She validated his feelings, while not necessarily agreeing with him.

Alma: "I know you have always had a lot of curiosity about a lot of things. So, it makes sense to me that you would wonder about masturbation. I understand that you have had fantasies that might be different than mine. You are a separate person than me."

She understood that as a couple they are differentiated (two different people). Just like Don had different appetites for foods than she did, Alma recognized that he could have different sexual fantasies as well. This did not threaten his love for her.

Her ability to express understanding, regardless of how hard it may have been for her to hear his fantasy, made Don feel safe and secure in their relationship. He felt he could tell her anything. He began to cry in the session, and told Alma he had never felt closer to her.

Using empathy, she tried to guess at his feelings.

Alma: "I can imagine that telling me this fantasy was embarrassing for you, but also that it made you feel relieved, and maybe a little turned on."

Don: "Yes, and I also feel a lot of love for you because you listened to me without judging me."

Alma: "So you also felt love for me because I listened to you without judging you."

Notice that Alma never agreed or disagreed to fulfill Don's fantasy. She simply allowed Don to talk to her freely, and really listened to him express his need.

They agreed that they would continue to explore Don's fantasies. This showed generosity and open-mindedness and made Don feel more secure about his sexuality. Don's gratitude and love for Alma dramatically improved for many sessions after this.

As a result of talking about Don's fantasy, Alma was able to talk about her fantasies, and share with Don erotic thoughts she had. She had never been honest about them because she was afraid Don would reject her if she did. This shame is deeply rooted in childhood, and can interfere with the ability to share erotic needs with our partners.

Adding Risk to Your Relationship

3

All of us want to feel safe and secure in our lives, and marriage and committed partnerships help us to feel that way.

Unfortunately, committed partnerships and marriages still last only about 50 percent of the time, with divorce rates changing little over the past fifty years. Yet, even with such a high rate of divorce, we still seek out marriage as an institution. People are waiting longer to get married, marrying at later ages, and choosing to live together first, but still marrying. More and more, we are marrying a second, and sometimes even a third, time. We still want partnerships, despite knowing that long-term relationships can sometimes lead to the demise of passion and erotic energy in those relationships.

It would seem that the longer we are connected to someone in a safe and secure relationship, the more honest and open we could be about our sexual needs. There would seem to be a connection between long-term partnerships and good sex. And yet, after about ten years of marriage or partnership, many couples complain that they feel "out of love" and no longer feel the passion they once felt.

Splitting Off Sexual Needs

When we are first dating, sex can be hurried or frenetic. The rush adds to the excitement. An element of getting caught can feel thrilling. The mile-high club (having sex on an airplane), elevator sex, or sex in unusual places where there is the possibility of being seen creates a feeling of excitement. The danger makes sex feel erotic.

Because erotic energy feels "dangerous," it can also feel exciting. But keeping the excitement alive is difficult. Our need for exciting and stimulating sex is normal. But after couples have been together for a while, they fear that talking about their erotic needs can corrupt the "safety" of the long-term relationship. So, in actuality, over time it becomes more difficult to talk about what we really want.

Before children come along, we may find that in our early relationship we enjoy long, leisurely weekends of erotic juiciness. Without children we have fewer constraints and lots of uninterrupted time to act out our fantasies. But after we have children, we split off our sexual needs, or bury them, hoping to take them out again when the kids are older, or when we are less tired.

Some of the ways we split off the sexuality from our relationship can include things like looking at pornography or visiting porn sites, having phone sex, chatting on the Internet, or having an affair. Or we can simply close down our sexual needs, splitting them off into a compartment within us, shutting down our sexuality. In some ways, couples can feel that these behaviors keep them in the relationship. It is a way to justify getting their needs met, and keeping the relationship at home safe and secure. They don't have to bring in any of their erotic needs, thereby keeping the home bond sacred and pure.

If we are in a partnership to feel safe and secure, and erotic sex is dangerous and forbidden, then being safe and secure certainly feels antithetical to passion. But splitting off our erotic needs does not help us be closer to our partner, and it doesn't help us get the sex we really want. This is the dichotomy of marriage.

Taking the Next (Risky) Erotic Step

One way to bring the excitement of "forbidden" sexuality into a relationship is to add an element of "practiced spontaneity," or *risk*. In other words, practicing spontaneous ways to keep the sexual relationship alive and vital can recharge the partnership. Ironically, spontaneity can be part of our relationship if we focus on a plan to put it there.

Ironically, spontaneity can be part of our relationship if we focus on a plan to put it there.

In the early stages of a relationship you may have found that the times when you were spontaneous and took risks were your hottest sexual moments. These more risky experiences may have come after a period of not seeing each other for a while. Maybe the times you were apart were the times that you felt a romantic longing for your lover, and perhaps fantasized about what it would be like when you were together again. Maybe you thought about what you wanted to do to your lover the next time you were in bed together. Fantasy and distance can create great erotic energy.

Talking on the phone, for example, is one way to recreate the feeling of that erotic longing. Talking on the phone can feel intimate and far away at the same time. Having sexy phone conversations can add erotic excitement to an already familiar relationship, making it feel young and passionate again.

The other added benefit of talking sexy on the phone is that because there is no eye contact there is a natural distance that is created between you and your partner. This can help those who are naturally more shy or reticent to say things in person. The phone allows for erotic freedom and can be a safe way for you to practice saying things out loud, including sexy things that you want to do to your partner. It can sometimes be easier to share these ideas when you don't have to look at your partner while saying them. Telling your partner on the phone the sexy things you want to do when you get home is great practice for what you can say later, in person.

The following exercise will build on the dialogue skills you learned in the earlier chapters and incorporate some sexier, and maybe even racier, language. Because you will have this conversation over the phone, the safety and distance will add an erotic element that will give you room to take some risks in what you say to each other.

By now you have a new form of communication, the Imago dialogue. You can tell your partner what you want, and all he has to do is listen. He can listen actively by mirroring, validating, and empathizing. You will continue building on this format throughout the book, creating a safe structure to talk about your erotic thoughts and fantasies.

So take risks! Do the exercise and use the sexiest language you can imagine. What words can you come up with that might make your partner blush? Use them! What words describe things you want to do? Will they make you blush? Go ahead… no one will see because you're on the phone!

EXERCISE
Phone Sex

For this exercise, you will need at least ten minutes of uninterrupted private time to call your partner on the telephone. Find a quiet place where you can comfortably make the call, where you know you will not be interrupted or overheard.

This call should be a surprise, so try to call your partner at a time when he or she is not expecting it. It works best if you call during a challenging time in the day when it is hard for your partner to talk openly—when your partner is at work or otherwise occupied. This will increase the tension and the feeling of erotic risk. (Make sure you are not truly putting your partner's job at risk by doing this, if the job entails recorded phone calls, etc.)

As in the previous exercises, we will be sharing and then mirroring. This is a basic dialogue skill and one we will use for many of the other exercises to come. Although you may have practiced it, you might still feel uncomfortable with the slow pace that this creates in your "conversation." See if you can appreciate the slower pace of the dialogue and notice how it brings you closer to your partner, allowing you to appreciate each word and nuance of emotion in what he or she is saying to you.

The words you use on the phone with your partner may feel awkward and forced. That's okay; say them anyway. Let the exercise feel awkward for now. Practicing erotic conversation is a great way to grow toward having better sex!

It doesn't matter if you call first thing in the morning or right before you get home. The earlier you call the more the tension will build toward the moment when you are together again. You can call once in a day or five times. During your call, try to allow your partner to really hear what you have to say, and leave enough room and mystery to think and fantasize about what will happen when the two of you get home.

Step One

Call your partner on the telephone. Tell her in detail what you are planning to do to her when she gets home tonight.

For example, you might have a fantasy of undressing your wife when she gets home. If you are calling her at work, you might say, "Hi, honey, I've been thinking about you," and then ask her, "can you just mirror that back for me?"

(If she can't mirror you—either because of her work environment or another reason—ask her whether she can stay on the phone with you, and if so, ask her to mirror you internally.)

Step Two

Continue the dialogue over the phone, taking your time, and relaying the smallest and most intimate details about how you plan to undress her when she comes home.

Listen while she mirrors you. She may have to repeat it a couple of times until she gets it. You might have to send it over again if she didn't get it all. Then tell her more.

Tell her, "I can't wait to sit you down on the edge of the bed and slowly slide off your shoes." Let her mirror you.

Tell her how you will then "slowly and very carefully pull each stocking off of her thighs." Then ask her to mirror that.

Then tell her, "And then I am going to touch your smooth legs and soft thighs. And I can't wait to pull your panties off very slowly, down your thighs and off of your legs ... "

And ask her to mirror you. She may be breathless by now, or feel silly and giggle. She might feel surprised at how uncomfortable it is to feel so erotic. Keep telling her intimate details of what you are thinking of doing. This may seem awkward and uncomfortable, particularly if you have never used this kind of language before.

Remember, you are on the phone, and she can't see you blush! Keep describing in detail what you want to do to her.

"And then I will slide my hands up your legs and very slowly touch you between your legs with my fingers to see how wet you are."

Then ask her if she's wet just listening to you! And then ask her to mirror you back.

(continued on page 50)

(continued)

Step Three

Finally, when you feel she has had enough, or if you want to leave her wanting more, you can ask her to validate and empathize for you. Say, "So, knowing me the way you know me, does it make sense that this is what I am thinking about?"

And let her tell you why it makes sense to her that you would want these things. It might sound like, "Yes, it makes sense that you would want to do these things. I know you love my legs and you would love to take my stockings off and touch my thighs. And I know you love it when I am wet for you, so I can imagine that you would love to put your hand on me to feel that wetness and how turned on I am."

Then you might ask her to empathize with you, or imagine your emotions. It might sound like, "And what do you imagine I might feel if we did all these things?"

And see whether she can guess your feelings. If she gets them, then just say, "Yes, you got me."

If there are other feelings as well, you can add them.

"Yes, you got me and I would also feel totally turned on, crazy for you, hot, and madly in love."

Step Four

Hang up and get ready! At this point you can decide how long you will take to get home, or to meet your partner. You might take your time, building the tension, and calling a few more times to add to your fantasy list. Or you might hang up the phone and rush home, to fulfill your fantasy with your partner.

Remember that going home might not seem as risky and exciting as being on the phone did. If you have children, make sure there is a babysitter or someone to take care of them for a few hours. If there are chores to be done or things like taking care of pets, etc., make sure you take care of what you need to and find time to focus completely on your partner and your relationship. You both deserve to have this time to yourselves, and to take your phone sex conversation one step further!

Adding Excitement to Sex

Remember, eroticism is a way to express love. It is through connection with each other that we find the ultimate union and can experience love in physical form, the ultimate sensual experience.

Sometimes we forget this. Or we feel torn about our erotic needs. This is because erotic fantasies are often loaded with anticipation and a feeling of being "bad" or "naughty." This feeling can add an element of excitement to sex. Erotic fantasy is often more edgy than the sex we have in real life because we may imagine things we have been taught are wrong or illicit and have erotic fantasies about them. Examples might include fantasies about having sex in a public place or masturbating in front of our partner.

The exercises in this chapter and the next one will help you explore the "naughty" part—the sexual and erotic self inside that longs to come out and play. That part of us wants expression, and it yearns to feel free and open to express its "bad" side. If we can be "naughty" in our relationship, with someone we feel safe with, then we can have the best of both worlds. We have safety, and we have risk. Eroticism can be explored freely when we feel safe, but only if we feel safe enough to take the risk to be "bad."

EXERCISE
When Being Bad Is Oh… So Good

In this exercise, you will share your memories and thoughts with your partner after you have written them down, so you will need a piece of paper or a journal. Building on the Imago dialogue, you will mirror what your partner shares, which will help him to mirror you when you talk about what you have written.

Remember, there is no right or wrong way to do this exercise. This is the beginning of practicing a new way of relating to your partner. It may feel awkward or embarrassing at first. That's always okay. Taking a risk sometimes means doing things we aren't comfortable with at first.

For this exercise, you will need at least thirty to sixty minutes of uninterrupted private time together. You will need a quiet place where you can first sit comfortably and write for about ten minutes. Next, you will need twenty to fifty minutes to dialogue with your partner.

(continued on page 52)

(continued)

Find a comfortable place to sit facing your partner, either in chairs or on a bed. Try to see if you can maintain eye contact for the entire exercise.

Step One

Using your journal and a pen, take a moment and remember something "naughty" or "bad" you did when you were first having sex with your partner. Did you have sex in a place where there was a risk of getting caught? Did you try new positions that you normally wouldn't perform? What kinds of risks did you take? Was there anything you did that made you feel particularly erotic at the beginning of your sex life together?

Write down any "naughty" things you can think of.

Step Two

Think about what "naughty" or "bad" thing you want to do to your partner right now. Remember, your idea of "naughty" may be different than your partner's. That's okay. Just write down something that makes you feel "bad" when you fantasize about doing it now with your partner.

Don't worry about what your partner will think or say—the receiver's only job is to mirror you. Your partner doesn't have to agree to do it, or have a conversation about it. Right now we are just practicing the early parts of the Imago dialogue.

When you have written down one "naughty" sexual thing you want to do with your partner now, let him know that you are done and ready to dialogue.

Step Three

Choose who will be the sender and who will be the receiver. The sender will "send" over what he has written about remembering something naughty from early in the relationship.

The receiver will simply repeat, or mirror, what the sender says.

An example might be the following:

Sender: "I remember having sex with you in the back of my convertible, outside on the street in front of your house."

And the receiver would simply say back, maintaining eye contact: "So, you remember having sex with me in the back of your convertible, outside on the street in front of my house. Is there more?"

The sender can say "yes" and send more or "no" and stop there. After the receiver has mirrored, the sender switches and becomes the receiver.

Now that you have shared your memories and fantasies with each other, how do you feel? Can you tell your partner what it was like to hear those things? Try not to judge what you heard, or disagree, or argue about them. You can ask questions, but try to just be curious for now. If it feels comfortable, move on to having that naughty experience! Make sure your partner wants to and is ready to take this experience into action.

If you are both intrigued and want to try this new (or old) risky behavior, then go for it. Or make a date to make your fantasy come true!

Just knowing that the time is coming when you will have fun and do something "bad" will build your erotic energy and excitement. You may feel more attracted to each other. It might even remind you of the old days—when you were first in love.

An Appointment with Passion

Another way to increase the readiness for passion is to make a date for sex! Some couples object to this because they feel like it takes the spontaneity out of the relationship, and therefore depletes the passion.

Actually, many times it does the opposite. If we know that sex is coming on Saturday night, we can plan for it! Remember, eroticism is in our minds—it is in our fantasy life. If we have some lead time, we can begin to use our imagination and our fantasies to create sexual tension, and by the time our "sex date" comes along, we have been looking forward to it for a while.

If you think back to when you were dating and had plans to meet, it is entirely possible that you knew you would have sex play that night. You were prepared in your mind and in your imagination. The anticipation added an element of erotic connection to the night. Sex dates do the same thing. They allow time for physical preparation, including waxing, shaving, buying lingerie, taking special baths, etc. They can also increase the time available to plan special surprises or appreciations for your partner prior to the date.

If you can schedule a sex date every week, on the same night, it can bring many benefits to your relationship. For example, even though one or both of you may not be in the mood for sex, a sex date means that you do it anyway. And the more you "do it anyway" the more you want to do it. Sex hormones increase the more sex you have. And the more your body and your mind get used to the idea and the rhythm of the regularly scheduled sex date, the more you will naturally anticipate the sex.

For women in particular, this long lead time can lead to a slow buildup, which corresponds with their sexual plateaus that physically lead up to orgasm. Women need to build up slowly until their bodies are ready for orgasm. Having several days lead time every week can really contribute to a buildup of passion before the date.

The sex date also adds an element of respect to the sexual aspect of the partnership. It makes sex a priority. It's what we mean when we say "relationships take work." Work means scheduling, making sex a priority, and doing it even if you don't feel like it. The great part of working on your sex life and scheduling sex dates is that you get to make your passionate partnership a priority in your life. Date night becomes more important than other things that might creep up in your schedule. This gives your partner the very clear message that your partner is important to you, and that a healthy and passionate sex life is a priority!

A Date with Desire

Ken and Dara, a couple in their late thirties, used their date night to revive their sex life, after their three kids and both their jobs had taken a toll on their energy and enthusiasm for each other.

Neither of them wanted sex to go to the bottom of the list, and yet after the kids and sleep, it began to lose its appeal. Without it, they both felt disconnected from each other, and frustrated. They argued more, and felt more conflict in their relationship. Because they knew that the erotic part of the relationship would keep them alive and connected, and they wanted to stay passionate toward each other, they created a date night, on Friday nights, every other week.

They got a sitter and rented a hotel room in their neighborhood. They had take-out food brought in, ate dinner in bed, and planned a different fantasy to act out each date night. One night they would watch soft porn movies on the hotel television. One night they dressed up in costumes and acted out a role-play fantasy. One night they lit candles and gave each other long, sensual massages.

They found that they both began anticipating their Friday night sex dates with glee and a secret determination to keep those nights a sacred part of their relationship. Both of them kept the nights a priority, working around babysitting difficulties, illness, money, and weather conflicts. They agreed that those nights got them through the early years of child rearing and kept their relationship alive and passionate, even adding a new level of eroticism for both of them that they had not known existed.

For date night, pick nights and times that are realistic, even if they still challenge your schedule a little. Some challenge is okay. Remember, date nights mean making sex and passion a priority. When you have your date nights picked out, mark them on your calendar… in pen.

Decide where you will go and what you will do. If you have kids, get a babysitter. Plan your outfit. Use your imagination to add any unusual or special elements to the night. Do you need candles? Do you need a blanket to have sex outside? Do you need to make a reservation? How can you surprise your partner on date night, remembering fantasies he or she may have shared with you in the previous exercises? Now have fun!

When Erotic Needs Split Off from the Relationship

When we are in a long-term partnership, and grow past the romantic love phase, it seems like the sex begins to change. Our passion for each other seems to wane. Our own sexuality might feel different. We are still physically driven to have sex with our partners but might find the frequency diminishes, and sometimes the emotional desire to be close to our partners decreases as well.

When this happens, our natural "Eros" needs, our passion, begins to split off from the relationship. Because our erotic needs are normal and natural, they have to go somewhere—they don't just disappear. If we don't work on getting our erotic needs met and dealing with these issues and challenges, we will act out some of our frustrations and our relationships may suffer.

Our needs can indeed be met when we understand what happened to them and what we can do with our partners to help feel erotic and alive again.

As noted before, the safer your relationship, the more your erotic needs may become split off from the partnership. This is not a sign that the relationship isn't going to work—it may instead indicate that you are invested in its survival, but just haven't figured out a way to integrate your erotic needs within your safe relationship.

There are specific ways to do this, and the exercises in this book can help.

The following issues explain the reasons that our erotic needs get shut off or split off from our relationships. As you read about them, try to identify whether any of these apply to you or your partner.

Madonna/Whore Complex

The Madonna/whore complex is a projection of roles or archetypes onto women that applies only to part of who the complete, sensual woman truly is. Women in our culture are often viewed as either the "Madonna" or the "whore."

This belief has roots in our most sacred stories. Mary Magdalene and the Virgin Mary are examples of this split. When women give birth to children, they become the "mother"—a pure symbol of wholesomeness and nurturing. They are viewed as pure and untouchable.

Sometimes this view of their lover as the "mother" makes it difficult for men to see their partners as the sexual and erotic women they once were. Now that they have borne children, men can see their partners as too "mother-like" to feel sexy toward them.

In our culture, we see women as "bad girls" if they want sex and "good" if they don't. Many women have difficulty integrating the sexual parts of themselves because they feel "bad" if they want sex. And being a mom and wanting sex can be very confusing for women. So they compartmentalize; that is, they put away their erotic needs in a little box deep down inside "until the kids are older." Being a mom and being sexy at the same time are hard roles to balance. It is hard to make macaroni and cheese during the day for the children and then go upstairs and put on the sexy garter belt at night!

When men start to see their partners as "mom," and not the women whom they have sex with, the erotic energy may dissipate. Sometimes men feel torn about their attraction for their partner when they are in this role.

EXERCISE
Exploring the Madonna/Whore Woman

For this exercise, you may need several nights, or dates. Find time when the kids are taken care of and you will not be interrupted. You will need a day or an evening where there is no pressure and you can take your time.

Know that for some women, these role-plays may bring up difficult feelings or emotions, but they will also bring out joy and sexual celebration.

You can divide this exercise and use different role-plays on different date nights. Be the good girl on one date, and the bad girl on the next. Keep your partner guessing!

Step One

Write down all the ways that you are a good mother or a good nurturer if you are not a mother.

Step Two

Now write down all of the ways that you a sexy, erotic woman.

Step Three

Share your list with your partner.

Step Four

Now play with the idea of "good girl/bad girl." How can you have sex as the "good girl" and how can you set up erotic play as the "bad girl"? For example, as the good girl, try wearing white, lacy lingerie, and become your softest, most nurturing and loving self. Make love with the lights off, in the missionary position, and see how sexy you can make that for your partner. Whisper in his ear, "I'm a good girl, you are doing such good things to me!" or maybe pretend to be nervous, scared, and virginal. Whisper in your partner's ear, "I am so scared… please don't hurt me … ."

And see whether your partner can whisper in your ear, "I love that you are a good girl, and I will be oh so gentle … ."

Step Five

As a bad girl, try dressing in black, in leather, and baring lots of skin. Have sex with your partner on top, and talk firmly in his ear as you are doing it—"I am a bad, bad girl, and I am going to do anything I want to you!" Play with that powerful, sexy self, and feel the bad girl come out to take control!

The Hunger for Sex versus Food

Women in general have a hard time recognizing what they want and asking for it. Frequently, women have been taught that hungering for sex is not okay.

Because we grow up in a culture where being thin is more important than being healthy, most adult women have been on at least two diets in their lifetime. Dieting often means denying physical hunger. It also means that many women who have been dieting most of their adult life have gotten out of touch with their bodies and the body's natural signal for hunger. Learning to listen to the body and its signals and desires can then be difficult.

Women sometimes experience their sexual needs as a feeling of hunger. When they feel a stirring in their body, they might not understand that this is a sexual stirring. They don't know how to identify what their hunger really is. This may be in part because girls are not taught what to do with their sexual desire.

Girls who begin dieting when they are young learn to turn off the small voice inside that tells them they are hungry. How many times do women stand in the kitchen in front of the cabinets, looking for something to fill a craving? Sometimes nothing seems to satisfy because the craving isn't always for food. It might actually, sometimes, be for sex.

Women may not recognize what it feels like to have a physical craving for sex. They have not been taught to listen to their hunger for sex, or to recognize their body's signals.

For women, it is easier to repress their sexual needs or turn them into self-destructive acts like compulsive eating or starving. Are women trying to prove how strong they are by not listening to any of their body's signals? Or are they just cut off from what they are really craving?

Because women have not been taught to recognize when they want sex, they don't really know how to ask for it. If they cannot recognize the desire for sex, they cannot recognize what kind of sex they want. And they therefore can't ask for it!

EXERCISE

Recognizing What Your Body Hungers for

This exercise is about increasing the awareness of your body. Keep focused until you can identify all the different feelings in your body.

For this exercise you will need at least fifteen minutes of uninterrupted time. A comfortable place to sit or lie down will help you get in touch with your physical sensations.

Step One

Find a way to sit or lie down that allows you to feel all the parts of your body. Close your eyes and take at least three deep breaths. Try and breath all the way down into your belly, softening your center to let in as much air as you can, and then making your exhalation longer than your inhalation.

Notice how your body relaxes as you breathe deeply.

Step Two

Start at your feet and notice what your feet are feeling. Are they tired, sore, or cold? Do they feel warm and relaxed?

Now move up your legs and notice what your legs feel like. Can you feel tingling or energy in your legs? You can touch your legs with your hands if you want, and feel the shape of them as they lead you to your center.

Now move up to your genitals and your reproductive organs. Can you feel what your genitals are experiencing right in this moment? Do you feel tingling or tightness? Relaxation?

Try to identify words in your mind that describe this whole area. Words might be "sexy, relaxed, tight, wet, tense," etc. Try to experience all the sensations there. Use your hands there to explore the sensations and think about what you are feeling.

Now move up your body through your back and belly. Notice how they feel, and move your awareness up to your chest. Do you feel yourself breathing? Do you feel aroused? Are your nipples responding to your thoughts? To your touch?

Now move your awareness up to your neck and face and hair. Notice how your face and neck respond to your breathing and to your touch.

(continued on page 60)

(continued)

Try to be aware of how you are feeling in this moment. Breathe deeply and notice where in your body you feel sensation. Are you hungry? Tired? Warm or cold? Do you feel aroused or stimulated?

Now you have a language to recognize your body and its responses. Keep this in mind the next time you are wondering what (or whom) you are hungry for.

"Parentifying" Our Partners

Another aspect of partnership that interferes with sexuality is the need for *dependence*. To some extent, we as humans are all dependent on each other. And yet the healthiest relationships include a sense of "differentiation," or the recognition that our partners are separate from us, and might not always want the same things as us.

Sometimes we treat our partners as extensions of ourselves. We assume that if we are hungry, they are hungry. If we are tired, then they must be tired. If we want to have sex, then our partner must as well!

However, our partners have their own erotic needs and interests. We make assumptions that if our partners loved us they would just "know" what we wanted—in the relationship and in bed. But this is not true! We cannot psychically divine what our partners want unless they tell us.

Living with a partner brings a set of issues unique to cohabitation. We "parentify" our partners by projecting onto them our needs. In other words, if you chase your partner around, nagging him to pick up his socks, then he will begin to see you as a parent figure, and not as a partner. If you boss your partner around, or try to have control over her behaviors, then your partner will experience you as parental. This means she probably will not want to have sex with you! Parentifying desexualizes the relationship.

In addition, if we add children to the family, our priorities change. Our need to create a safe environment for kids becomes paramount. We want safety and security for our children, so the heightened need for security in the household supersedes the need for eroticism. The childbearing years are, for most couples, the hardest time of the relationship. These years may coincide with the conflict phase and stress the partnership to its limits, and with good reason.

Having kids is very stressful. The job of being a parent is physically and emotionally exhausting. Sometimes the end of the day means the finish line for parents of young children, when the need to sleep feels more important than having sex with the coparenting partner.

Trusting that this is a phase of the relationship is important. This time will pass, and the kids will grow up. The time for passionate connection will return. Meanwhile, working on that continued connection in your relationship is very important.

EXERCISE
Hot Night Out

This exercise is different from date night. This is a one-time night out that is expressly for your stress relief and to remember that you are both adults and that there is more to your relationship than being parents. Remembering that there is a grown-up connection between you can revitalize a parenting relationship that may have become desexualized and exhausted.

Make this a special night. Make it an escape. Make it a hot night out that you take for a treat. And do it as often as you think you need to restore that feeling of passion in your relationship. Get a babysitter for an evening.

Plan on the kind of sex you want to have on your night out. Are you craving a relaxed, sensual night, where you spend lots of time on massage, talking, and taking a long hot bath together?

Maybe you need to have more edgy sex to break free of your roles as parents. Tying each other up with silk scarves or using a silk scarf as a blindfold can be a fun way to add some excitement to your hot night out (later exercises will help you explore these types of erotic elements in more detail). For now, decide on one element that you will add to your night. The following are some suggestions: bring along massage oil, order or rent pornography, order room service and feed each other fruit or other sensual foods, or take a bath together.

If you have an overnight babysitter, enjoy a night's sleep together!

The Shame that Keeps Us from Going "There"

There may be a deep erotic well inside of you that you find you have trouble accessing. You might sense that you are a passionate person who wants to explore many aspects of your sexuality, but are not sure how to do that.

Shame contributes to the splitting off of sexuality and erotic needs. Appreciation can go a long way to helping your partner heal from shame.

We all have parts of ourselves that we hold back. Sometimes we might feel embarrassed about our needs, or our curiosities. We might even feel ashamed of what we feel or want. Shame can keep us from feeling free and alive. Working through that shame, with the help of your partner, can free passionate energy and allow more intensity into your erotic life. So how does shame happen?

Webster's Dictionary defines shame as "a painful emotion caused by consciousness of guilt, shortcoming, or impropriety. A condition of humiliating disgrace or disrepute. Something that brings censure or reproach. Something to be regretted."

Shame is a learned feeling, and it comes from many places. It has its roots in our religious organizations, in our government's desire to control sexual practices and relationships, and through our own fears that we are somehow different than everyone else.

We also receive messages from our parents about what sex is about. Can you think of what your parents taught you about sex? What is one word your parents might have used to describe sexuality when you were growing up?

What is one word your parents would have used to describe their own sexual relationship, if you could guess? How do you think these feelings and beliefs affect you now as an adult? How do you think they affect you as a sexual person in a relationship?

Shame contributes to the splitting off of sexuality and erotic needs. Our need for sex and passion does not disappear, it just splits off. It can split off into pornography, internet relationships, affairs, sexual addiction of all kinds, and other problems. When there is no appropriate channel for our erotic needs, the energy has to go somewhere. That split-off energy sometimes has no outlet when there is intense shame involved.

The hard part of the sexual relationship when there is shame is that it separates us from our partner. How do we talk to our partner about our sexual and erotic needs when we have shame about them? Shame happens when one's fantasies are imagined to be harmful to another. When we feel shame it can be hard to share what we really want.

However, research shows that people are much more open to hearing what we say when we start with an "appreciation."

Many times in the later stages of our relationship we fail to mention the positives and start nagging our partners about what makes us unhappy. We criticize and let our partner know how unhappy we are. But we don't tell them what we appreciate.

Behaviorists tell us that to extinguish a negative behavior we should ignore it, not exert pressure to change it. To get more of a positive behavior we should appreciate it!

Reminding our partners of what we appreciate about them will create more of that behavior. This works when we talk to our partners about our sex life. When we want to have a conversation about our erotic needs, the last thing we want to do is shame our partner. We want to build up their confidence in themselves so that they are more likely to respond to us in a positive way.

Appreciation can go a long way toward helping your partner heal from shame. And it can also be a way to feel safe to share the things you want in a sexual relationship.

As you try this next exercise, remember what you have done in the previous exercises, and how it felt to have your partner mirror back everything you said. You will, by now, have had an experience of really being heard and seen by your partner. Knowing how this has helped you to feel safe and connected, you can give this experience to your partner to help him feel those things as well.

EXERCISE
Appreciating Your Partner Sexually

This exercise includes writing and sharing. Have something to write on and a pen or pencil. You will write a short list and then share what you wrote with your partner. Have a comfortable place to write and enough light to see.

Find a comfortable place to sit or lie down for at least thirty minutes. Make sure the kids are taken care of and you have total privacy. Create an atmosphere of sensuality by turning the lights low, lighting candles or incense, and turning on soft music. Allow yourself to make eye contact with your partner, sitting close enough so he or she can see your eyes, and reach out to hold hands.

Know that this exercise may make you feel embarrassed, or even bring up some shame. You might feel awkward or silly. This may make you want to run away, or hide. Take a deep breath when you feel this way. Notice how your pulse quickens and your heart races. Remember that his happens during sex, too, and can be an exciting and sexy part of the exercise. It's okay to feel nervous. Try to stay with your feelings and honor them.

Step One

First, take out your paper and pencil and think about the things you appreciate that your partner does in bed. List three of these things.

Step Two

Next, list three things you would like more of.

Step Three

When you are both ready, decide who will be the sender first and who will be the receiver. Share your answers with your partner. For example:

Sender: "So, one thing I really appreciate that you do in bed is give great oral sex."

Receiver (mirrors): "So one thing you really appreciate that I do in bed is give great oral sex."

Repeat until all three things have been mirrored.

Step Four

Validate and empathize with one another. For example:

Receiver (validating): "So, it makes sense that you would like the way I perform oral sex because you are really turned on when I do it, and I imagine that when I do that it makes you feel really excited because it always makes you orgasm."

Step Five

Switch. Receivers become the senders and send three things they appreciate that their partner does in bed. The receiver mirrors these three statements, then validates and empathizes with them.

Step Six

Repeat the process, with the senders sending over the three things they would like more of, and with the receivers mirroring them after each statement, followed by validation and empathy.

Notice what happens when you are through with sharing this exercise. What do you feel toward your partner? How are you feeling about what you shared? If you are feeling any embarrassment, share it with your partner now using the Imago dialogue. For example:

Sender: "I am embarrassed about admitting that I like oral sex so much."

Receiver: "So you are embarrassed about admitting that you like oral sex so much. Is there more?"

Just mirror and ask whether there is more until the embarrassment has been talked through. Now switch if the receiver has any embarrassment about what the sender shared.

Notice what happens now that you have shared your embarrassments. What do you feel toward your partner? How are you feeling about what you shared? What are you feeling in your body? Do you feel any sexual stirrings or physical longings for your partner?

The Difference in Arousal Levels

Most women have a long lead time when it comes to passion. Men need to know that if they want to have sex on a Saturday, they should probably start on a Wednesday!

This is because women have many arousal plateaus that they need to go through before they reach their peak. Before they ultimately are ready to orgasm, they need to be aroused for a while. Most men, however, have one arousal plateau. They need to be touched, preferably directly on their penis, to create a peak physical arousal.

The good news for women is that because their arousal levels rise slowly, they also come down slowly, which is what enables women to have multiple orgasms. What men need to know about women's long lead time is that they need to start foreplay days ahead to prepare a woman emotionally and physically for sex.

One way that men can prepare women for sex is to connect physically before an actual night of sex. Coming up behind your partner and kissing her on the neck unexpectedly, and then walking away, without expectation, adds an element of sexiness without pressure. Phone calls and text messages that tell her you are thinking of her in erotic ways, notes left under her pillow, or whispered fantasies in her ear in the car while she's driving are all good ways to lead up to a hot erotic night that might not officially begin for several days.

EXERCISE
Sensual Full-Body Contact

One way to begin to build up passion is to enjoy physical contact in a new way. Feeling the body of your partner and being mindful of how it feels against you can increase sexual feelings for each other.

For this exercise, you will need at least forty minutes of uninterrupted time together. In this exercise you will be totally naked with each other. There may be some awkwardness or discomfort at first, but the easy part is that you start back to back, not face to face. Know that being naked is a natural part of sexuality, and that your comfort level in your body will contribute to your erotic connection with your partner. The more comfortable you are in your body, the sexier you will feel.

You can do this exercise with the lights on or off. Try it first with the lights on low, or with candles lit. Make sure the room is warm enough so neither of you gets too cold to stand together naked. Make sure you have a comfortable floor to stand on.

Make sure the kids are taken care of and you have privacy.

Step One
Stand back to back with your partner, preferably naked. Notice what parts of your body are touching. See whether you can get more of your body parts to touch. Can you press tighter against each other? Is there a way to press up against each other's whole body?

Step Two

Now turn around without losing contact. Touch each other's body as much as possible as you slowly turn around.

Step Three

Now feel the front of your bodies touching. See whether you can get more of your body parts to touch. See whether you can press together and get your whole bodies to touch. Can you press tighter against each other? What other parts need to touch to add more togetherness? What parts feel the most alive?

Step Four

Tell each other exactly where you think your partner can move closer to you. Tell your partner where you like to feel him close to you. Ask your partner to rub against any parts of you where friction feels good. Close your eyes and feel the texture of each other's skin.

Step Five

Now separate slowly. Feel each body part leave the contact of your partner's body. Notice what the space feels like.

Step Six

Reconnect. Take your partner's hand and place it where you want more contact. Press his or her hand using all of yours—palm, fingers, the pads of your fingers—on that area. Connect with all of your hand. Feel the heat and energy from your partner's hand. Move your hand closer and make more contact.

Step Seven

Slowly remove your partner's hand and feel the disconnect.

Step Eight

Switch.

Step Nine

Continue moving your partner's hand over your body. Move your hands over your partner's body now. Feel the heat and energy coming off your partner's body. Notice which areas of her body are cool, warm, soft, or rough. Notice with curiosity and openness and without judgment the different private parts of the body and also the more public parts that show every day. See whether you can appreciate the parts in a new way, as if you are seeing them with your hands. Feel the passion and the energy rise.

Holding an Appreciation Night

In general, women need to feel emotionally connected before they have sex, and men feel emotionally connected after they have sex.

A couple can never share too many appreciations. This next exercise will help you to feel connected, and help women feel the emotional readiness to be open to sex.

EXERCISE
Appreciation Night

Make an appointment with your partner to hold an appreciation night at a time that works for both of you.

Remember in the previous appreciation exercises you learned to mirror back everything your partner says, without agreeing, refusing, explaining, or denying. Just be a "flat" mirror, which means to reflect back exactly what your partner says, no more and no less.

In this exercise we will also practice **summarizing** before we empathize and validate. The first receiver will summarize what he or she has heard.

Find a comfortable place to sit or lie down for at least fifty minutes. Make sure the kids are taken care of and you have total privacy. Create a sexy atmosphere by lighting candles or incense, putting on soft music, or having a sexy movie playing in the background.

Try to make eye contact with your partner, sitting close enough so that you can reach out and touch if it feels appropriate in the moment.

Know that this exercise may make you feel embarrassed, awkward, or silly. Take a deep breath when you feel this way. Notice how your pulse quickens and your heart races. Remember that this is part of the excitement of the exercise.

Step One

Decide who will be the sender and who will be the receiver. The sender will share the following three appreciations with his or her partner, one at a time:

- One thing you appreciated about your partner when you first met

- One thing you appreciate about your relationship now

- One thing you appreciate about sex with your partner

Step Two

After the sender sends over the first appreciation, the receiver mirrors back. It may sound like this:

Sender: "One thing I appreciated about you when I met you was how outspoken you were about your feelings for me."

Receiver (mirroring): "So one thing you really appreciated about me when you met me was how outspoken I was about my feelings for you."

Do this until you've sent over all three appreciations and had each one mirrored back.

Step Three

The receiver now summarizes all three appreciations.

Receiver: "So one thing you appreciated about me when we first met was how outspoken I was about my feelings for you, and one thing you appreciate about our relationship now is (for example) how attentive I am to your needs, and one thing you appreciate about sex with me is how I always make sure I give you an orgasm before I have one. Did I get that?"

Sender: "Yes" (or no, if the receiver has missed anything).

Step Four

The receiver validates what the sender has said.

Receiver: "It makes sense to me that you would appreciate those things, knowing you the way I know you, because of … . Did I get that?"

Sender: "Yes, you got that" (or add what the receiver might have missed).

Step Five

The receiver empathizes with the sender.

(continued on page 70)

(continued)

Receiver: "And I can imagine that having all those things makes you feel ..." (say any emotions that you think your partner may be experiencing).

Sender: "Yes, you got me."

Step Six
Switch.

Notice what happens when you are through with sharing this exercise. How are you feeling? Do you feel softer toward your partner? What are you feeling in your body? Do you feel any sexual stirrings or physical longings for your partner? Do you feel sexier? Turned on? Share with your partner what the exercise brought up for you.

Ravishment versus Rape

Over the past few decades, women have made great strides in working against sexual violence and abuse. The rape of women and the prevalence of violence and sex in the media, movies, rock videos, and society in general has led to a societal backlash of "no means no."

Feminists, lawmakers, police forces, and others have led the way to educate a male-driven society about the difference between sex and violence. Our laws now protect the victims of sexual violence and allow for broader representation, giving women a stronger voice and taking the violence out of sex.

In America we have feminized sex, which is a good thing, because it educated both men and women that rape is a violent act, not a sexual act. And yet, even though we've made progress, something has slipped through the cracks. Maybe we have confused sex for both men and women and mistakenly taken the passion out of sex.

For example, we have begun to teach men about the positive aspects of intimacy and sex. We have shown them how to touch our face, and be emotionally available and loving, which is wonderful! And yet women spend billions of dollars each year on bodice-ripping paperback novels, where some big, strong man throws the woman down on the bed and tears off her dress.

Maybe we have confused sex for both men and women and mistakenly taken the passion out of sex.

So what do women really want? Perhaps their desires include both tenderness and ravishment.

Being ravished means being swept off your feet, having your partner be crazy with love and desire for you, and being carried away by the moment. Being ravished can be a moment of pure and sublime bliss, because it allows for total surrender and trust.

Being ravished is a trust exercise, because it demands a ravisher and a ravishee. There must be a "yes" or permission from the one being ravished. This is what separates it from rape. And also what makes it hot and erotic. When the ravishee gives permission to be ravished, he or she is allowing someone else to take control, which allows the one being ravished to feel in control!

Letting go and having fun can mean acting out a sexual ravishment scene, as in the next exercise. This can be the beginning of role-playing and a way to experiment with the feeling of being vulnerable, and of being in control. Switching back and forth allows for both partners to experience the delight of how that can feel, and what it feels like to be the one letting go and being totally taken over by the desire of the other. And playing the role of the lover doing the ravishing can be a titillating experience of being in control and directing the other's pleasure.

Would you rather be ravished or be the ravisher in bed? Decide who will go first in this next exercise.

EXERCISE
Ravishment

Find a time where you and your partner will be free to act out your most erotic ravishment fantasy. Start with the idea that one of you will be totally in control, while the other will be totally naked (literally), and vulnerable to the erotic moment.

(continued on page 72)

(continued)

Set the mood by lighting candles, or by having a date night first. Come home and don't waste time. Start immediately, without waiting for permission. Remember, you have already gotten permission when you each decided who would be naked and who would be the ravisher. Now is the time to play!

Keep in mind that this is all in the spirit of erotic play and that you can laugh and giggle at any time. You don't have to keep up the role-play at all times. Experiment with how much you want to play the role, and take a breather if you have to.

If the ravishee at any time says "no," then stop and take a break. But remember to tell each other another word that might be fun to play with, like "stop," that the ravishee can say during the heat of the moment, but not really mean it.

This can add an element of danger that feels real, but is really playacting. (In a later exercise we will talk about safe words and why they are so important.)

Step One

Choose which partner will be naked tonight and which will be the ravisher. Those doing the ravishing will keep all of their clothes on. The ravisher can build up to taking the ravishee's clothes off slowly, torturing him or her with the exquisiteness of the subtle desire that is created by the waiting game. But remember, ravishment really means making the other person feel he or she is being taken over. Rough kissing, gentle hair pulling, stretching clothes, and yanking them off are fun ways to get into the make-believe of the ravishment fantasy.

Start any way you feel comfortable. Remember that the ravisher is in charge and will take off the ravishee's clothes in any way desired.

Step Two

When and if the ravishment turns into sex, the ravisher gets to decide whether to start slow or go fast and quick (remember, the ravishee has given permission for this to happen). Having sex with much of the ravisher's clothes on will keep the feeling of being in control paramount. Opening key clothing areas is, of course, permitted.

Know that next time, you will switch. But for this evening or afternoon, stay in the role until you are all the way through the exercise, or until you have had sex for the evening and can de-role.

Step Three

Afterward, talk about what it was like for you, and what you appreciated about being in the role of ravisher, and what you appreciated about being in the role of ravishee.

Reacting to Fantasies

Talking about our fantasies is risky business. For some, it might feel like sharing a private and intimate part of ourselves that we have never shared before. For others it might feel like something that we just don't talk about. And yet telling our partners about our most private thoughts is a way to feel connected and intimate with them.

Having the experience of being heard in a safe way by our partners is a way of helping them heal as well as a way to help us heal. The feeling of being held, being truly heard and listened to, and being seen for who we really are can heal us from the wounds of our past.

Many times, the one sharing the fantasies feels such a sense of gratitude and relief just for the opportunity to be heard that he begins to experience a new connection with his partner. True intimacy is achieved in those moments and remembered afterward.

Sometimes the telling of a fantasy alone is enough to create a heightened sense of erotic stimulation and connectedness within the sexual relationship.

Sometimes, as the receiver of this information, hearing about your partner's fantasies can be difficult. What if the fantasy involves something you are not comfortable with, or feel threatened by?

One way to deal with hearing a partner's fantasy that makes you uncomfortable is to simply mirror your partner. Just sitting with him allows your partner to express himself fully. Sometimes his fantasies are just fantasies, and he may never really want to take them into action. Perhaps he has wanted to tell these fantasies for a long time. Imagine how safe he would perceive you to be and how warm and loving he might feel toward you for simply listening to his fantasies.

When we first hear a fantasy, it can be a little surprising and sometimes create tension and uncertainty. We can feel unsure of whether our partner wants us to live out this fantasy, and sometimes unclear about where the fantasy comes from. Maybe it makes us wonder whether our partner has always wanted this, and perhaps has felt dissatisfied up until now. All these feelings are simply a story we make up based on our initial reaction to hearing the fantasy. With some time to digest, and hearing more about what our partner is thinking, it can become clearer to us, and we may begin to empathize.

It might make sense when we give ourselves the space to think about it, or to listen for more information, how our partner might want this. It might not make sense from our perspective, because perhaps we don't share the same fantasy. But this is what makes a relationship healthy and exciting. We are differentiated in our needs. What we want is many times different than what our partner wants. We don't have to be turned on or excited by the same things.

Learning to appreciate what our partner thinks and fantasizes about can be a key element in seeing our partner as sexy and alive.

EXERCISE
Sharing and Summing Up

Take some time together, perhaps on a date night, or create an evening where you have at least thirty minutes of uninterrupted time together, to review the exercises you have done so far in this book.

Spend some time talking to your partner about how the exercises have made you feel. Tell your partner what you have appreciated about him or her for doing the exercises with you, and talk about one thing you have learned about yourself from doing the exercises.

You may feel differently about your relationship now. Can you tell your partner? You might feel more anxious or a little scared that you have stretched into new areas. You may feel more excited and passionate toward your partner, and more excited about your relationship. You might also feel hope about the future of your relationship, honoring that there is an ongoing passionate connection available to you both, just by talking about your most intimate fantasies and appreciating each other.

Step One
Decide who will be the sender and who will be the receiver. The dialogue should start off like this:

Sender: "These exercises made me feel sexy."

Receiver (mirroring): "These exercises made you feel sexy."

Sender: "Particularly in the exercise about pressing our bodies together."

Receiver (mirroring): "So that particular exercise made you feel sexy."

Sender: "You got me."

Receiver (validating): "It makes sense that you would feel that because I know how much physical closeness means to you."

Sender: "You got me."

Receiver (empathizing): "I can imagine that doing those exercises also made you feel emotionally closer. Did I get that?"

Sender: "Yes, you got it."

Step Two
Switch.

Step Three
Follow the dialogue pattern in Step One, only the sender starts off with the following:

Sender: "One thing I learned about myself was (for example) that I really enjoy pleasing you."

Receiver (mirroring): "One thing you learned about yourself was that you really enjoy pleasing me."

Sender: "Particularly in the exercise about sharing our fantasies."

Receiver (mirroring): "So in that particular exercise you learned (for example) that you really enjoy pleasing me and that taught you something about yourself."

Sender: "You got me."

Receiver (validating): "It makes sense that you would feel you learned that because it sounds like you have learned that somtimes pleasing me makes you feel good too."

Sender: "You got me."

Receiver (empathizing): "I can imagine that learning that made you feel (for example) interested in learning more about yourself and finding out new ways to have better sex. Did I get that?"

Sender: "Yes, you got it."

Step Four
Switch.

(continued on page 76)

(continued)

Step Five

Follow the dialogue pattern in the above steps, only the sender starts off with the following:

Sender: "One thing I appreciated about you doing these exercises with me was how open you were with me."

The receiver then mirrors, validates, and empathizes with the sender.

Step Six

Switch.

Step Seven

Follow the dialogue pattern in the above steps, only the sender starts off with the following:

Sender: "One way I feel differently about our relationship is (for example) that I feel like I can tell you anything."

The receiver then mirrors, validates, and empathizes with the sender.

Step Eight

Switch.

The Payoff of Sexual Empathy: Passionate Closeness

Sexual empathy provides the safety and connection that allows for the exploration of fantasies. It means trying to understand how another person might want something different sexually than what we want.

Sexual empathy is also about perception. Do we know how empathetic our partner is? How understanding would they be if we were to tell them our most secret sexual fantasy—do we know or are we just guessing? And are you, as a partner, sexually empathic? Does your partner perceive you as someone willing to explore his or her sexual fantasies?

The payoff in being sexually empathic is huge. The power in the relationship is always held by the one with the most sexual empathy. Being the partner who can be open and understanding regardless of the topic means that you are perceived by your partner as being open enough in the relationship to talk about anything. If your partner knows he can tell you anything, then passion doesn't need to get split off outside the safe confines of the relationship.

Sexual empathy leads to improved communication and sexual generosity. When we know our partner can hear us, listen to us, and not judge our deepest fantasies and desires, there is a greater likelihood that these desires will become a reality.

Working together to increase sexual empathy prevents the need to go outside of the relationship to get your sexual needs met. It channels the erotic energy *into* the relationship. This increases the energy and loving feelings between partners, and it improves communication, sexual safety, and respect in the relationship.

The power in the relationship is always held by the one with the most sexual empathy.

When Empathy Is Lacking

Let's take two scenarios based on what could happen with and without sexual empathy in a relationship. Average husband and typical wife go to a couple's therapy session. They are encouraged to communicate with each other about their sexual needs. Average husband tells his wife he has a fantasy he would like to share with her. A low sexually empathetic response would be something like this.

Average husband: "Honey, I have a fantasy of seeing you dressed in sexy lingerie and waiting for me when I get home from work."

Typical wife: "Oh sure, like I have nothing better to do."

After a conversation like this, where one partner uses sarcasm, the partner who took the risk in sharing his or her fantasy will feel misunderstood and put off. We use sarcasm and defensiveness with our partner because we don't know how to empathize. Because of our own feelings, we might find it hard to respond to our partner's desires with understanding and compassion. We can't put ourselves in our partner's shoes, because we resist trying to understand his feelings.

Even if it doesn't make any sense to us that our partner wants to see us dressed up, it might make perfect sense to us that he might want that. If we can understand where he is coming from, we have an opportunity to be empathetic and show we care about his feelings and desires.

How Imago Can Help

Using the Imago dialogue, we can get past some of our resistance, and instead of deflecting our partner's requests and desires, we can respond in a way that feels empathic and understanding. When our partner feels our empathy, even if we don't agree to do anything, there is room for more satisfying sexual possibilities.

With the Imago dialogue, showing empathy starts by mirroring what our partner has said, which gives us a caring and respectful way to respond to our partner when he expresses a fantasy. Many times, having the structure of the dialogue helps us to hold our "reactivity" when we hear something that surprises us, or something that we don't understand.

"Reactivity" is the behavior, such as sarcasm or distancing, that shows up in our relationships when we react to our partners in a way that may hurt their feelings. Our reactivity is a response to something that hurts or angers us. If we don't take a moment to try and understand where our partners are coming from, we are more likely to go into a reactive and defensive mode. When we pull away from our partners, it can feel like we are doing it to protect ourselves from hurt, yet they will perceive it as abandonment or rejection. If we attack our partners when we are afraid or angry, then our partners will feel intruded upon, and they may become reactive in response.

This creates an unhealthy cycle of pursue and withdraw. When one person withdraws and the other pursues, no one is really making a connection. And we probably aren't getting the sex we want!

What Sexual Empathy Sounds Like

Giving a sexually empathic response to our partners when they share a fantasy means only that we mirror back what they have said. This gives time to think about what they are asking before there is a need for a response. It also allows us to really take the time to listen to their fantasy.

This feels much safer to our partners than when we attack them or withdraw from the relationship. Sharing a fantasy can make our partners feel vulnerable and exposed, and this can be a big risk. If we can help our partners feel safe while exposing their most private and intimate thoughts and desires, they will see us as a caring and empathic lover.

A sexually empathic response might sound like this:

Average husband: "Honey, I have a fantasy of seeing you dressed in sexy lingerie and waiting for me when I get home from work."

Typical wife: "So, okay, let me see if I got this ... you have a fantasy of seeing me dressed in sexy lingerie and waiting for you when you get home from work?"

In a sexually empathic relationship, all we have to do is mirror back what is being said using the Imago techniques. As stated above, this response gives us time to think about what our partner is saying and time to react. We don't have to rush into action before we are ready. There is time to decide about acting out the fantasy later. Right now, having the dialogue about sex is the most important thing, as it will increase the sexual empathy in the relationship, allowing for the development of trust and safety.

As this ongoing trust is created in your relationship, a new type of energy may emerge between you. Feeling safe and open with your partner can be the beginning of a new type of erotic connection. Your ability to be verbal about sex and share with your partner your deepest desires and fantasies creates a space that allows for further experimentation and risk. Risk can't happen unless you trust your partner to receive your efforts with empathy and understanding. Your partner will in turn be more likely to move to an action phase, helping you move your fantasies into reality.

EXERCISE
Exploring Sexual Empathy

This exercise will build on the dialogue skills you learned in the earlier chapters and incorporate more validation and empathy.

For this exercise, you are adding new and exciting elements to your dialogue and telling your partner what you want to do to him or her. By now you have a new form of communication, the Imago dialogue. All your partner has to do is listen, using the Imago dialogue skills. He or she can listen actively by mirroring, validating, and empathizing. This type of empathic conversation creates a safe structure in which to talk about your erotic thoughts and fantasies.

Using the Imago dialogue, tell your partner the following:

- What you always wanted to try sexually

- One thing you would like to do for your partner sexually

- One thing you would like to do sexually while your partner watches

These statements might feel a little riskier than in earlier dialogues. Doing the sexual empathy exercise will make you aware of how to talk about and risk sharing your true feelings and desires. So take some risks! Do the exercise and use some of the sexy language you have practiced in previous exercises.

For this first exercise, you will need at least forty-five minutes of uninterrupted private time with your partner. Find a quiet place where you can talk comfortably, either sitting up or lying down together. Make sure you face each other and make eye contact when you share this dialogue with each other.

As in the previous exercises, we will be sharing and then mirroring. Although you may have practiced these dialogue skills already, you might still feel uncomfortable with the slow pace that this creates in your "conversation." See if you can appreciate the slower pace of the dialogue and notice how it brings you closer to your partner, allowing you to appreciate each word and nuance of emotion in what he or she is saying to you.

In addition, you will be validating and empathizing with your partner, adding a new level of understanding and safety to the conversation. You may have to stretch to mirror and validate your partner's desires, and with practice, the more difficult language will become more comfortable. Soon you will have a safe way to talk to your partner about your fears. This is a great place to create the empathic relationship you will need later on as you take more risks together.

Step One

First, choose who will be the sender and who will be the receiver. As stated above, senders will tell their partner the following:

- What you always wanted to try sexually

The receiver will simply repeat, or mirror, what the sender says. It is important in an empathic dialogue that you don't add any of your own reactivity, and mirror exactly what your partner sends over.

An example might be the following:

Sender: "What I have always wanted to try is to have sex together in the shower."

The receiver simply mirrors back, maintaining eye contact, "So, what you have always wanted to try is to have sex together in the shower."

There are only two responses receivers need to make at this point—either "please send that again" or "Is there more?" The sender can say "yes" and send more or "no" and stop there.

(continued on page 82)

(continued)

Step Two

Senders then say, for example, "One thing I would like to do for you sexually is give you a back rub." Receivers mirror back what the senders said.

Step Three

Senders then say, for example, "One thing I would like to do sexually while you watch is masturbate." Receivers mirror back what the senders said.

Step Four

After the sender has sent all three desires and the receiver has mirrored them back, the receiver summarizes all of them by saying, "So what I heard you say was … ."

Step Five

The receiver then validates each statement, starting with, "It makes sense to me you would want to try … knowing you the way I know you, I can understand why you would desire that." This format makes validation easier.

Step Six

Now empathize, which means to guess at what you think your partner would feel if she had these desires and fantasies fulfilled. For example:

Receiver: "And I can imagine that if you did those things it would make you feel … (add feelings). Is there more?"

Step Seven

Now switch and your partner will have a turn to summarize, validate, and empathize.

If now is not a good time, or if further dialogue is needed to find empathy, then ask for another time to talk further about your desires and fantasies. Making a plan to keep talking until you feel openness and trust in the relationship. There is no rush. Just hearing about each other's sexual and erotic desires might add enough spark and excitement that making love spontaneously is definitely a possibility!

What Prevents Sexual Empathy?

Sometimes we want to be sexually empathic and, for whatever reason, cannot. One reason this happens is that our own personal fears and anxieties keep us from being sexually empathic toward our partner. If we feel shame about our own curiosity, it becomes difficult to be empathic with our partner.

We all fear being judged. Our inner fantasy life is often so personal and many times so secret that just the thought of sharing these feelings with another person can create anxiety and shame.

We are ultimately afraid that we will lose our connection with our partner over our deepest sexual needs. We may have a desire to tone down our thoughts and fantasies because we don't want to hurt the other person.

And finally, we use something called "projection" to justify how we think the other person will feel and react to us if we share our sexual fantasies. We project how we feel onto our partners: "If I feel this way, then so will he. If I think that certain sexual acts and desires are 'weird,' then so will my partner." Most times, in actuality, we have no idea how our partners will react, even when we have known them for a long time.

Sexual Empathy Contributes to Long-Term Happiness

Couples with a higher level of sexual empathy have a greater likelihood of staying together in the long term because they are more satisfied. Increasing sexual empathy in the relationship develops deeper connections. Sexually empathetic couples process and communicate their fantasies in healthy, relaxed ways and consequently maintain lasting satisfaction in their relationships.

Couples who identify what they are erotically curious about increase the feeling of sexual empathy in their partnership. They learn to normalize their curiosity and fantasies and can communicate with each other about their desires.

When couples explore their erotic curiosity with each other, sharing their fantasies safely, they can learn how to make all of their dreams come true and really have the sex they want.

Sexually empathetic couples process and communicate their fantasies in healthy, relaxed ways and consequently maintain lasting satisfaction in their relationships.

Our erotic needs include a desire for safety and trust, but also a craving for deep connection and intensity. Some levels of "safety" in a relationship may feel like boredom or being stuck. This is different than being in a sexually empathetic relationship, where it is safe to share feelings about sex.

Communication exercises where couples can learn to ask for their erotic needs to be met and explore fantasies together help solidify the freedom in a relationship. The capacity to tolerate and talk about the anxiety that hearing another's fantasy might bring up makes a relationship stronger.

How to talk, touch, and improve the sex and sensuality in a relationship, and being present for the other, are the goals of the erotic partnership.

When we learn how to be authentic with each other, we find a renewed intimacy in our relationship.

Taking More Risks

This next exercise will flex your fantasy muscles. You are now getting more comfortable talking to your partner about sex. Now you have a structure in which to ask for specific things you like. Now you can begin to get in touch with your own inner fantasy life.

Educating your partner about your fantasy life is the only way to give your partner the opportunity to give you what you want. You are teaching your partner how to love you. Give your partner the tools to do that, and he will feel more successful at it, and you will feel like you are getting the sex you want.

EXERCISE

Flex Your Fantasy Muscles

For this exercise, you will explore your own internal fantasy world first, and then share these thoughts with your partner. You will need a quiet place to sit down and write, along with a pen and paper or a journal. Take about thirty minutes of uninterrupted quiet time to think and describe in detail your thoughts.

You will need another sixty minutes of quiet private time with your partner to dialogue about what you have written. These two parts of the exercise can be done at two separate times or at the same time. You might want to have this dialogue on a date night, when you can concentrate on each other and listen to each other's inner fantasies.

Step One

First, get out your paper or journal, and answer the following questions. Try to include as much detail as you can, such as where you would be, what you would wear, what your partner would be doing, and so on.

- Write down one sexual thing in bed that you love to do.

- Write down one sexual thing that your partner might want to do.

- Write down one sexual fantasy you have that you haven't told your partner.

Step Two

Now ask for the time to share with your partner what you have written. Find a comfortable place to sit or lie down where you can make eye contact with your partner as you share what you have written about your fantasies.

Senders "send" over their desires in their first statement. Receivers simply repeat, or mirror, what the sender says. Take turns going through each step, sending and mirroring. It is important in an empathetic dialogue that you don't add any of your own reactivity, and simply mirror exactly what your partner says.

An example might be the following:

Sender: "One sexual thing that I love to do in bed is to be on top."

The receiver simply mirrors back, maintaining eye contact:

Receiver: "So, one thing that you love to do in bed is to be on top."

After the receiver has mirrored, the sender switches and becomes the receiver.

(continued on page 86)

(continued)

Step Three

After you've both shared and mirrored, summarize what each other has said. Receiver: "So what I heard you say was (summarize all three desires)." Ask your partner to remind you if you've forgotten part of what he or she said.

Step Four

Next, validate what each other has said. Using the sentence frame "It makes sense to me ..." makes this easier. How does it make sense to you, knowing your partner the way you do, that he or she would like these things and want to do more of them with you?

Step Five

Next, empathize with what your partner has said. Remember, it might be a stretch to do this, but you are an empathic partner now and you can listen in this active way. You don't ever have to commit to living out your partner's fantasies until you are comfortable.

Receiver: "And I can imagine that if you did those things it would make you feel (add feelings). Is there more?"

Step Six

Now switch and your partner will have a turn to summarize, validate, and empathize.

You can move on from here if you are both comfortable, and each of you can choose one thing your partner has expressed a desire for. Remember that you are giving your partner a gift of living out a fantasy. This generosity comes from the sexual empathy you now have for your partner, a deeper understanding of his or her thoughts, feelings, and desires.

If now is not a good time, then ask for another time to talk more about your desires and fantasies. Making a plan to keep talking until your partner understands you can create openness in the relationship. Just hearing about your sexual and erotic desires might add enough spark and excitement that making love spontaneously is definitely a possibility!

Bridging the Sexual Communication Gap

Taking erotic communication to the next step, we can use the Imago techniques we have learned so far to help bridge the separation that sometimes exists in sexual partnerships.

Men and women have different communication styles, and within a relationship partners have differing comfort levels talking about sex. How honest we are with each other about our sexual needs is dependent on what we have learned about sex and our bodies, as well as the rules and customs with which we grew up. It is also contingent on how much we trust our partner to listen and validate our desires.

In our society, there is a lot of confusion when it comes to sexuality and sexual relationships. This confusion makes it difficult for us to identify our sexual needs and even harder to talk about them. We are unsure about how to ask for what we want sexually, what words to use, and what is acceptable for discussion.

Being honest with ourselves about our desires is not as clear-cut as it may appear at first glance. If we were honest with ourselves about what we craved, then we could be honest with our partner about our desires. However, many times we aren't sure.

Being sexually honest with our partner means taking the risk to share what is going on in our bodies. It means telling our partner what feels good and what might feel better. It means having a language to describe what may not be working and what would work better. It means having an open dialogue and a level of comfort with each other to talk about our sexual needs. This can help us get the sex we want, and it can help us give our partner what he or she really wants in bed.

Unfortunately, figuring out what our partner wants in bed can sometimes feel like adolescent fumbling in the back seat of a car. We stumble around our partner's body until we hit on something that seems to work, and many times we repeat that same move and style every time we make love, because we have found the "right button to push." If our partners want something different or want to try sex a different way, it can be hard for them to be honest with us without worrying that they will hurt our feelings.

EXERCISE
Sexual Honesty Questionnaire

Use the questionnaire below to gauge you and your partner's sexual honesty.

Answer the questions below, using a scale from 1 to 5, with 1 meaning never/not at all and 5 meaning always/very much so.

Rate your answers to your questions and share them with your partner. There is no right or wrong way to do this exercise, so answer quickly and without judgment.

1	2	3	4	5
Never	Sometimes	Many times	Usually	Always

I talk freely about sex with my partner.

1 2 3 4 5

I think it is important to our relationship to be intimate.

1 2 3 4 5

I am satisfied with our sex life.

1 2 3 4 5

There are things I would like to try if my partner was open to the idea.

1 2 3 4 5

I have thoughts and fantasies about new things to do in bed.

1 2 3 4 5

I am confident I can ask for what I fantasize about.

1   2   3   4   5

I feel good about my body.

1   2   3   4   5

I would like help from my partner to indicate where he/she likes
to be touched.

1   2   3   4   5

I would like help from my partner to indicate where her clitoris is
located.

1   2   3   4   5

I would like help from my partner to indicate where her G-spot is
located.

1   2   3   4   5

My partner and I talk freely about any sexual dysfunction in
our relationship, for example, premature ejaculation, difficulty in
maintaining or achieving erection, or not ejaculating.

1   2   3   4   5

My partner can achieve orgasm through clitoral stimulation.

1   2   3   4   5

My partner can achieve orgasm through vaginal stimulation.

1   2   3   4   5

My partner can achieve orgasm through vaginal and clitoral
stimulation.

1   2   3   4   5

I would like assistance from my partner to locate spots
along the vaginal wall and the outside labia that feel good
when stimulated.

1   2   3   4   5

I know what the perineum is and where it is located on
my partner.

1   2   3   4   5

(continued on page 90)

(continued)

I know what the male prostate gland is and how it is stimulated in my partner.

1   2   3   4   5

I am open to anal stimulation from my partner.

1   2   3   4   5

I would like to experience anal sex, either for the first time or more often.

1   2   3   4   5

I would like help from my partner to indicate how she would like her clitoris stimulated.

1   2   3   4   5

I would like help from my partner to indicate how she would like her vagina stimulated.

1   2   3   4   5

I would like help from my partner to indicate specifically the ways in which he enjoys having his penis stimulated.

1   2   3   4   5

I know where my partner's scrotum is located.

1   2   3   4   5

My partner enjoys having his scrotum stimulated.

1   2   3   4   5

I would like help from my partner to indicate how he would like his scrotum stimulated.

1   2   3   4   5

I have a sincere desire to talk more openly with my partner about our sex life.

1   2   3   4   5

Add up your score. If you have a lot of 4s and 5s, you are more open and ready to be sexually honest with your partner. If you have more 1s and 2s you are ready to work on opening up to your partner in safer and healthier ways.

Types of Arousal

Many times our partner's erotic fantasy life is different from our own because their body is different, as are their arousal levels and points of intensity.

Arousal levels differ among women, too, depending on their sensitivity, hormone levels, and psychological openness to the experience of sexuality. Men have differing levels of arousal depending on age, mood, and energy level.

We also vary as people depending on what stimulus creates arousal in our bodies. Some of us are visual, with a high level of turn-on based on seeing things like our partner's naked body. Some of us are tactile, which means that touch, of a varying sort, can arouse us to stimulation. Some people are aural, meaning they get aroused hearing sounds and words.

Figuring out what our arousal points are and learning about our partner's are part of the wonderful erotic discovery possible through communication.

Ask whether your partner is more visual, tactile, or aural during sex. Help your partner identify which area is the most intense. You might think you know what turns your partner on. And you may be right, but now is your chance to find out.

EXERCISE
Your Partner's Senses

This exercise can be the beginning of the sexual honesty that leads to long-term passion. Learning to be honest with each other is key. Sexual honesty is about engaging our partners in conversation about what turns them on.

First, find a time that will allow you enough uninterrupted privacy that you and your partner will feel comfortable exploring each other's senses. Warm up the room by raising the heat, lowering the lights, and creating an atmosphere of sensual discovery. Make sure you set up things in the room that your partner can see and smell, such as fresh flowers. Add something sensual your partner can hear, like jazz, classical music, or light rock. And also add something in the room that feels wonderful against the skin, such as silk sheets or soft pillows.

(continued on page 92)

(continued)

You will also need some props for this exercise. Find a soft feather or clean feather duster, an ice cube, a hairbrush, and anything else you think might feel sensual against your partner's skin. Find a blindfold or a silk scarf.

Step One

Decide who will be the sender and who will be the receiver. Receivers should lie comfortably on the bed and remove as much clothing as they are comfortable with. Senders should ask receivers whether it is okay to tie the blindfold over their eyes. Then get comfortable, and dazzle your partner with sensual delights.

Step Two

Focus on your partner's sense of hearing by whispering in his ear. Whisper the things you are planning to do to his tactile senses, through the skin. This might sound like:

"I am going to gently touch your skin ... ."

Then take the feather and lightly tickle and brush the skin with it.

Take the ice cube and slide it over his warm body until it melts.

Then take the brush and very gently scratch your partner with the bristles.

The idea is to give him a heightened tactile experience, while whispering in his ear for his aural pleasure.

Step Three

Now slowly take off the blindfold and let him see what you are doing to him. This will add visual stimulation.

Step Four

Now ask him what he liked the most. "Do you like when I talk to you? Do you like when I touch you? Do you like to watch me touch you? Tell me what you like the most ... ."

If you want to keep going and make love at this point, save the "switch" part of this exercise for next time.

Step Five

Switch.

Navigating Arousal

Helping your partner learn the "arousal map" of your body is important to sexual connection. An "arousal map" contains the patterns and sensitivity in your body that are unique to your physical self. Your partner has his or her own arousal map, too.

No one gives us a map to each other's body when we meet and fall in love. Part of the joy of an erotic relationship is exploring this landscape together. Without directions, we can wander joyfully and find places we like, yet still risk missing some of the more important and delightful places on our lover's body. With interaction, we can go back and forth together, exploring, learning, and growing as a sexual couple.

What Sex Ed Didn't Tell Us

Growing up, we learn in health education classes about the egg and the sperm, but we don't receive the "manual" for the opposite sex's body. As young people, we can be confused about how the opposite sex feels in his or her body. We might know how the internal organs work from health class or anatomy, but we don't learn about how the opposite sex reaches arousal levels or orgasm. This is something we fumble with later on as we grow into relationships.

As adolescents and adults, our confusion about our partner's body might be resolved subtly over time, as we explore and delight in each other's differences. (Same-sex couples have this experience as well. Exploring another person's body is intriguing, even if it has the same parts as ours—because the other person still has differences in arousal points and levels.) But most of us are still unsure about how to fully engage our partners sexually, unless they tell us how.

Growing up, we are not only confused about the opposite sex but also about our own growing bodies and newly developing sexual desires. When we mature and engage in erotic relationships, we begin to discover our sexuality, and if we learn to be sexually honest with our partners, we give them a way to bring us the pleasure we desire, and we open a dialogue to learn to express our own needs, learning more about ourselves in the process.

Learning how to talk about sex can be a hit-or-miss process. We might find a book or helpful partner to encourage us, but there is not a lot of information or training available to learn how to talk about sex with our partners. Lots of books discuss sexuality, but not how to talk about it with the people we are having sex with.

Our culture does not make it easy to talk about sex. We can see sex in the media, in magazines, and in the movies, but no one seems to be able to talk about it openly and honestly.

The Imago dialogue process of mirroring and validation can help bridge this gap and also any differences in our communication styles. Sometimes it's hard to verbalize our needs, and having someone listen in this empathetic way can make it easier to say what may feel awkward or uncomfortable. Listening to our partner use these dialogue skills gives us a new level of mastery over sexual communication.

How Other Cultures Approach Sexual Education

In some cultures, boys are initiated into sexuality by an older, more experienced woman, who shares the ways of eroticism with them so that they may pass it on to less experienced girls.

In other cultures, boys are introduced to sex in brothels and by prostitutes, paid for by their families. In today's age of AIDS and other sexually transmitted diseases, these practices may be less common than in the past. Many cultures are now similar to ours, in that young people fumble and grope as an introduction to sexuality, where once the elders of the society may have been more involved and supportive in the sexual development of their youth.

A Pattern of Dysfunction

If our relationships are complicated, then talking about sex can be the same as talking about anything else in a relationship—difficult. Whatever dysfunctional style of communication we have adapted in our partnership will most assuredly be acted out when we talk about our sexual needs.

Talking about sex can sometimes wound at a deeper level than other discussions. Because most people have some kind of insecurity around sexuality and performance, talking about sex with your partner can be a sensitive and difficult challenge. There is a risk of hurting each other's feelings, bruising egos, and using sarcasm or defensiveness to prevent open and honest sharing. We might not mean for this to happen, but we can get stuck in a pattern of relating to each other that makes it hard to reach a new level of openness. Many couples don't know where to begin to talk about sex honestly and with a level of vulnerability that helps them feel connected and intimate.

Whatever dysfunctional style of communication we have adapted in our partnership will most assuredly be acted out when we talk about our sexual needs.

Here is an example of what can happen when couples try to talk about sex. Sometimes other issues get dragged into the discussion along with sex.

Pete and Pam were not happy with their sex life. They began to talk about sex together one night after a long day fighting about money. Instead of using the Imago dialogue as a guide, they got into their regular pattern of relating to each other.

This pattern had been established long ago in their relationship. Pam had a long-standing resentment against Pete because she felt that he didn't understand that she needed to invest money in her business. She saw spending money as a necessity for the growth and expansion of their family. Pete saw Pam's spending as unnecessary. He felt that she should not invest any of their hard-earned capital in her business until it was established.

Pam took Pete's withholding financial support as being emotionally withholding. She felt this was a sign that he did not believe in her. Pete felt Pam disregarded his feelings about money and saw this as a lack of respect for him. Neither Pam nor Pete had insight into his or her own issues around money and spending, nor did they explore their deeper needs for acceptance and love, which were left over from their childhoods.

They both craved a deeper sexual connection, which would comfort them and make them feel more connected. Particularly after fighting about money, they both wanted an erotic experience that would make them feel more intimate with each other. For example, Pete wanted to share his fantasies with Pam.

One night, they thought that talking about sex might get them through their resentments that had been building all week. Pam asked Pete to talk about what he might be interested in trying. Finally he shared, cautiously at first. He told Pam, "I would like you to dress up in leather clothes during sex."

Pam immediately responded by saying, "Well, that's not going to happen because you wouldn't let me spend the money on leather clothes!"

Pete immediately shut down.

A Different Way of Sharing

If Pam and Pete had used the Imago dialogue and been able to mirror their fantasies, they could have slowed down this process, allowing time for receptivity and not reactivity. They could have experienced their conversation very differently. The Imago dialogue can hold a space that can be experienced by both as being generous and supportive.

Another way that conversation could have gone would be:

Pete: "Is now a good time to have a dialogue?"

Pam: "Yes."

Pete: "Is now a good time to talk about sex?"

Pam: "Yes, okay."

Pete: "I have a fantasy I would like to share with you."

Pam: "You have a fantasy you would like to share with me."

Pete: "One thing I really appreciate about you is the way you look in clothes."

Pam: "One think you really appreciate about me is the way I look in clothes."

Pete: "And one thing I have fantasized about but never shared is to see you dressed up in leather clothes."

Pam: "And one thing you have fantasized about but never shared is to see me dressed up in leather clothes. Is there more?"

Pete: "Yes, and specifically to have sex with you while you are wearing a leather thong."

Pam: "So specifically you have thought about having sex with me while I am wearing a leather thong. Is there more?"

Pete: "Just that it would mean a lot to me because I know this would be a stretch for you."

Pam: "So this would mean a lot to you because you know it would be a stretch for me. Is there more?"

Pete: "No, that's it."

Pam (validating): "Knowing you the way I know you, Pete, I understand you like to see me dressed up; you have always liked that. So it makes sense to me that you would want to see me in leather. And I know you like thongs, and would appreciate it if I stretched for you, since that is really not my thing. I can imagine that you would really appreciate it if I wore that for you."

Pete: "You got it!"

Pam (empathizing): "And I can imagine that if you got those things, if I were to wear leather and a leather thong while we had sex, that you would feel really turned on, and very loved, since it would be a stretch for me, and you would know I would be doing this just for you."

Pete: "Yes, it would be very sexy."

Pam: "So for you it would be very sexy."

Pete: "Yes."

Pam: "Did I get all your feelings?"

Pete: "I would also feel grateful."

Pam: "Oh, okay, and grateful."

Pete: "Yes, you got me!"

Pam, you'll notice, does not commit to acting out Pete's fantasy, nor does she judge him. She mirrors him, validates, and empathizes. This allows Pete to express his feelings honestly, and allows Pam time to absorb what he is asking. She can decide at another time whether she will actually take him up on his request.

She might think about it for a while, or fantasize about it herself, or even talk to him about it again at a later time. She could even talk to her girlfriends about it.

The Differences in Dialogue

Men are intrigued by women's conversations. Men want to understand not only how women's minds work, but also what they share with each other when men are not around. More important, men want to know what women actually say to each other about sex. Do they share details? Do they compare notes? Do they compare *them*?

Most men are amazed to hear that women talk about sex more often than men do, and with much more detail. Women, in groups, have a tendency to talk much more graphically about sexuality than men. Men, when in groups, often talk about women objectively and in generalized terms.

"Oh, yeah, last night was great, we had great sex ... ."

Or they look at women in the bar and comment, "Look at the breasts on her."

Women, while in groups, also objectify men, but they share intimate details of their own sexual scenarios. Women talk graphically about what happens in bed. For instance, a woman might explain what a man did to her sexually, describing her own multiorgasmic experience, but not necessarily detailing the man's performance.

The drive women have to share their feelings about relationships stems from both their history and their natural approach to problem solving. For example, women have spent eternity in community. Joined in the ancient, sacred bonding ritual of womanly sensual arts, women throughout the ages have gathered in red tents, in quilting bees, around the hearth, and at summer camps. During sleepovers, around the kitchen table, around the birthing bed, women have shared intimate details of their sex lives, opened up about their feelings, and talked about their relationships.

Women's natural tendency to express their emotions is part of their capacity for problem solving. Women talk until they have diluted the emotion attached to a problem. Men have a tendency to problem solve by finding solutions to problems, and therefore find women's capacity to repeatedly talk about a problem confusing and redundant.

EXERCISE
Learning the Language of Arousal

Learning how to communicate with your partner about the arousal levels in your body begins with identifying your own arousal patterns. You'll need a language to communicate this to your partner. Finally you also need a way for your partner to understand and translate what you are saying.

In this exercise, your partner will help you find the parts of your body that trigger the greatest levels of arousal, and will help you pinpoint the areas where you like the most concentrated touch. Your partner will also help you figure out what type of touch you like the most in those areas. How wonderful that you have someone to share this information with! Remember to appreciate your partner for his or her willingness to go on this exploratory journey with you.

(continued on page 100)

(continued)

For this exercise you will need at least sixty minutes of uninterrupted time. Make sure the children are taken care of and that your phone is turned off. Make sure the room you are using is quiet enough to be able to hear each other speak in a low tone of voice. Set the atmosphere by lighting candles, putting on soft background music, and making the bed with soft or silky sheets.

You can do this exercise with sexy and comfortable clothes on, or you can be naked, either taking turns or both of you disrobing before you begin.

In this exercise, your partner will touch you and you will respond verbally, using a number system to specifically identify how sensitive each section of your body surface feels. Numbers 1 to 10 will reflect how something feels as your partner touches you, with 1 meaning there is hardly any sensation and 10 meaning that the arousal and sensitivity level is at its peak.

Step One

Decide who will be the sender and who will be the receiver, and remember you get to switch, so you will each have a turn. Receivers will be the first to be touched and to express their reaction to each touch. You will use the number system to have a language to accurately describe the sensations and to give your partner clear information about the sensitive arousal map of your body.

Receivers should lie down in a comfortable position that they can sustain for at least thirty minutes. Senders should find a comfortable place to sit or lie with their prone partner, where they can reach all parts of their partner's body with little effort.

Step Two

First, receivers should tell their partners how much they appreciate them for doing this exercise with them. It might sound like: "I really appreciate you helping me find the sensitive areas of my body and helping me find a way to express that information to you."

Your partner, the sender, can mirror this back. "So you really appreciate that I am helping you find the sensitive areas of your body and helping you express that information to me."

Step Three

Now ask your partner to help you find the parts of your body that are most sensitive to touch. The sender now gently touches each area of the receiver's body, choosing small or large areas and caressing each spot until the receiver identifies a number of sensitivity.

Start on the outer parts of the body, furthest from the center of the torso. For example, starting with the hands or feet and moving inward will increase the arousal and sensitivity for the receiver as the touch gets closer to the more sensitive genital and nipple areas.

Receivers should relax, close their eyes, and feel each touch and caress. As the sender gently touches and caresses every part of the receiver's body, the receiver responds with a number from 1 to 10 to show how sensitive that area is. For example, the sender may touch the receiver's ankle. The receiver relaxes into the touch and decides how sensitive the area is, with 1 being little sensitivity and 10 being highly stimulated and aroused.

After being touched, the receiver might say, "That's a 4."

The sender then mirrors back, "So this is a 4."

Then the sender moves on to another area of the receiver's body.

The sender may want to try adjusting the touch and intensity of the caress. Perhaps the light touch on the receiver's ankle is a 4, and then the sender deepens the stroke and makes it a more massaging caress, and the receiver now shares that this feels like a 6. The sender mirrors back this information.

After varying the intensity of the strokes, from tender and gentle to firm and assured, vary the speed. Most people do not like simple repetitive movements over the same area for a long period of time. This can feel irritating.

Notice what speed or variety works the best to increase the level of sensitivity.

Notice that as you progress from the outer parts of the body to the inner parts of the body (closer to the center of the body) that the sensitivity level may increase.

Step Four

Now try to identify specific feelings associated with being touched on certain areas of your body. The sender should touch you gently or firmly in different areas. Senders should try to remember what the receivers responded to in the first part of the exercise. Did they feel more sensitive with a lighter stroke or a firmer caress?

The receiver can now say an adjective or descriptive word describing how it feels to be touched in each area. For example, if the sender touches the receiver's knee, the receiver could identify a feeling or reaction, such as, "That feels nice and soft."

The sender mirrors: "So that feels nice and soft."

(continued on page 102)

(continued)

If the sender touches a genital area, or more sensitive skin, the receiver might say, "That feels wonderful."

The sender then mirrors, "That feels wonderful."

Senders might try to think up words beforehand so that they have some in mind when the receiver begins to touch them.

Step Five

When you are through with each part of your partner's body, front and back, then switch.

(Another variation on this exercise: Combine this exercise with another. The receivers should be totally naked while the senders remained clothed. Receivers take turns identifying their levels of sensitivity by number, and then use feeling words as the sender touches different areas of their body. Save the "switch" for another night.)

If this exercise leads to lovemaking or erotic connection, great. If not, that's okay, too. Know that you have just discovered a huge amount of valuable information about your partner's arousal and her body's map of sensitive areas. You can use this information next time you make love or anytime you need a language to describe your body's response.

Step Six

Talk about any feelings that came up for both of you, and how it felt to do this exercise.

Step Seven

End with an appreciation for each other, both as the sender and as the receiver.

This exercise is a great way to work through some of the inherent shame attached to expressing and communicating sexual responsiveness. It also allows for a deeper level of intimacy and connection with your partner. Intimacy is a great aphrodisiac, and it can help keep the passionate part of your relationship alive for years to come.

Behind a Curtain of Shame:
Erotic Art History

We are all affected by our culture's view of sexuality, and we integrate this into our sex lives. Erotic connection is a normal and healthy part of a love relationship, and yet it is the most private and intimate part of connection.

A woman came into my office recently suffering from a feeling of distance in her relationship. She wanted to be closer to her partner, but was afraid to tell him how she felt and what she needed, and this made her feel sexually and emotionally distant from him.

On a recent business trip to New Mexico, she discovered that she came by this fear naturally, and that it was prevalent throughout our society and not just in her relationship. She learned from the experience and was able to take this trip home with her, "pulling her own curtains aside," and be more honest and open about her sexuality with her partner.

She told me the following story:

"I was in Taos recently, and wandering along the plaza, I stumbled on the La Fonda Hotel, hidden behind old green wooden doors since 1820. Wandering in out of the dust and hot sun, I found a small white sign that said 'D.H. Lawrence Forbidden Paintings, $3.'

"I crept further into the dark lobby, where a woman sat behind glass where there was a small opening at the bottom of her window hollowed out for sliding in money. I felt like I was at a peep show. I paid my $3 and the woman came out from behind the glass and led me into a back room.

"I was the only patron there to see the show, despite it being the peak of tourist season. I felt like I was about to enter into the secret world. (D.H. Lawrence was the author of *Lady Chatterley's Lover*, a drastically erotic novel for its day, published in 1928.) I wanted to be alone to see his paintings, but it was obvious that the guide was not going to leave me alone with the exhibit. She stood next to me and handed me a small piece of paper describing the paintings.

(continued on page 104)

Behind a Curtain (continued)

"She then told me to turn and face a large wall in this otherwise nondescript room filled with dining tables and a podium. She slowly pulled on a long gold rope, which opened worn velvet curtains that filled the wall from floor to ceiling. The heavy golden material parted dramatically, revealing nine large oil paintings. I glanced down at my one-page program. The paintings dated back to the 1920s, when Lawrence, known as a writer, had painted them in Europe. The paintings were confiscated in England for their erotic content. He was able to move them out of the country by promising they would stay in America. His benefactor was the owner of the La Fonda Hotel.

"I moved toward the paintings and their primitive shapes. I saw a range of naked buttocks, thighs, pubic hair; male-female parts. The paintings drew me in. The colors were somehow New Mexican desert colors, although he painted many of them in Italy.

"I realized that Lawrence had been a sexual rebel in his time, surrounded by negative publicity for *Lady Chatterley's Lover.* I smiled. The paintings were so benign compared to the pornography of today. If these paintings were done by a contemporary artist, they could hang safely and uncensored in any New York gallery today.

"When I got ready to leave, the guide standing by my side slowly closed the heavy drapes over this piece of 'erotic' art history. I asked her about the curtains.

"'Are they there to protect the pieces from dust and light? Or are they there to hide the content of the art?'

"She answered, 'Well, the governor was here last week, and the paintings are somewhat ... .' She hesitated. I knew she was thinking, 'They are somewhat erotic.'

"Obviously, the paintings were not for public consumption. These erotic works would be hidden forever."

This story is an illustration of how erotic and beautiful the world is. All of our great artists and writers have understood the sensuality and eroticism of the world, and captured the interplay of lovers through their art.

My Client also realized that her own erotic life had been behind curtains of her own making for years, and now she was ready to open them up and share herself more honestly with her partner.

Censorship, sexism, views of women, economics, and politics have all played social roles in how we view eroticism and sexuality throughout our culture and how we create art depicting it. They have also shaped our beliefs about sex and kept us from being able to talk about it. Like golden curtains drawn over our fantasies, we hide our most private thoughts, even from those we love.

What would it be like to open the curtains and reveal the beauty of your own inner erotic life? Can you visualize yourself as someone who stands in the face of shame and explores his or her own sexual honesty?

The Differences between Male and Female Arousal

When we talk about arousal and our partners' bodies, we also include a discussion about the differences between men and women. There are similarities in sensitivity and orgasm, but there are also significant differences.

Because we don't always understand the differences between the sexes, there can be a lack of understanding in couples and a gap in sexual communication. It is easier to communicate what we need and want with our partners if our partners understand the differences between our bodies.

It takes women an average of eight to twenty minutes of direct clitoral stimulation to achieve orgasm, and yet when men were surveyed they thought it should take women no more than four minutes. This is not surprising in an age when women are faking orgasms at an average rate of seven out of every ten. If women fake an orgasm after four minutes, doesn't it reinforce for men that women only need four minutes of clitoral stimulation to orgasm?

EXERCISE
Mutual Sexual Awareness

The following exercise is a great way to begin to understand the differences between your body and your partner's. Your arousal cycle may be different from your partner's. It may take longer for your partner to get to a peak arousal phase where he or she is ready for orgasm. Understanding how your partner masturbates can teach you a tremendous amount about his or her sexual response cycle.

There is a lot of shame and embarrassment in our society around masturbation. Religious and cultural prohibitions about it have made the act of self-pleasure secret and hidden. Some people may feel more inhibited about masturbation than others. Women are sometimes more embarrassed about masturbating in front of a partner than men are, but differences in personality and personal sexual history have more to do with comfort levels than gender does. If you have grown up with prohibitions against masturbation, it might be hard to share this most personal of acts with another person.

Masturbating in front of our partners is like giving them instructions. It is a fast and wonderfully erotic way to increase the intimacy between the two of you. It gives you a physical language of sexual expression that tells more about your body than words can. Watching you touch yourself in ways that give you pleasure may be so arousing to your partner that it becomes an erotic encounter as well as a learning experience. It takes a lot of sexual generosity and understanding to give this gift of erotic connection to your partner.

First, before we can masturbate in front of our partner, we may need to find a mutual language that helps us break the ice. Getting over the discomfort and awkwardness around masturbation starts with a conversation. Communication about masturbation can be a turn-on, and it can be a way to connect to your partner. Now, with your Imago dialogue skills, you have a way to talk with your partner about what might otherwise be an uncomfortable topic.

For this exercise, you will need thirty minutes of safe, uninterrupted time. Because this may bring up some embarrassment, or even shame, privacy is essential. Find a place where you will not be interrupted and where there is a comfortable place to sit or lie down facing each other. Have this conversation in a safe and respectful way by giving each other the time and space to talk, and mirror back what the other has said. This is a great time to use validation and empathy in your dialogue. It will help your partner feel understood, and is the first step toward feeling safe.

Step One

Decide who will be the sender and who will be the receiver. Senders will talk for fifteen minutes about masturbation, and everything they can think of about the subject of self-pleasure. The receivers will mirror, always asking, "Is there more?"

For instance, ideas about masturbation might include how you feel about it, how often you do it, how you do it, what you were taught about it, and so on. Make sure you take the full fifteen minutes.

Step Two

Receivers mirror back what the senders have said, after each sentence or chunk. If they send too much, the receivers should ask them to send it over in smaller chunks so they can make sure they got it all.

Step Three

Receivers summarize, validate, and empathize. For example, the receiver might say, "So let me see if I got all that (summarize here to the best of your ability everything the sender has said about masturbation). It makes sense that you would feel this way about masturbation, knowing you the way I know you, because ... ."

(continued on page 108)

(continued)

Then check that out with the sender.

Receiver: "Did I get that?"

Sender: "You got me" or "Yes, and I want to make sure you heard the part where I said ... ."

The receiver mirrors back if there was a part the sender wanted to make sure was heard.

Now empathize. It might sound like, "So it would make sense to me from everything you said that you would feel (include feeling words here like "removed, scared, anxious"). Are there other feelings you have that I didn't get?"

Sender: "No, you got me" or "Yes, I also feel ... ."

The receiver then mirrors back any other feelings the sender has.

Step Four

Then you switch and the receiver becomes the sender.

Does it feel more likely that you would now feel comfortable enough with each other to masturbate in front of your partner? If so, make a date to do so.

Plan on a night where you will be undisturbed for an evening. Set the stage for an erotic evening. Take a long hot bath, wear sexy lingerie, light candles, and put soft sheets on the bed. Then pile up comfortable pillows, make sure you have lots of lubricant, and sit across from each other, where you can watch your partner while he or she watches you.

Moving from Sexual Curiosity to Erotic Action

6

Erotic curiosity is about thoughts, fantasies, and desires of a sexual or erotic nature. All mammals are sexual, but we are the only mammals that "eroticize" sex because we have the power to use our imagination to create erotic thoughts and images, which we use to fuel our passion.

Everyone has this capacity, although sometimes it may be difficult to get in touch with our fantasies. Some people engage in an active and erotic fantasy life, and some of us shut down our capacity for fantasy, and even get so rusty at it that we forget how. A healthy and active fantasy life is part of being a healthy and active human. Keeping the imagination alive helps keep our sex life alive and awake.

As we explore our erotic imagination and fantasy, this knowledge can help us communicate to our partner what we find exciting and stimulating. Using the Imago dialogue, we have skills that allow us to talk about our inner life and feel more intimate and connected to our partner.

There is a spectrum of normal human erotic curiosity. Understanding our personal spectrum of erotic thoughts can help us discover our fantasies and begin to make them happen.

Our erotic imagination includes three things—**curiosity, fantasy,** and **erotic action.** These three areas are all on an Erotic Curiosity Spectrum. The Erotic Curiosity Spectrum is a way to describe thoughts, fantasies, and desires on a continuum, from simple thoughts about sexual experiences to actions.

Erotic Curiosity Spectrum

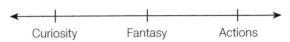

Curiosity   Fantasy   Actions

At the left end of the spectrum are erotic thoughts about things we are curious about. These may include sex acts, erotic games, wearing sexy clothes, or wondering about what it would be like to have sex with other people, including friends, colleagues, or movie stars. Being erotically curious about something or someone doesn't necessarily mean we have full-blown fantasies about it; these are sometimes just passing thoughts or images. Maybe we have read about a sex act or have seen something in a movie that intrigues us, but we don't think much about it, or give it much energy. Still, there is a curiosity and a wondering.

Anything on your own erotic curiosity spectrum is normal for you. What you think about in the privacy of your mind is your own personal, fantastic movie theater on the screen of your imagination. What you do about your thoughts and fantasies are called erotic actions.

In the following exercises you will begin to explore your erotic curiosity, and then share your fantasies with your partner. Discovering these parts of yourself, you may find that your sexual desires become more intense. You will also be able to differentiate between what you would like to keep at a fantasy level and what you would like to take into action. Beginning to share these thoughts and feelings with your partner may feel scary or uncomfortable at first. Using the Imago dialogue, including mirroring, validating, and empathizing, can make it safer.

EXERCISE

From Sexual Curiosity to Erotic Action

There are several parts to this exercise, and you can do them all in one sitting, or you can do one part of the exercise and then leave it for a few days. There is no right or wrong way to do this. The important thing is that you explore some of your own inner fantasies and then share them with your partner using the Imago dialogue process.

You will start off with a writing exercise, which you do on your own. You are exploring your own erotic curiosity, and later you will dialogue with your partner about the things you have written.

Before you begin, find something to write on and a pen or pencil. You will need a comfortable place to sit and quiet time to think where you will not be interrupted.

These exercises will wake up your imagination and help you discover your deepest desires.

Step One

Write down three sexual things you are curious about, have wondered about, or want to know more about.

Step Two

The things that you wrote about in step one will naturally lead to thinking about your sexual fantasies.

The higher the level of curiosity, the more likely that there will be a fantasy about that erotic need. In other words, something you are curious about may eventually be something you fantasize about. Erotic curiosity can lead to fantasy.

Fantasies are thoughts and pictures in our minds that turn us on. They can be of people, sex acts, or erotic scenes. Things that make us feel sexy and erotic fall into this category.

For this part of the exercise, you will continue with a personal writing exercise, and this you do on your own. You are beginning to explore your personal erotic fantasies; later in this exercise you will have the opportunity to share this in a dialogue with your partner.

Before you begin, find something to write on and a pen or pencil. You will still need a comfortable place to sit and quiet time to think where you will not be interrupted.

Write down three things that you fantasize about.

1. Sometimes I fantasize about ... .

2. There are times I get turned on when I think about ... .

3. One thing I think is really hot is ... .

Sometimes we share these things with our partners, letting them in on our fantasy life. And many times we keep our fantasies a secret. These fantasies may come to mind when we masturbate or when we have sex with our partners, but we don't necessarily talk about them.

(continued on page 112)

(continued)

Sometimes we find enough security in our relationship and we do talk to our partners about our fantasies, but we still don't act them out. They stay on a fantasy level only and serve as erotic energy or fuel for our sexuality.

Step Three

This next part of the exercise is about taking our fantasies into action. First write down fantasies you have that you might want to make come true. For example:

"My fantasy that I want to take into action is for me to hang on a swing from the ceiling and make love to my partner while suspended."

Then think about any props you might need, or special setting, or how you might need your partner to participate. Examples might be as follows:

Three things I need to make that happen are

1. I need to buy the swing.

2. I need my partner to help me screw it into the ceiling.

3. I need encouragement from him to make it happen.

Hold on to your answers and to your newfound clarity. Be excited and congratulate yourself that you have gotten this far! You are on the road to getting the sex you want.

Step Four

This next step is about sharing the fantasy that you want to take into action with your partner using the Imago dialogue. There is no need to commit to these things as you are listening to your partner express his or her desires.

This is different from an action plan; you don't have to agree or disagree at this time. Instead, the Imago dialogue offers a way to hold our partners in an active listening place, so they feel listened to and their desires are honored.

Expressing your desires and sharing the things you want to do with your partner can be a risk. You might be worried that your partner will not understand your desires, or will have different fantasies than you. You should hope so! Having a variety of desires and fantasies keeps a relationship exciting, and the thrill of discovering your partner's most secret fantasies can be incredibly erotic.

You may feel anxious about being so open, and this may make you feel vulnerable. Being vulnerable is good! It creates more intimacy. The more risk you take in trusting your partner with this valuable information, the more intense the connection will be between the two of you. Remember, hearing about your partner's fantasy can be a turn-on for you and telling his fantasy can be a turn-on for him. Do not underestimate the power of sexual communication. It is an erotic life force that creates new energy and aliveness in your relationship.

Make sure you will have privacy for this exercise, and you may want to set up the room you are in for potential lovemaking after you are through. Turn on low lights or candles, and put on sexy clothes or lingerie. Take a bath or shower and shave before this exercise. Light incense or put fresh flowers close by. Using all of your senses will heighten the intensity of the sensual experience for both of you.

Find a comfortable place to sit for at least forty minutes or longer with your partner. Sit or lie down close enough to each other so that you can read notes that you made in the previous part of this exercise. If you are sitting across from each other, make sure you make eye contact. Sit with your knees touching as you face each other. The close proximity will increase the feeling of intimacy and connection.

Decide who will be the sender and who will be the receiver. The sender goes first.

Sender: "One thing I have fantasized about and would like to make happen is handcuffing you." (Describe your fantasy in as much detail as you can. What does it look like, feel like, smell like, taste like, sound like?)

Receiver (mirroring): "So one thing you have fantasized about that you would like to make happen is handcuffing me. Did I get that?"

Sender: "Yes" or "Let me make sure you got this part … ."

Receiver (mirroring): "Is there more?"

Sender: "No, you got it" or "Yes, and another thing is … ."

Sender: "Three things I would need to make this fantasy happen are a, b, and c."

Receiver (mirroring): "The three things you would need to make this fantasy happen are a, b, and c. Is there more?"

Sender: "No, you got it" or "Yes, another thing is … ."

Receiver (validating): "It makes sense to me that you would fantasize about … Knowing you the way I know you, it makes sense that you would want … ."

Receiver (empathizing): "And I can imagine that you would feel … if you were to have that fantasy come true."

Sender: "Yes, I would feel that" or "Yes, and I would also feel … ."

Now the sender and receiver switch.

(continued on page 114)

(continued)

When a fantasy is shared with your partner, it can raise the heat and passion between you, just by talking about it. Once a fantasy is out in the open between you, it can become something you talk about often, or just use on special occasions.

Step Five

Now comes the action plan. Find a quiet place for you and your partner to talk, facing one another. Decide who will be the sender and who will be the receiver.

Sender: "I would really like to make this fantasy happen within the next day/week/ month (choose a specific time frame)."

Receiver: "So you would really like to make this fantasy happen within the next day/week/month."

Sender: "Yes, if we did that it would make me feel ... ."

Receiver (mirrors): "So if we did that it would make you feel ... (validates): It makes sense to me that you would want to do this within a day/month/year. (empathizes): I imagine that if we did that you would feel ... ."

Sender: "You got me" or "I also want you to know I would feel ... ."

As you close this exercise, add an appreciation at the end and then switch. This is a wonderful way to end an exercise that might be a high risk for both of you. Appreciation is a very validating and emotionally responsive reaction to any high-risk sharing. It gives a nice closure and adds an important element that can become an ongoing part of your conversations.

Now that you have shared the fantasy that you would like to take into action, begin to create that reality. Don't wait for your partner to provide the catalyst for your fantasy. Begin to explore what you need to make the fantasy happen.

Over the next few weeks, begin to think about your fantasy as something that you are coming closer to. Let the erotic tension build as you look forward to making it happen.

The Consequences of Making Fantasies Come True

Acting out a fantasy or curiosity can be great, or it can be painful for you or others. Actions can be healthy or not, depending on your relationship and how they affect your partner. Our actions always have consequences.

If we have a fantasy about having an affair and act it out, for example, this action usually affects all those involved. (See more about affairs below.)

What we choose to take from fantasy to action should be determined by our personal boundaries and a sense of integrity. An example of this might be a fantasy that is common to both men and women—the ménage à trois, or threesome. Both men and women fantasize about adding a third person to their lovemaking at some point in their relationship. Taking this fantasy into action may have many consequences. And sometimes the reality is not as good as the fantasy!

Threesomes can be exciting and sexy, but the reality is that they can also be messy, awkward, and emotionally threatening. Talking about this fantasy without acting it out can spice up your sex life, with no negative consequences to the relationship.

Being clear with your lover that you have a fantasy you would like to share but are not ready to take to the action stage can actually make it easier to share the fantasy. When you tell your partner about your fantasy, you can always preface the conversation with a request. Indicate whether you would like to keep the fantasy as a fantasy or whether you want to act it out. Knowing that your partner will more clearly understand where your fantasy falls on the Erotic Curiosity Spectrum can prevent feeling pressure to act it out before you are ready. For example, you might be more likely to share your fantasy of being suspended from the ceiling during sex if you are not worried that your partner will run out right away and buy hooks to hang you from!

(continued on page 116)

The Consequences of Making Fantasies Come True (continued)

Sharing your fantasies with a lover falls on the right, or more active, side of the spectrum. When you choose not to share some of your erotic curiosity with your partner, then these thoughts fall on the left, or passive, side of the spectrum.

Erotic Curiosity Spectrum

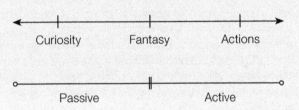

Submissive versus Dominant

Also on the erotic curiosity spectrum are two general categories—receptive and directive. Our thoughts and fantasies run toward a preference to be receptive or controlled in bed. Being under someone's erotic control falls on the submissive side of the spectrum.

Or we might have thoughts and fantasies about being more dominant or directive and like the idea of being able to be in erotic control of our partner. Both of these categories function as their own erotic spectrum, with many variations of control, and the erotic power plays of submission and domination can be acted out in many ways.

Erotic Curiosity Spectrum

Curiosity Fantasy Actions

Passive   Active

Receptive   Directive

Submissive   Dominant

Controlled   Controlling

Consider what's on your erotic curiosity spectrum. Are you more turned on by thoughts of being receptive, sexually controlled, and submissive? Sexual submissives might enjoy thoughts of being told what to do or being spanked.

If you are sexually directive and enjoy thoughts of being in control sexually, you may have more dominant fantasies, including being on top during missionary sex, blindfolding your partner, or "ordering" your partner to perform oral sex.

This part of the exercise will help you decide which fantasy you want to make happen in your relationship. Any thoughts that have moved from curiosity to fantasy, which you now would like to begin to explore, can be included in this "action" area. These fantasies can be reasonable, where all the practical aspects of acting out the fantasy seem simple and obtainable, or they can be complicated and take planning and communication to make them happen.

In both cases, taking a fantasy into action can be thrilling and exciting—or somewhat disappointing. Sometimes things are best left as fantasy. And for others, acting out your most private thoughts and desires can be the pinnacle of joy and connection in your relationship.

A Catalyst to Move Fantasies into Action

Moving fantasies from the imagination end of the spectrum to the action end of the spectrum can be a big leap for some couples. It might be very comfortable to have a fantasy that stays in the imagination. Perhaps you share this with your partner. Being clear with him or her that you are just sharing a fantasy is different than asking your partner to help live out that fantasy in real life.

Sometimes we need a catalyst to have our fantasies come to fruition. That catalyst might be anything that pushes us from curiosity to fantasy to *action*.

Many times we need a stimulus to help us act out our fantasies. A catalyst might mean being in the right place at the right time. Or it might mean our partner makes something happen for us that convinces us to move forward into action.

An example of this type of stimulus is reflected in the following couple's case.

Anne came into my office complaining that her sex life was dull and un-imaginative. She shared that she always had orgasms, but that she felt bored with sex and wanted to try something new with her husband, Tim.

Using the erotic curiosity exercises, she wrote down the things that she was curious about, the things she fantasized about, and the fantasies that she wanted to take into action.

Through this exercise she discovered that she was curious about dressing up in costumes and role-playing during sex. She always wondered how people made those things happen, and she was wondering whether she would have the energy and courage to present this curiosity to her partner.

She wrote down her thoughts and realized that she often fantasized about dressing up in a maid's outfit. She thought about this for several days and nights, and fantasized about what it would be like to be waiting for her partner when he came home from work at night, wearing a black and white maid's costume and holding a dustpan. She found herself turned on by these fantasies. Anne then decided she wanted to take this fantasy into action. But, she wasn't sure she could make it happen on her own.

She shared her fantasy with her partner, Tim, and using the dialogue process he was able to mirror, validate, and empathize. Still, Anne couldn't move her fantasy into action. She was delighted that Tim could talk about it with her, and for a while that added a new energy and enthusiasm to their lovemaking.

One day she came home from her job and found on her bed a maid's outfit, complete with feather duster and dustpan. The skirt was short, and there was a ruffled apron and a tight top with a name tag that said "Anne" pinned to the front.

This was the catalyst she needed. She was able to put on the costume and play the part of the maid, and she waited for her husband to come into the bedroom that evening, where she was dressed in costume and able to act out her fantasy.

EXERCISE
Be Your Own Catalyst

After you have discussed your fantasy, find one thing that represents your fantasy—let this be something of your own choosing.

Perhaps it is a piece of clothing, an accessory, or a sex toy. Buy this item, bring it into your home, and keep it in your bedroom to remind you of your fantasy.

Giving the Go-Ahead
Sometimes we need permission to act out our fantasies.

It is hard for women in particular to ask for what they want sexually. Because of the guilt and shame attached to sexual desire for women, it can be hard to own the need for sex. Some women say they don't have the self-esteem or the confidence to ask for their erotic fantasies to be fulfilled. Even if they are curious about

(continued on page 120)

(continued)

something, they might not feel they have the right to ask for it. It is important for women to own their desires, to state them clearly, and to let go of the guilt and shame about asking for what they want.

It can also be scary for men to ask for their desires and fantasies to be fulfilled. Men are sometimes more articulate about asking for action than they are about expressing emotion. Women can sometimes speak more freely about their feelings, but find it difficult to talk about what they want in bed.

Asking our partner to help us take our fantasies from imagination to action can be hard for both sexes. Getting permission first, or waiting for a catalyst to make something happen, can ensure that we have an easier time with it. But the most direct way to begin to live our fantasy sex life is to share with our partner what our fantasies are and which ones we want to make happen.

EXERCISE
Commitment to Focus

Committing to working on one fantasy can bring focus to our relationships. It gives erotic energy a chance to grow and develop. The fantasy becomes the catalyst for change in the relationship. And committing to creating this new fantasy together gives the partnership a common goal and a focus on growth.

For the following exercise, you need a piece of paper and a pen. Think about one sexual aspect of your partnership that you want to focus on for a finite period of time. Decide how long you want to completely focus on that one aspect. For example, this could mean having intercourse every night for a certain, limited amount of time. It may mean that you try all the exercises in this book over a long weekend.

Share your idea with your partner and listen to your partner's idea. Is there a common goal that you can both work toward?

Decide what your commitment will be to each other and sign the sexual contract below:

I, [insert name], am totally committed to our sexual relationship for the next [insert specific time frame]. This includes being totally faithful, and focusing all my energy on pleasing you. I am committed to exploring your erotic fantasies for this amount of time. I will also [fill in blank].

Leave the contract somewhere you can both see it. Check in periodically (e.g., daily or weekly) to see how you are doing. Are there consequences in your partnership for not living up to your commitments? What are they?

Why Fantasies Happen

Fantasies happen for a reason. Fantasies are a direct result of our anxieties and fears. We work out our anxieties through our sexuality.

What we fantasize about is also many times our psychological edge. An "edge" is the place at the end of our comfort zone. It is a line where we feel comfortable on one side, and uncomfortable on the other. But we will be stuck if we stay where we are. Picture a plant growing against a windowpane, searching for fresh air and sunshine. The "edge" for the plant is the window. It would like to move beyond its comfort zone, but may not know how to get there. Pushing against our edge in our sexuality means moving into the places where we initially feel uncomfortable, but ultimately more whole and fulfilled.

In our sexuality, we all have psychological needs. For example, we have a need to feel safe, a need to feel loved, and a need to feel excited and turned on. We also have psychological fears, such as the feeling of being trapped, the fear of heights, or the fear of abandonment.

We fantasize about things that are on our psychological edge. Many times our sexual fantasies are also our psychological and relational fears. This psychological anxiety can make sex tantalizing. If we are excited about something that causes us stress, we experience it as a thrill. Think of a roller coaster or skydiving. They may feel dangerous and scary, but we are also highly stimulated and excited when we do those things. Sometimes our fantasies give us that "rush" as well.

When Forbidden Acts Become Fantasies

We seek mastery over our fears though our sexual fantasies. This is an interesting way that our minds work to heal us of our greatest anxieties. Through seeking pleasure and stimulation, we can turn something scary and negative into something arousing and beautiful. The forbidden becomes fantasy, and we have the power through our imaginations to have a sense of control over our deepest worries. We can control, in our minds, who does what to whom, how long it lasts, and how it ends. This gives us sense of mastery over the things we feel we have no control over.

These forbidden aspects of desire make our fantasies rich and alive.

Forbidden acts can become fantasies, and with enough safety and communication between partners, they can become part of our sex life.

An example of how our anxiety becomes fantasy is illustrated in the case below. Notice how acting out the fantasy actually heals Tara of her persistent and chronic fears.

Using Sex to Overcome Anxiety

Tara came into my office complaining of anxiety. She suffered from claustrophobia, a fear of small spaces. When asked if she had any other fears, she admitted she also had entrapment fears in her relationships. If she felt emotionally "trapped" in a commitment to a partner, she would react by feeling some panic, clenching her teeth, and sweating. This was the same response she experienced in elevators. After many years, she was finally in a relationship with a man she was able to commit to and not panic when she felt trapped.

Tara's concern was that she was having sexual fantasies that were disturbing to her. The erotic fantasies she had were about being trapped! She felt herself being turned on by thoughts of not having control during sex, such as being tied up, handcuffed, or held down. She fantasized about her boyfriend playing a dominant role during sex and ordering her to lie down and take her clothes off. She had fantasies about being restricted. It felt counter intuitive for her to feel erotically charged over being trapped, while at the same time having entrapment fears. She wanted desperately to tell her partner that she had these thoughts, but didn't know how. Her shame was too overwhelming.

She was confused about why she felt turned on by something she found so disturbing in the rest of her life. It was understandable that Tara would feel confused about her fantasies. What was distressing to her was also a turn-on. Her confusion was about whether she should seek pleasure in this way, given that this same area brought her such distress. What she needed to experience was how her fantasy of being trapped could actually decrease her fears and anxiety.

Her intuition (and her therapy) told her that if she could begin to talk about her fears, they would lessen. She trusted her partner, Bill, and wanted to talk with him about her fantasies. She also understood that to feel totally fulfilled, she would like to take this fantasy into action with Bill. After doing the exercises on erotic curiosity, she began to explore what she had written. She wrote about the things she was erotically curious about, what she fantasized about, and what she wanted to take into action. She knew she would need Bill's support and understanding and found she was anticipating a dialogue with Bill about her fantasy. She waited for the right moment with great trepidation and also a heightened sense of erotic stimulation.

Soon Tara found the time to share her fantasy with her partner. Bill had done the exercise on erotic curiosity as well, and he was excited to share his fantasies with Tara. Tara went first, and was the sender. Bill listened to what she had to say. He did not try to comfort her as she talked, but just mirrored everything she had to tell him.

Tara: "So, I know its crazy, but I have this fantasy that you will tie me to the bed. And that I won't be able to get out. And you will have sex with me while I am trapped there. I know that's awfully strange, since I have such a fear of being trapped!"

Bill: "So, let me see if I got this. You have a fantasy that I will tie you to the bed." Bill gazed into Tara's eyes as he mirrored back to her and she visibly relaxed in her chair. "And you think about what it would be like to not be able to get out. You want me to have sex with you while you are trapped there on the bed. You think it's awfully strange to have this fantasy since you have such a fear of being trapped. Did I get it all?"

Tara: "Yes, perfectly."

Eventually, Bill and Tara did act out this fantasy. Bill tied her to his bed with silk scarves. She felt excited and could feel her heart race and her pulse increase. She also experienced some anxiety mixed in with sexual excitement. Bill and Tara had sex while she was tied up. She experienced a deep and profound orgasm.

The next day, as she got on to an elevator, she felt some anxiety, but also to her amazement, she felt pleasure. What she hadn't expected was that acting out her sexual fantasy would change the experiences in the rest of her life.

Her body remembered that being "trapped" wasn't all that bad. She had worked through some of her entrapment fears by acting them out in bed.

This makes sense. Tara did something she was afraid of, which was now connected to deep pleasure. She was able to control her entrapment by asking Bill to do it, by giving him permission to tie her up, and by letting him have sex with her while she was bound. She could have stopped the game at any time, and she knew that Bill would honor that. She had created a scenario that gave her power over her fears. Her anxiety was now something she had control of.

The act of working out this fantasy in life actually connected a pleasure stimulus to the anxiety, in a safe and erotically charged moment, with a loving partner. This created a positive connection in her mind with a positive physical experience, and the feeling of being trapped in other areas of her life could now be experienced differently.

The Fear Factor

Fear is a powerful motivator. It keeps us stuck and locked into patterns of relating to others that is not always in our best interest. We may freeze and cut off parts of ourselves that need expression, or we may act out in ways that are defenses against being overwhelmed by our fear.

There are healthier ways to deal with our fears. We can use the Imago method to communicate and express our fear. Imago gives us the language to share our anxieties and hope for a better way.

The following case example describes a couple exploring fear in this new way. Although it feels risky to share with a partner something we are afraid of, this can actually increase our intimacy and connection with our partner. Sharing our fears lessens their intensity, and it also helps us look at fear in a new way.

Jenna and Mark had been in couple's therapy for a few sessions when they started talking about their sexual fantasies. They also talked honestly about their fears. Jenna's worst fear, because of her childhood, was the psychological fear of abandonment. This manifested itself in her persistent fear that her husband was going to leave her for another woman. This was not based on anything he had actually done. Mark constantly reminded her that he was faithful and loved her deeply.

Jenna's fear of abandonment was also her most secret sexual fantasy. She found herself fantasizing about her husband having sex with another woman. She wanted to watch him while he went down on another woman, giving her an orgasm through oral sex. She thought about this often but was too afraid to tell her husband, for fear that he would act it out and fall in love with the other woman, and then leave her, as she had always feared.

Jenna was balanced on the precipice of fear and erotic energy. Her fantasy was for her husband to have sex with another woman. It was not to participate sexually with the two of them, but to watch the woman having oral sex with her husband. This felt like a psychological edge because it contained "danger" for her.

As mentioned previously, an "edge" is the place where we most resist change. We all have boundaries, socially and sexually. Our edge is also the place where we need to grow the most. When we push our edge, even just slightly, we grow into areas that are new for us, which allows us to experience more joy and fulfillment.

Sometimes pushing our edge can be a real stretch. The way we grow sexually by slowly pushing the boundaries of what we are comfortable with. These stretches also help us to push our edges and grow into the people we need to be.

Stretching into places that hold anxiety for us is many times exactly what our partner is asking us to do. Sometimes those places are the hardest for us to grow into. Stretching for our partner could mean sharing our deepest thoughts and feelings. It might mean sharing fantasies we have kept secret. It could even mean trying something new in bed because it's important to our partner. If our lover asks us to do something that feels like too big of a stretch, we can ask for a smaller stretch.

Jenna was pushing her edge by telling Mark about her fantasy. This was a scary and uncomfortable place, but she felt that in doing so she would grow closer to him and be a more confident sexual being.

Jenna and Mark were able to talk about the fantasy she had of watching him with another woman. They used the dialogue process to talk about it. Mark listened to Jenna describe her fantasy of seeing him in bed with someone else, and he mirrored back everything she said. After every revelation, he asked her, "Is there more?"

Because of his encouragement, Jenna was also able to share her confusion. She asked Mark to understand that although she thought about it, she was not convinced she wanted to bring her fantasy into the action phase.

When Mark listened to Jenna's fantasy and her fears, he validated her by saying things like this:

Mark: "Jenna, knowing you like I know you, it makes total sense to me that you would be nervous about taking that step to live out your fantasy. I can understand that this must be so difficult for you to talk about, since you have expressed your fears about me leaving you for someone else."

When Mark went on and empathized with her feelings, Jenna seemed to relax in her seat.

Mark: "I can imagine that talking about this makes you very nervous. It must be scary to confess these thoughts and fears. I also imagine that if you were to act out this fantasy you might feel very conflicted. It might turn you on, but also make you feel slightly insecure. Is there more?"

Jenna: "You got me. That's exactly how I would feel. And yes, it makes me nervous and uncomfortable to talk about these things. It also, to be honest, turns me on a little."

Mark: "Oh, okay, so it makes you nervous and uncomfortable to talk about these things, but it also turns you on a little? Did I get that?"

Jenna: "You got me." She giggled.

Mark: "Is there more?"

Jenna: "Well, I hope that we can agree to keep this fantasy just a fantasy for now."

Mark: "So you want to keep this fantasy just a fantasy for now."

He agreed, but he asked if they could talk about the fantasy again.

Sometimes fantasies can stay fantasies and not move to the action phase. Instead, the fantasy can be integrated into their lovemaking. For example, during sex Mark could whisper in Jenna's ear as they are having intercourse,

"If there was another woman here, I would go down on her and you could watch … ." This would let Jenna play with the fantasy over time without feeling threatened.

As a result of sharing and playing with this fantasy together, Jenna realized that she no longer had the fear that Mark would leave her. She felt more connected to him and felt safer in their relationship than ever before. Mark was turned on just by hearing her fantasy. He was also so flattered that Jenna trusted him enough to share her fantasy with him that he felt more intimately connected to her.

If Jenna decided to take the fantasy to the action phase, she could live out her greatest fear and experience erotic pleasure. Over time she might deal with her fears about Mark differently. What she was most afraid of also gave her an erotic charge. Mark felt that someday they could safely act out her fantasy and still stay connected.

This couple confronted a fear that was also a fantasy, and the energy that was released from this sharing created a whole new dynamic in the relationship. They were able to work through jealousy and possessiveness and see them less as a threat to the relationship and more as a way to express tension and fear, and then work it out through sharing their deepest desires with one another. This case is also an example of how using the dialogue works for most, if not all, of our sexual issues in our partnerships.

Discovering Where Your Fantasies Fall on the Erotic Curiosity Spectrum

Below is a list of common fantasies that fall on both ends of the erotic curiosity spectrum. Sit with your partner and fill out this exercise separately, but in the same room.

Go down the list, and mark each item with a number from 1 through 5. When you are through, share your responses with your partner.

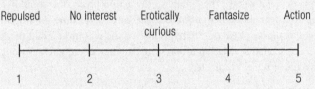

Repulsed	No interest	Erotically curious	Fantasize	Action
1	2	3	4	5

1. One means you are repulsed by the idea.
2. Two means the idea holds no interest for you.
3. Three means you are erotically curious about it.
4. Four means you have fantasies about it.
5. Five means you would like to turn this fantasy into action.

Examples of fantasies:
- Watching two women have sex
- Watching two men have sex
- Having sex with a man and a woman
- Having sex with your partner and another couple
- Multiple partner sex
- Having sex with a group of strangers
- Being seduced by an older woman
- Watching your partner masturbate
- Masturbating in front of your partner
- Being dominant with your partner
- Being dominated by your partner

- Giving Oral Sex
- Recieving oral sex from your partner
- French kissing partner after a blow job
- Partner swallowing after a blow job
- Sex with a prostitute or stripper
- Sex with a celebrity
- Sex with someone you know (not your partner)
- Receiving anal stimulation
- Having anal sex
- Tying up your partner and having sex with him or her
- Forcing your partner to have sex
- Being forced to have sex
- Being filmed during sex
- Talking dirty
- Double penetration
- Watching pornography with your partner
- Acting out pornography scenes with your partner
- Anonymous sex with a stranger
- Sex with an old boyfriend/girlfriend
- Sex with two women
- Sex with two men
- Sex with a group including your partner
- Sex with a group of men
- Sex in front of your partner with someone else
- Being dominated by your partner
- Being spanked
- Having toes sucked
- Sex with vegetables or fruit

(continued on page 130)

Discovering Where Your Fantasies Fall
on the Erotic Curiosity Spectrum (continued)

- Sex with food (e.g., whipped cream)
- Sex with vibrators and dildos
- Masturbating with vibrator in front of your partner
- Sex outside or in public places

Domination Fantasies:

- Dressing up in leather
- Role-playing with costumes (e.g., stripper, cowboy, doctor)
- Wearing boots or high heels
- Tying up your partner
- Putting handcuffs on your partner
- Putting a collar on your partner
- Pinching your partner with clothespins
- Using a cane, riding crop, or whip to threaten
- Using a cane, riding crop, or whip to inflict sensation
- Blindfolding your partner
- Having your partner lick your boots
- Urinating on your partner
- Sex doggie style
- Playing the master role
- Sex slave fantasy

Submission Fantasies:

- Dressing up in plastic
- Dressing up in rubber
- Dressing in women's clothes (for the man)

- Being urinated on
- Playing the slave role
- Being handcuffed
- Being tied up
- Being strapped down
- Wearing a collar
- Having your hair pulled
- Submitting and thanking partner
- Being caned or whipped
- Being spanked

Talk with your partner about what came up for you, what it feels like to hear his or her answers, and how you feel now that you have read and talked about your fantasies.

How Exits Take Us Away from Our Relationships

We all have behaviors that take our focus away from our love relationship, and sometimes we use these behaviors as a way to avoid intimacy or connection. "Exits" are ways in which we avoid being "present" or actively involved in our relationship. If we choose these "exits" we have to be aware of the consequences.

Some examples of exits include the following:

- Drinking excessively
- Using drugs
- Eating compulsively
- Shopping compulsively
- Over focusing on the children
- Spending excessive time at hobbies
- Using the computer or watching television to excess
- Watching pornography
- Having affairs
- Getting involved in Internet relationships
- Spending time in chat rooms
- Working too much
- Going out with friends
- Traveling
- Reading

Many of these exits could be behaviors that feel healthy and are not necessarily negative. Things like hobbies and focusing on our children are important and necessary, and they also help us grow as individuals. Some of these exits are behaviors that are fine in moderation, but when they are used to avoid intimacy, they can become problematic.

Affairs: Exits and the Invisible Divorce

Searching for a partner outside of our primary relationship can take us away from building on the relationship we have. Sometimes an affair can be an "exit" or an "invisible divorce." Often it can be a way to avoid the issues in our current partnership.

Feeling passion in your relationship means being thrilled that you want what you have. Energy going out of the relationship to other potential partners can drain the energy we have to focus on each other. Safety sometimes includes an understanding that no other sexual partners will be involved. For most couples, this safety in the relationship allows for open exploration of erotic fantasies.

An affair can take away our feeling of trust. However, an affair does not necessarily mean the relationship has to end. Most people have affairs not because there is something lacking in their relationship, but because an opportunity presents itself.

Making a choice to close your "exits" can increase the power flow into your current partnership. Instead of draining the focus off of our issues, the extra energy can help us figure out what we want. If there are people, places, or things that are draining your energy, can you identify them?

Read the list on page 131 and see if you can find what your exits are. Are there any exits you use that you can add to this list? Think about which of these you might be willing to modify or give up, at least temporarily.

More specifically, can you identify what exits you use to avoid focusing on your sexual partnership? Perhaps watching TV at night, reading in bed, staying at work late, drinking at night, or going out with your friends all interfere with the intimacy in your life.

Can you make a commitment to your current partner that for a finite period of time you will focus all of your energy on your emotional and sexual relationship? For a limited amount of time can you commit to closing at least one of your exits?

Is there one thing that you might be willing to give up for a month? For six weeks? Share these things with your partner and make a commitment to close one of these exits for a finite period of time. This will give you more energy to increase the passion in your partnership. It may also bring up other issues that you might be avoiding in your life. Maybe now is the time to look at them.

EXERCISE
Exit Contract

Use this contract to help you close one or more of these exits:

I, [name], am totally committed to closing the exit I use to avoid intimacy. The exit I will close is [name a specific exit]. I commit to closing this exit for the next [include specific time frame].

Signed _____

Now that you have taken this giant step toward change, what exactly do you want to focus on? What issues do you have that need to be looked at? What can you commit to doing for a finite period of time that will help work on this issue in your partnership? Perhaps you and your partner just want to work on improving your partnership on an erotic level. What is one thing that you think will help you do that?

Closing exits is about not doing something. Commitments are about doing something differently. Commitment means only that you make a decision. Think about what decisions you can make regarding your exits and where you can push your edge. Think about what your partner would appreciate now that you know more about his or her fantasies. What fantasies would you like to commit to working on?

Closing exits and committing to focus totally on the erotic aspect of your partnership creates a new safety in your relationship. The irony is that safety must exist to create an environment where vulnerability, fantasy, and risk can happen. This allows for greater passion and erotic sex. However, safety is sometimes antithetical to erotic sex. If erotic sex is illicit or forbidden, even in your imagination, then safety is not necessarily a turn-on! And yet safety needs to happen for partners to go to a deeper level sexually. Greater passion means greater depth and greater connection.

How to Safely Explore "Dark" Fantasies

Sometimes safety is being able to live out your deepest and perhaps darkest fantasies. Sometimes fantasies fall on the dominant side of the erotic curiosity spectrum, and sometimes they are on the submissive side. They may contain thoughts about bondage, domination, or submission.

For instance, many people have a picture in their minds of "S&M" or "sadism" and "masochism" as anonymous and involving black leather, full-face masks, pain, and torture. Another common picture of S&M is the dominatrix in black leather boots with a whip torturing the defenseless submissive tied to the floor.

These notions may all be true, but bondage, discipline, and sadomasochism, or BDSM, is more often about a range of play that includes varying levels of sensation. There is a wide range of true BDSM interests and participant levels. Partners play roles in the dominant/submissive (dom/sub) world of sexual play. Acting out scenes is a form of role-play where each partner feels safe enough to step into a part and act it out for each other.

In BDSM play, one partner is in the dominant role of "bossing" the other around for the pleasure of being in control. The submissive is giving "permission" to be used in that role. The dominant is acting out the role as a gift to the submissive partner. The other partner is submissive, taking pain or "punishment." This role-play can be foreplay or include penetration and orgasm.

The polarities of good and bad roles play with energy and power, transferring it from one person to the other and back again. These two ends of the spectrum can create a strong attraction or repulsion.

Acting Out Light Fantasies

Light fantasies are romantic and sweet scenarios that make you feel sexy. These fantasies may be more traditional than dark fantasies, but they are not necessarily better or worse. Some examples of light fantasies might include the following:

- Sensual massage with aromatherapy lotion
- Taking a warm bath together
- Making love on a bed of rose petals
- Making love by candlelight
- Listening to soothing music while making love
- Tickling each other with feather dusters
- Wearing lacy lingerie
- Using ice cubes
- Shaving one another
- Slow dancing in the dark

All of these fantasies can be combined with sex or experienced alone. Being mindful and in the moment adds passion to light moments. Breathing in to the moment and focusing completely on your partner can bring a heightened arousal of all your senses. Focus on what you smell: the candles, the bathwater, the rose petals, your partner's skin. Focus on what you hear: soft music, your partner's breathing, etc. Focus on what each of your senses is telling you, and give yourself permission to be totally relaxed in the moment.

Creating a Safe Word

Before a BDSM role-play, both partners should always commit to a "safe word." A "safe word" is a word decided on beforehand that is not something that one might normally say in the course of the play. This is a way to say "no" or "stop." Creating this word helps both partners feel more comfortable playing their roles.

One is likely to moan or scream things like "oh, God," "no, don't," or even "stop." But these words may be part of what keeps submissives in their role, and only part of the act. A real "safe word" would be something totally out of the ordinary for that moment, like "cherry pie" or "frog." It doesn't matter what the word is, as long as you both agree to it before the games begin.

Dominants need to know that they can continue the game, trusting submissives to end the play when they need to. The sexual tension that is created during the games should be part of the energy that grows between you. Remember that starting out at a high sensation level is not pleasant, and that most of us need to build up slowly to tolerate pain as well as pleasure. Working up to more intense sensation is the goal.

You might include toys in your BDSM play, such as handcuffs, blindfolds, leather cuffs, and collars. Sex toys include dildos, vibrators, anal plugs, and nipple clamps. Games include spanking, whipping, caning, and pinching the body with clothespins.

EXERCISE
Sexual Sending and Receiving

In this exercise, you will need at least sixty minutes of uninterrupted time and privacy. Create a sexy environment by darkening the room, lighting candles, and putting fresh flowers by the bed. Put clean, soft sheets and blankets on the bed or floor where you will be. Put on soft, sexy music in the background. Take the time to create an erotic environment you will both enjoy. This is a way to honor your sexual relationship and bring a level of integrity and respect to your lovemaking.

Find props before you begin. You will need several long silk scarves. Take the phone off the hook and begin.

Step One
First, decide who will be receptive (receiver) and who will be directive (sender). Senders should start by kissing their lover softly and slowly, and then become more assertive in their kisses. Lift your partner's arms above her head and continue kissing her on her neck and chest.

Step Two

Gently and seductively, tie her hands above her head with a silk scarf, being careful not to cut off circulation. Tie another silk scarf over her eyes. Continue to kiss, lick, and nibble her body with her hands tied and eyes blindfolded. Make love to your partner without asking how she wants it. Love her in ways that you know will please both of you.

Step Three

Afterward, take off the silk scarves slowly and hold your partner quietly for several moments. Give her a chance to come down from the experience and reconnect with you. Discuss what the experience was like for both of you.

Step Four

Next time, reverse roles.

Playing the Game

Spanking is a very intimate form of "light" BDSM. It is more intimate than other types of BDSM because there is lots of bodily contact. It also triggers the release of endorphins, the feel-good brain chemicals released under stress.

Spanking, done with an open hand or palm, can be a way to inflict a sensation that becomes pleasurable for the submissive partner, and it gives the dominant partner a feeling of control. There is also a temporary visual mark left on the buttocks. The pinkness is sometimes called "pinking" the submissive. Always remember that gentler is better! Start slowly and lightly.

To begin, the submissive person can be lying down, kneeling, or tied up with rope, handcuffs, or scarves. The dominant person should decide how the submissive will be restricted, being very careful not to cut off circulation. Remember that as the submissive pulls on the ropes or cuffs, they may get tighter, so allow for some room to prevent blood flow restriction.

(continued on page 138)

Playing the Game (continued)

Make the restriction part of the game. Dominant partners, or "tops" should take their time, making sure that the submissive partners, or "bottoms," feel every moment of the tension that is building as they get more and more helpless. The rope or cuffs can be slid over the submissive's body parts, so he experiences the delightful titillation of knowing what is to come when he is restricted.

A blindfold works well to heighten the sexual tension and leave the submissive guessing about what's coming next. Differing levels of sensation can be created now. Slowly, the top can begin teasing by touching, pinching, or squeezing all parts of the bottom's body. Levels of pain can be increased as the bottom becomes more used to the sensation. The slight pain of gentle pinches or taps can be increased as the bottom gets more turned on.

Using a small whip or cane, the top can inflict gentle whipping or caning, starting softly. Remember, this is all about sensation. A harder stroke or a stronger squeeze will be perceived in the same way. As the endorphins increase and the bottom becomes more accustomed to the teasing pain, then harder strokes can be used.

Some strokes will leave a mark or redness on the body, and this can be a turn-on for the top. Alternate between harder and harder sensations and softer, soothing strokes.

The top can whisper in the partner's ear all the things she wants to do to him. This can make the bottom swoon with anticipation.

The top can be in control and have power over the partner in this way. The bottom in this game can relax and let go, knowing the top is in charge. This allows the bottom to totally relax and enjoy, and it gives both roles the erotic connection they may be looking for. The direct connection between demanding what you want and getting what you want is a powerful feeling. Erotic requests made with clear instructions and permission increases the feeling of control and safety for the bottom.

This permission often allows both partners to feel empowered. Without having to manipulate to get what they want, they can act it out. And this game can be acted out over and over again! The capacity to be fully present for the game and to escape reality by going totally into sensation is the lure of BDSM.

Use caution with this exercise. It takes very little pressure to create a sensation. The back of a brush, a riding crop, or a bamboo rod can all create the sensation of a hard spanking or "caning."

Always remember to choose a safe word before you start. Remember, whichever role you're in, you both carry great responsibility in creating safety while tolerating greater levels of intensity.

For this exercise, you will need at least sixty minutes, and lots of privacy. Make sure you will not be interrupted, either by children, the phone or other distractions. Safety and security are particularly important in this exercise.

Be highly tuned in to the needs of the submissive. Show empathy by mirroring their sounds or mirroring their words in your mind. Listen carefully to their breathing and their sounds of pleasure or fear. Be particularly sensitive to feelings that come up before, during, and after this exercise. This may push partners to the edge of their comfort zone, and extra affection may be in order after you are through. Be prepared to be affectionate and loving when you are through, and do this in any way that makes you feel appreciative of your partner. Stroke her physically, being soft and comforting with your hands. Talk softly in her ear and reassure her that you love and care for her, and that she is safe. This experience can be very powerful, because it is a high intensity exercise and can bring up confusion for many couples.

The most important part of this exercise is to have fun with it! Remember that playing erotic games is part of finding joy and intensity in your sex life. This is a role-play game as well as a game of sensation and intensity. Experience the pleasure of being the "top" and also the power of being the "bottom."

Talk after this exercise if you need to, or drift into sleep, knowing that talking later may feel important and necessary.

Caning

To do this exercise, the bottoms, or subs, should be bent over a table, ottoman, or the other person's lap—somewhere that they can be comfortable for a while.

Starting slowly, tap the buttocks with a rhythmic percussion. Increase your speed before you increase the intensity. Eventually, the buttocks will adjust to the sensation and some numbness might result. Harder caning will produce a greater release of endorphins and the bottom may experience more painful strokes as pure sensation. You can alternate your strokes with harder slaps of the cane and break the pattern, creating tension as the bottom or sub waits for the next tap.

Always stop when the bottom, or sub, says his or her safe word.

When you are ready, help the bottom come out of the experience gently.

Remember to go slowly to help the bottom transition from the intensity of the experience. Show affection and support in a low and calming voice.

If this exercise leads to sex, enjoy it! Have fun with the endorphins that have been released, and remember that all sensations can be pleasurable.

The Submissive

Submissives temporarily give up control of their worlds during sex. There is a freedom in having someone else take erotic control of the body.

For some, being submissive during sex or BDSM play can be a healing experience. Allowing someone else to take the control gives subs permission to totally let go, to surrender. Letting someone dominate completely allows that surrender, stretching beyond the openings of the body and into the psychological strongholds of the mind.

For women, the need to surrender during sex is connected to the physiological need to "let go" in order to orgasm. Women often have a more passive role in sex because they have to physically open their bodies to let in the male partner. This creates the need for more total relaxation and surrender to the male. Being submissive or playing a submissive role allows women to let go and surrender to the process.

For men who have experienced the pressure of having to be in control over the course of their careers, being submissive can be a temporary relief from the burden of constant responsibility.

Try the next exercise if you haven't explored being submissive or want to learn more about yourself and what it would be like to be in that position.

EXERCISE
Submission Is in Your Mind

Find a place for you and your partner to sit or lie down comfortably for twenty to thirty minutes. Find a pen and paper to answer the following questions. After you are both through, you will move into a dialogue and discuss your answers. Remember that the dialogue allows for intense listening and validation, and is not about agreeing to anything at this time.

Step One

Write down a few sentences that describe what it would be like for you to be submissive in bed. For example: What would happen? What would it look like? Can you describe it? What would you be doing? What would your partner be doing? How? Who would do what?

Step Two

Now write about what it would be like to be dominant in bed, using the questions in Step One.

Step Three

Now decide who will be the sender and who will be the receiver. Senders go first and share their fantasies with their partner. Receivers mirror back what the sender says. Senders share with their partner which fantasy they are the most curious about. The receiver mirrors, validates, and empathizes with the sender.

Step Four

Switch.

Balanced Sexuality

Healthy sexuality is a balance. But for those who suppress their needs, either in the masculine (directive) role or in the feminine (receptive) role, the repressed needs and energy actually grow stronger. We all have both male and female energy, aspects of our personalities and our sexuality that, when in balance, bring a sense of wholeness and peace. Have you ever tried to hold down your feelings? Eventually they come up, and sometimes they sneak up without warning.

The need for balanced sexuality may include a desire to be in both roles, with a preference for one. Perhaps being told what to do takes the pressure off. Being in the submissive role can help you let go of performance pressure, physically and psychologically.

Male or female, acting out a submissive role, surrendering to someone else, can bring a heightened sense of control. Submissives actually have control over the scene. They can relax into the experience, and then go back to their normal way of relating after the role-play is over. They can take back their control and their illusion of power after the session.

Acting out an erotic game by playing with power and control can sometimes create anxiety. Letting go of control by being in sexual submission pushes our edge and increases stress. Pushing our edge forces us to deal with our fears. The stress combined with eroticism forces the body into a heightened state of arousal, releasing a combination of brain chemicals commonly found in people in a "fight or flight state." This stress in the mind creates anxiety and erotic tension at the same time. Overriding this response, and allowing the body to find pleasure in the submissive role, may rewire the brain to live with stress in a different way outside of the scene.

In other words, if in the moment the submissive experiences some panic but then has an orgasm, then the panic becomes linked in the brain with pleasure. When slight sensations of pain are experienced during BDSM play (for example, pinched nipples), then that slight pain becomes connected to pleasure. This confuses the senses and breaks down resistance. When the submissive experiences the confused sensation of being out of control along with erotic pleasure, the pleasure gets linked in the brain. The body holds a memory of the pleasure/pain response it experienced during the BDSM session.

One doesn't need to always act out the BDSM play. Sometimes fantasy can bring us to this place. Going to the pain/pleasure places in the mind can begin to connect pain and pleasure with the areas in ourselves where anxiety lurks.

The Dominant

Dominants in a sexual or erotic game get to feel a heightened sense of control over the world. They are able to experience being powerful, which can increase their sense of self-esteem. Dominants get to be the director. They get to write the script, act the part, and direct the scene. They also have the responsibility of keeping the submissive safe and turned on.

Dominants are responsible for keeping the submissives in their role. Tops develop a keen sense of intuition about their partner's erotic state. Erotic intuition is a heightened level of awareness where all the senses are engaged, including our sixth sense, or intuition. The top's supersensitivity to the bottom's experience engages all of the senses.

 Tops get to play the double role of bringing the bottom to the edge of danger and also keeping the bottom safe. They get to inflict discomfort or anxiety on their partner, while also bringing them pleasure.

When dominants can cause pain and pleasure at the same time for their partner, they can become more comfortable and secure in their partnership, outside of the dominant/submissive roles. Dominants actually lose the fear of hurting their partner outside of the BDSM play.

Most men at some time have fears of hurting their partner, emotionally and/or physically. This can create an oversensitive, walking-on-eggshells type of partnership. When dominants feel what its like to play at "hurting" their partner, they begin to understand not only their own power but also the strength and flexibility of their submissive. The range of feelings depends on how fragile they see their partner and how encouraging the submissive is.

If submissives ask to be "disciplined" using pain or control, they are giving permission to their partner that allows for a new freedom of expression. Creating sensation, intense on any level, can be a gift from the top to the bottom.

This freedom and power creates a sense of strength in the world. Knowing that their submissive partner trusts them enough to let them play at being dominant can be a way to feel more committed to the relationship. There is a high level of trust necessary to play the BDSM game. When partners trust each other to stay in the role, and to get each other out when necessary, then all sensation, painful or pleasureable, becomes intense.

The following exercise involves intense role-playing. Find at least ninety minutes or longer where you will not be interrupted. Also, find a safe and comfortable place to act out this role-play. Make sure your phones are off and you will be able to stay in the role for the duration of the exercise.

Set up the room where you will be according to the exercise. If you are the dominant partner for this exercise, be in charge of arranging the furniture, the lighting, and the music in the way that you want it. Take charge of your surroundings, just like you will take charge of your partner.

Tips for Domination Fantasy

Female dominants should dress in black leather or rubber. Use straps and buckles to enhance the outfit, and leave skin and body parts showing. Wear high heels or leather boots. Use a riding crop to "threaten" your partner. "Demand" that he assume positions where you can be in control. Whip him gently, telling him with a forceful voice to get on his knees. Threaten, but do not cause, pain. Have him wear a collar, blindfold, or handcuffs. Tell him what you want him to do to you.

Male dominants should dress up in chaps, a tie, or leather. Tie her hands with scarves or use handcuffs. Talk to her from behind where she can't see you. Blindfold her with a scarf. Keep your clothes on while she strips naked. Tell her how hard you are. Talk dirty. Tell her everything you are planning to do to her before you do it.

Remember that this is erotic play, and it should be fun. If at any time one of you feels uncomfortable, make sure to call a "time out" and ask for a break. Talk about any anxiety or difficulty you are experiencing, and then decide together whether you will continue now or another time. Knowing ahead of time that you can drop the role-play can help both partners trust the BDSM play and relax into it.

Feeling Sensation and Stimulation

All sensation can create a heightened level of arousal. Our physical bodies do not distinguish between different types of arousal. If there is a heightened state of stress, whether it is fear, pain, or pleasure, we react with all our senses.

We become intently focused on the stimulus that is causing us stress. We hear more intensely, we see more clearly, and we smell things we wouldn't normally notice. We observe the passing of time differently. Everything slows down during intense moments of arousal. (Think about what happens during a crisis, such as watching a child run out into the street. The experience of time seems to slow down. Everything feels like it is going in slow motion.)

Any heightened physical state will raise our energy and force us into hyper-arousal. This happens when we are scared, stressed, and sexually aroused. The more aroused we are during sex, the slower and more sensual the dance.

Acting out issues around dominance and submission using bondage and control as erotic play can bring up all of our and our partner's "issues." Experimenting with varying levels of sensation can trigger positive and negative psychological baggage from our childhood.

And yet working with pain, control, and power can help heal us from childhood wounds and memories. With a supportive and understanding partner and by talking through feelings, we can heal from memories that may still be influencing us as adults today.

Understanding and Responding to Physical Sensations

This exercise will help you communicate what feels good and give you a language to understand feedback from your partner. It also gives you a way to focus completely on how to give your partner pleasure.

You can use this 1 to 5 number system during sex. If your partner hits areas that feel like a 4 or 5, tell him or her. Feedback is important for great sexual communication.

EXERCISE
Rating the Touch

While sitting comfortably across from one another, senders hold the receiver's arm so that the forearm is face up. Receivers can close their eyes and relax.

Using a scale of 1 to 5—with 1 meaning "I don't like that" and 5 meaning "I love that" (3 would mean okay)—give the sender feedback on the way he touches your forearm. The sender can start with slow, soft touches to the wrist area.

As the sender moves up the arm to a different spot, the receiver gives a 1 to 5 response. The sender changes the type of touch from light scratching to deeper rubbing.

When the receiver gives a higher number response, the sender can continue that pressure and sensation until he finds a touch that results in a 5 response.

Being focused on our partners is like a slow, sensual dance, where you follow their steps, or lead them in the dance, becoming perfectly in tune with their rhythms and their breath. The generosity of being totally present and focused on your partner brings a sense of connection and togetherness.

A Case Example of Control and Light Bondage

Mary and Robert came to therapy to create a deeper and more intense connection. They had been drifting apart as a result of Robert's busy work schedule, and they hadn't had sex in months.

After several sessions they felt reconnected and had made love every weekend for a month. They worked on being able to talk about fantasies, and they had done some exercises at home. One day they came into my office describing a recent sexual experience they had.

Mary described the night before. They had talked about a fantasy that Robert had never shared with her before.

Mary: "He wanted to be tied up."

Robert (smiling): "It was just a fantasy with some light bondage. I always wanted to try it, but never had the nerve to tell Mary about it. I was afraid she would think it was weird, or I was weird."

Mary: "So, anyway, that night, as a surprise, I waited in the bedroom undressed. I was trying to be generous and initiate for once. I was waiting up for Robert to come home. Of course he was late, but that's another story. So he finally comes home and sees me and takes off all his clothes and jumps in bed.

I pulled out some silk scarves that I had hidden under the pillow, and flipped him over, and tied his wrists to the headboard."

I asked her how she was feeling at that point

Mary: "Well, I felt awkward and uncomfortable at first. I am usually the one who waits for Robert to initiate sex. But I wanted to give him his fantasy. He wanted me to be in control. And I wanted to try it for once. So, anyway, he was tied up to the bed. He looked nervous but excited."

I asked Robert how he felt at that point.

Robert: "Oh, I was totally turned on. I had a huge erection and thought it was so cool of Mary to do this for me. But I was slightly embarrassed by the whole thing. Surprisingly, her confidence made me relax. She seemed like she was really into it."

Mary: "Yeah, but then he freaked out."

Robert smirked.

Robert: "Yeah, I did."

I asked what happened.

Mary: "Well, I was on top of Robert, sitting on him, and I bent down to kiss him. That's all I did."

Robert: "Yeah and I freaked."

Mary: "Yeah, he said, and I quote, 'You're freaking me out!' So I got totally angry. I was taking this big chance to try something new and he really hurt my feelings."

Robert: "Yeah, I know, but then she left me there, tied up and walked away!"

Mary laughed.

Mary: "I came back and untied him eventually."

"So what do you think happened, Robert?" I asked.

He described what came up for him. He had experienced an overwhelming feeling of panic once he felt that Mary was in charge and that he had no control. Robert was not as comfortable being *out of control* as he thought he would be. As much as he fantasized about Mary taking initiative and letting her take control, he felt anxious and "freaked out" when she took over.

Mary had felt angry and hurt, not only because she felt rejected, but also because she worried that she had done something wrong. They talked about what control meant to each of them and how it played out in their relationship.

Robert began to talk about his family business, and how his father was overly involved. He talked about how controlling his father was in the business. Robert realized that because of the resentment toward his father, he was anxious when someone else was in control. It was important for Robert to feel like he had power and control over his life.

When Mary realized that the issue of control had more to do with his childhood issues than about her, she softened toward him. They decided that they would try it again, inching Robert closer to his fantasy without making him anxious.

The next night Mary tied one of Robert's wrists to the bedpost, and lay down by his side. Robert experienced his fantasy in a manageable way. He felt more and more that his issues around control were being healed this way. They continued to work together to help Robert with his anxieties.

Robert continued to be the more dominant, directive partner in their sex life, but with Mary's help he was able to realize the other side of his erotic spectrum and push his edge. He felt he was growing as a person and as a sexual partner. Sexually they were able to work through it and begin to heal from their own childhood wounds.

How to Be
Sensually
Generous

7

"Generous: Characterized by a noble or forbearing spirit: magnanimous, kindly; liberal in giving: open-handed ... ."

—*The Merriam-Webster Dictionary*

Sensual generosity is the desire to give sexually for the pleasure of giving. It's an advanced skill used to channel more sexual energy into a relationship. The bonus of being sensually generous is that generosity begets generosity. The more we give, the more we receive what we want in our relationship.

Being generous toward your partner means allowing your partner to experience the moment without the pressure to reciprocate. Sometimes, sensual generosity means giving yourself over to your lover. However, being willing to give over your body to someone else can feel risky. It may be hard to trust that you won't be hurt or judged when you let someone in, let someone see, and let someone touch. Allowing yourself to feel vulnerable is an act of generosity toward the other person.

Generosity also means being open and willing to hear and experience the other person's fantasies—and possibly participating in those fantasies. It necessitates empathizing with someone else's feelings and understanding how our behavior affects our partner. Generosity requires you to have insight into your own issues and where they come from, and then have the generosity to change, sometimes in ways you would prefer not to.

In other words, our capacity to give to our partner and expect nothing in return can be limited, depending on how comfortable we are with generosity.

Most of us would like to think that we are generous and giving people, especially in bed, and yet we may wonder whether what happens in bed feels "fair" sometimes.

Allowing yourself to feel vulnerable
is an act of generosity toward the other person.

Keeping score about who gives more and who takes more detracts from a relationship. Partners who fear and worry that they won't get their needs met, perhaps because of past experiences, may hold back their generosity, hoping that they will get the time and attention they have long desired. On the other hand, partners who feel they always give—like a martyr—may hold back, hoping that this will get them the love and the sex they want.

It actually works the other way around. The more we give, the more responsive our partner becomes, and the more we can receive.

Our "Imago," or the "image" of the person we seek out in relationships, is a conglomeration of character traits that we hope will give us what we long for. We can end up disappointed and frustrated when our partners don't act like we want them to. It can be hard to give without the fear that we won't receive.

George and Martine—When Giving Means More

The beauty of choosing our Imago match is that by giving our partners what they need, we actually grow into the partner we need to become. For example, George and Martine came to my office for couples counseling because Martine felt neglected and ignored by George.

Martine came from a loving family, but had felt ignored by her father because he traveled often for work. She had chosen George as a partner because she saw that George focused on her needs. He was a generous sexual partner, always trying to please her in bed. But she wanted more. She felt invisible with him. He also felt that she withheld sex from him as punishment if he didn't give her enough attention. He wanted her to be more assertive in bed and to sometimes take charge. Martine said she wasn't in the mood for sex when she didn't feel connected to George.

Martine's growth gift in her relationship was to move toward what George wanted from her. He wanted her to take charge in bed. He felt her need to be seen would be met as a result.

Martine was able to push her growth edge. She was able to move into the area where George wanted her to grow and not be focused on how she wanted George to change. She was able to take the risk and initiate sex several times, being more assertive in bed. She pushed herself to grow in the way that George needed, and she put her own needs aside.

When she did this, she realized that she was actually getting more of what she wanted from George: attention and appreciation. She felt special and cherished by George, which is what she had needed as a child. Her growth was moving her into the areas where she most needed healing. And it was through her sexual generosity with George that his need to feel loved from Martine was fulfilled.

Getting Past "Not Being in the Mood"

Sometimes giving sex to our partners when we don't want to can feel like a chore. But caring for them—and being sexually generous—sometimes means we do things we don't want to do because we know it will bring pleasure to our partner.

When you aren't in the mood for sex, there are still things you can do for your partner that can help him feel pleasure. Being sensually generous might mean reaching out and touching your partner, even if you don't want to make love or have intercourse.

Sometimes pushing yourself to have a piece of lovemaking, but not the whole pie, can satisfy both of you. Giving or receiving manual stimulation—sometimes all the way to orgasm—is one example. Another is just experiencing the pleasure of touching your partner and enjoying the moment.

Having quick sex to satisfy your partner's needs can be a way to show generosity and stay connected, even when you are not in the mood to have a long lovemaking session.

In addition, mutual masturbation is something that can satisfy both of you, and it serves a dual purpose. When we masturbate in front of our partners, they learn what feels good by watching our technique. They see what we do to bring ourselves to orgasm and can use this information at another time to connect more deeply with our pleasure. It can also be a turn-on for them to watch us touch ourselves.

As noted previously, one way to be more interested in lovemaking is to consciously set the stage for sex by making a date night. It can also be a reminder that taking the time for sex is a priority in the relationship.

EXERCISE
Creating Rituals around Sex

Lighting candles, giving massages, and creating other such rituals around love-making can increase the mood. A ritual is something we do with concentrated mindfulness, to create an "occasion" for sex.

In this exercise, decide who will be the sender and the receiver. The receiver's job is to relax and receive pleasure, and the sender's job is to make the experience as sensual as possible. Without expectation of anything in return, experience the joy that being generous can bring you, as the sender, as you feel your partner's receptivity and pleasure.

Plan a night for sex. Make sure that your partner is available and that you have ample, uninterrupted time. You should both have the opportunity to go directly to sleep when you are through. Make sure the room is warm and lit with candles or low lighting. Pull the drapes, put on sexy music, and create scents with rose petals, fragrant candles, or incense.

Take a long, hot bath with fragrant bath oil.

Put soft sheets on the bed. Add extra pillows for comfort and sensuality. Have a lubricant and massage oils handy by the bed. Choose sexy lingerie or underwear that has texture and softness to it.

When your partner comes into the room touch him slowly, gently pulling him into the mood and allowing him to adjust to a slower, more sensual tempo.

Step One

Give your partner the gift of a full body, sensual massage. Reassure your partner that there are no strings attached to the massage. Give the massage freely, without expectation that sex will happen as a result or that there will be reciprocation of the massage.

Begin by spreading the massage oil on your partner's back and then out to the extremities. Make sure you use enough pressure so that your partner feels your fingers in the muscles. Ask your partner whether he or she would like softer or harder strokes. Try not to ask, "Is it okay?" Instead, be specific, always offering your partner the chance to direct you to make it harder or softer.

Then let your partner relax into the massage without talking. Use broad hand strokes and simple massaging motions with your palms.

Step Two

Now try squeezing different body parts with the flats of your hands. Hold muscles or body parts gently, letting the warmth from your hands relax your partner's muscles.

Step Three

Now scratch gently with your fingertips and nails. Trace the outline of your partner's body with your hand, from the base of the neck to the perineum. Part his or her buttocks softly, taking each one in hand and stroking deeply. Rub the insides of the thighs with long, deep strokes upward, bringing energy to the genitals.

Remember to breathe while you massage. The receiver can let out any sighs or moans or signs of appreciation for the experience.

Step Four

Now speak softly about how much you appreciate your partner's body. You could whisper things like, "Your skin is so soft," "Your shoulders are so strong," or "I love your thighs." If your partner tries to talk or thank you for the compliment, respond by gently whispering "shh."

Step Five

Continue until your partner falls asleep or the massage naturally moves into lovemaking.

Sharing One Another

We need to be open to sharing ourselves with another person, which is what creates true intimacy and connection. Letting someone else "in" emotionally can sometimes be harder than letting someone "in" to your body.

The next exercise will allow you to experience the connection with your partner in a deep and nonverbal way. Our eyes are the windows to our soul, and the left eye, in Tantric yoga, is considered the receptive eye. Gazing into your lover's left eye helps you focus on that person and look deeply into the true self. Receiving your partner's gaze can be a way to open up and allow him or her into your intimate space.

For this exercise, you will need a warm room, with no distractions. Make sure there is quiet or soft music playing in the background. Carve out uninterrupted time for yourselves, and set up the room for a full sensual experience. Put fresh flowers by the bed, turn down the lights (but not to total darkness), and put down soft blankets to sit on.

EXERCISE
Intimacy or "In-To-Me-See"

This is an exercise you do sitting up and facing each other. Sit as close together as possible—one classic way to sit is with the female partner on top of the legs of the male partner, with her legs wrapped around behind him. Both of you are sitting on your buttocks, but your legs form a cocoon that surrounds the both of you. This way you can be in close physical contact, and you will be more likely to feel your partner's belly when he or she breathes.

If this is not physically comfortable, sit as close as possible with legs overlapping, and find a position that you can maintain for several moments. Remember you can always shift around throughout the exercise if you feel uncomfortable.

Step One

Relax your shoulders. Breathe deeply and into your belly. As you breathe, try to register your partner's breathing. Notice when your partner inhales and exhales. See whether you can coordinate your breathing so that you both breathe together, at the same time.

Step Two

Gaze directly into your partner's left eye; the left eye is the receptive eye. See whether, with each breath, you can welcome your partner nonverbally into your body. Breathe your partner in as you gaze into his or her left eye.

Keep the breathing up for at least fifty breaths. You don't need to count out loud, but try to let yourself truly relax into the breathing.

Step Three

When you are ready to stop, take a final deep, cleansing breath and exhale with an audible sigh. Smile at your partner.

Step Four

Take a last deep breath in and ask your partner whether now is a good time to share. Using the Imago method of mirroring, share with your partner what it felt like to breathe together. Try to talk about any emotions that came up for you, including feelings of love, sadness, happiness, and anger.

This might sound like the following:

Sender: "When I was breathing with you, I felt deeply connected to you."

Receiver: "When you were breathing with me, you felt deeply connected to me."

Sender: "Yes, and I experienced many emotions. I felt deep love for you, and I also felt some sadness."

Receiver: "So you felt deep love for me and also some sadness."

Sender: "Yes, I felt sadness because I have missed you these past few weeks. But then I felt joy that I have you here now and that I love being with you."

Receiver: "So you felt sadness because you have missed me these past few weeks, but then you felt joy that I am here now and that you love being with me. Did I get that? Is there more?"

(continued on page 158)

(continued)

Step Five

Switch.

Step Six

When you are done mirroring one another, share one thing with each other that you appreciated about this intimacy exercise. For example:

Sender: "One thing I really appreciated about this exercise with you is how intimate and connected it felt."

Receiver: "So one thing you really appreciated about this exercise with me is how intimate and connected you felt."

Step Seven

If now is a good time to make love, you may find yourself naturally moving into pleasing each other. Or you may drift off to sleep in each other's arms.

How "Faking It" Hurts a Relationship

Sometimes generosity means being receptive to pleasure. Being blocked from receiving pleasure can be caused by many things—guilt around sexuality, poor body image, low self-esteem, or an inability to express our feelings. All of these things are important to recognize so that we can change how we receive pleasure, not just for us, but for our partners!

Our feelings about ourselves can interfere with our capacity to receive pleasure. Low self-esteem, for example, is expressed sometimes in the fear that "if you really knew me you wouldn't like me." Low self-esteem prevents us from letting our partners get close to us, because we fear that they won't like what they see.

One of the ways to improve self-esteem is by recognizing the parts of ourselves that our partner appreciates. Sometimes asking for those appreciations from our partner can help reinforce our positive traits. Yet, finding this self-confidence in ourselves is important. Our partners will find us infinitely more desirable and interesting if we believe the positive things about ourselves—self-assurance and confidence are very attractive in a partner.

Self-esteem is sometimes affected by how we feel about our bodies. Body image issues are chronic in our society. For women, the perceived failure to uphold the ideal body type personified by models and advertising images can create a feeling of dissatisfaction and even embarrassment about their body.

Only a small percentage of women will ever uphold the body type of a fashion model. And yet the majority of women compare themselves to this standard. Knowing that your body is unique and beautiful because of its size and shape helps improve body image distortions.

For men, body image is often tied up with performance. Men perceive themselves as being less than or better than, depending on their body shape and penis size. Penis size is not a direct correlation with sexual satisfaction in women. When men understand how to be sensual and sexually generous, they can heal from the anxiety around whether their penis is large enough.

Interestingly, when we care about our partners and are attracted to them, we focus on the areas we like and appreciate. This is part of sexual attraction. Most of the time, our partners focus on the parts of our bodies they adore and cherish. And yet the fear that we are unattractive prevents us from feeling comfortable in our bodies when we make love.

It is important to share these feelings with our partners. If you share your fears and insecurities with your partner, he or she will be less likely to take it personally when you hold back during sex. If you keep your clothes on, keep the lights off, or hide yourself in general, your partner may perceive this behavior as a wall between the two of you, and your partner might take it personally.

Being generous means reassuring your partner that your self-protection is not about him or her. Sharing your insecurity can reassure your partner and also help you to work on your own self-image.

Allowing Yourself Pleasure with Your Partner

It can be hard to receive reassurance from your partner. It can also be hard to receive pleasure because of it. Blocking pleasure from your relationship keeps the partnership from getting to the next level of intimacy and connection.

Although many women fake orgasms, they need to recognize that this is not a generous act.

Consider this example. A couple came into my office for sex and relationship counseling and described their relationship as "full of stress and without pleasure." Both partners wanted their partnership to be a place where they felt comfortable and secure, as well as alive and passionate.

The couple described their love life as "boring" and not particularly satisfying to either of them. When I asked them how often they had sex, they said they made love several times a week. I asked whether the female partner had orgasms.

"Not when we have sex," she said. "I can give myself an orgasm when I am alone, if I do it myself. But with him, I really can't come. And I don't think it's a big deal. I can have sex without an orgasm; it's fine."

Her partner, when asked, said he loved to give a woman an orgasm. He insisted he was "totally into it." He said he had been able to give women orgasms in the past without difficulty. I asked how he did that, and he said that his partners had always described to him exactly what they liked and wanted. He went further to describe his feelings about giving a woman an orgasm. He said he "got off on it."

I wondered, how many men feel the same way? When I surveyed the men in my practice and talked to male friends, each one told me that his number one priority during sex was to give his partner an orgasm! I explored this further and realized that men feel successful, powerful, and turned on when their partner reaches orgasm.

Talking to the couple in my office, I empathized with the woman and validated her feelings. I also told her that making sure she had an orgasm was not really about her, but about him. If she were to be generous enough to teach her partner what she needed to climax during sex, she would be giving him an incredible gift! The gift for men is to help them feel powerful in the relationship.

She said she had always felt that her orgasm was "not necessary" and didn't want to "burden" her partner with her needs. He disagreed with her and said her orgasm was "very" necessary, not just for her, but also for him! (This is illustrated later in this chapter with Don and Julie.)

Leading the Way

Generosity of spirit—giving to the other—and generosity with one's own body sometimes mean letting someone else experience the landscape of the self.

Although many women fake orgasms, they need to recognize that this is not a generous act. It is actually a setup for their partners to misunderstand their sexual needs. It prevents their partner from fully understanding what it means to give pleasure. This deprives them of the opportunity to be generous.

Our partners have no way of understanding how our bodies work unless we tell them. Even when two women are in a sexual relationship, they need to communicate how to stimulate each other. All bodies are different and can have slight variations in the ways that they respond to stimulation.

We make assumptions in relationships that if our partners really loved us they would be able to read our minds. Actually, they can't understand what our sexual needs are unless we tell them! And most of us don't come with instructions, so how can our partners know what works unless we teach them?

The following exercise will help women communicate with their partners about what they desire sexually. It is a direct and easy way to help women find a language to describe their sexual needs. Using this exercise can help decrease the fear that sometimes prevents women from being verbal about what they like in bed.

With this language, and with the Imago dialogue, women can learn to express their deepest sexual desires, and also teach their partners exactly what they need in order to reach orgasm.

To get the sex you really want, you have to help your partner know what that means. Remember that when we use the Imago language we can express our feelings and be heard. Our partner can listen in an active and direct way. This takes away the feeling of being judged for our needs and desires.

EXERCISE
Clitoral Clock

To do this exercise, you will need a quiet place where you will not be interrupted for at least sixty minutes. Set up the room (preferably with a bed) so that both of you will be warm, relaxed, and comfortable. Find soft music, fresh flowers, incense, or candles for the room. Make sure your phones are off and that there is sufficient light to see, but that the room is softly lit.

For the following exercise you will also need a lubricant. Any water-based lubricant will work, or use vegetable-based massage oils. (Please note that any scents or warming additive in personal lubricants can cause urinary tract infections and should be avoided.)

Make sure that as the sender your hands are clean and your nails filed or cut short. Keep in mind that the female vulva, including the clitoris, is tender and delicate but can withstand a lot of pressure to bring to orgasm.

The female partner, the receiver, can disrobe and lay in a comfortable place on the bed. Make sure the position is one that is comfortable for a long period of time, and gives access to the sender to touch and see the genitals.

Receivers should let themselves be in a receptive mode. Take deep breaths and allow your body to relax. Feel the opening in yourself as you spread your legs. Make eye contact with the sender and ask for any kiss, touch, or holding that you need before you begin.

Senders should be in a position to see and touch the receiver's vulva. Check with the receiver to make sure she is comfortable and whether she needs anything before you begin. Always warm up your hands before touching naked skin by rubbing your hands together rapidly or blowing warm air into your palms.

Step One

Start by touching the receiver's legs, rubbing your hands over her calves and over the knees and up onto the inner thighs. As you feel your partner relax, open the lubricant and spread it on your fingers as well as her vulva, paying particular attention to the clitoral area.

Using lots of lubricant, warm up your partner's clitoris and vagina with soft stroking and gentle rubbing. Then, imagine the clitoris as a clock, with twelve o'clock being the top portion of the clitoris closest to the belly. Using a well-lubricated finger or two, move clockwise in a small circular motion from the twelve o'clock to one o'clock position and around the clitoris, back to the twelve o'clock position. Do this slowly and repeat it several times.

Step Two

Now have your partner comment on each "time" position and tell you on a scale of 1 to 5 how that position feels to be stimulated and how intense the feeling is. Here, 1 means nonresponsive or uncomfortable, 2 is slightly pleasurable, 3 means "okay, starting to feel good," 4 is wonderful, and 5 is the best and will create an orgasm if it is continued. If you are the sender, tell your partner what time position she is in and wait for a response. This may sound like:

Sender: "This is one o'clock. How does that feel?"

Receiver: "Oh, that's a 4!"

Continue around the clitoris to each time, telling your partner where you are and asking how it feels for her on a scale of 1 to 5.

Step Three

Continue the slow circular motion using different strokes and pressures, and explore other areas of the vulva, always asking the receiver for feedback, using the 1 to 5 scale.

Step Four

Continue until you can bring your partner to orgasm. Keep in mind that even if your partner is at a 5, you may need to back down occasionally to a 3 or 4 level of stimulation. Bringing her back up and then back down can prolong the pleasure and make the orgasm more intense.

Also note that stimulation to orgasm can take anywhere from eight to thirty minutes for women.

The Scorekeeping Sabotage

In relationships we might find ourselves using sex as a way to keep score. We might add up the times we initiate sex, or we might keep track of how often we are the givers. Perhaps we become supersensitive to how often we are the instigators of creative sex, which our partner receives grudgingly and, many times, unwillingly.

Scorekeeping in our sexual relationships can also be a result of keeping score of who does the most household chores, or how often our partner makes an effort to connect with us. When sex is used as a way to even the score, our relationships suffer. Partnerships are not always equal.

Many times I meet with couples in my office and the session turns into a discussion of "who gave who what." One example might be a woman who comes into my office and resents her partner because he often expresses his desire for more oral sex. "He talks ad nauseum about blow jobs," she says. "That's all he wants. And yet, does he give me oral sex as much as I want it?"

She is keeping track of who gave whom oral sex, and how many times. She also wants to know:

"Do I really have to do it, and how come that's all he wants, and when do my needs come first, and why should I do that for him?"

What she really wants to know is: "How can I give him a blow job when I am so mad at him?"

What he really wants to know is: "How can we ever get over all this stuff so we can finally have sex?"

If women need emotional intimacy to be in the mood for sex, men need sex to feel intimate emotionally. What happens when there is a standoff? Eventually no one is intimate and no one is having sex!

If your resentments are getting in the way, here is an exercise to help work through them so that you both can have the sex you want.

EXERCISE
Locking Up Resentment

Sometimes our resentment can get in the way of being a sexually generous partner. If we use this containment exercise and learn new ways to communicate our resentment using the Imago techniques, we can get past our resistance and allow our sensual generosity to create a more connected partnership.

Step One
Imagine an antique trunk on a shelf in your closet. The trunk has a beautiful old padlock and brass straps around it. Visualize yourself putting all your resentment and frustrations in the trunk. In your mind, lock the trunk. Notice whether you feel more in the mood to have sex with your partner.

If not, explore whether there are other resentments that you might not have locked away. If so, add them to the trunk.

Step Two

Now put the trunk back on the shelf. Close the closet door in your imagination. Walk away!

You can take down the trunk anytime and feel free to pull out the resentments later. When you are ready to have a dialogue with your partner about your resentments, you can use the Imago techniques to communicate your feelings, but notice whether now, in this moment, you can let go of them.

Step Three

Tell your partner three things you appreciated about him or her when you first met. Have your partner mirror back everything you say.

Step Four

Now have your partner tell you three things he or she appreciated about you when you first met. Mirror everything back.

Notice whether you feel more connected. Take note: are you open to giving or receiving sexual pleasure in this moment? If not, appreciate the moment of connection with your partner.

Giving Up Control

In addition to holding on to resentments, we can also have difficulty being generous because we want to remain in control. Control issues keep us from letting go and moving toward our partners and giving them what they ask for.

The following case example illustrates how control plays into our sexual relationships and gives clear ideas about letting go and moving toward what our partner wants from us. In this way, we grow as individuals.

Melissa and Jason came into my office complaining of "difficulty" in their marriage. The sex was acceptable, but not what either of them really wanted. They had no experience talking about what they needed, and did not understand the language necessary to talk about erotic needs. They both wanted to learn how to reconnect.

One afternoon in their session together, Jason appeared withdrawn. Melissa was on the edge of her seat and looked tense and angry. Her fists were clenched and she crossed her arms over her chest.

Jason: "I think Melissa is withholding sex." He looked angry and hurt. His face was set in a grimace and he avoided making eye contact.

Melissa: "All Jason wants is oral sex! All he wants is a blow job, and he wants it the same way every time."

I asked Melissa what she wanted.

Melissa: "I want to feel connected to Jason. When I give him oral sex I feel disconnected and distant from him. It also hurts my jaw and I get cramped from the same motion over and over."

Jason: "So, Melissa, what you are saying is that you want to feel connected to me, and that giving oral sex makes you feel disconnected and it hurts your jaw."

Jason mirrored what she said, without offering a solution. Sometimes therapists will change the subject and instead of focusing on the sexual issues they will try to shift the focus to the emotional distance in the relationship. Helping a couple talk about sex can be a quicker way in to the relationship. To make some concrete changes in the relationship, why not go straight for the issue that is presenting?

If things change in the sexual relationship, the rest of the relationship can change. It can take many weeks of therapy to change a behavior like "taking out the garbage." And yet, when couples leave a session promising to take out the garbage, they come back a week later in the same pain and frustration they were in when they left. When changes are made in their sexual partnership, real intimacy and connection happens. So I asked Jason to continue mirroring the sexual content of what Melissa was saying.

Jason: "And so what you are saying is that you feel like all I want is a blow job and I want it the same way every time."

Melissa: "Yes, it's boring down there by myself! Nothing is happening for me and you just go into some trance and stop talking to me."

I asked Jason whether there were ways he could stay engaged with Melissa during oral sex.

Jason: "Sometimes oral sex is great for going into a trance. And sometimes, to be honest, I just want to come, and get a release. But if I know she hates doing it, I can't relax, and then it takes me longer to come."

I asked Jason to describe in detail what she did that felt good. Melissa mirrored everything he said. His appreciation of her softened her anxiety.

She relaxed into the session, and even smiled as he described the details of what she did with her tongue that brought him intense pleasure.

Melissa: "Thank you, Jason. I really do want to make you feel good if I can. But I am so lonely down there by myself!"

Jason mirrored Melissa and asked her what she needed. They came up with several ways he could make physical contact with her while she was giving him oral sex.

They agreed to try several things. He would put his hands in her hair and touch her shoulders while she was giving him oral sex. This would help her feel connected to him during the sexual act. This would also give him more of a sense of control, and possibly help him ejaculate sooner during oral sex, which they both identified as a desire that they shared.

Jason also decided that he would try to be more verbal during oral sex. He would talk to her as she was doing it, and tell her exactly what he liked about what she was doing. He would use phrases like, "That feels great when you lick me" or "I love when you suck hard like that."

During this dialogue in the office, as they mirrored back and forth, Melissa made more eye contact with Jason and he gazed into her eyes and held her hands. Their bodies were relaxed, and they were no longer angry or frustrated with each other. Melissa even described that she felt aroused by the conversation, and that it "turned her on" to hear what Jason wanted during a blow job.

The final part of the dialogue was about Melissa's desire to feel aroused while she was giving Jason oral sex.

Melissa: "I think I would feel more connected to you, and to the whole experience, if I was turned on. I just can't get into it sometimes."

Jason: "Can you keep eye contact with me during a blow job?"

Although that seemed difficult for both of them, she agreed to try. Jason also brought up another fun option.

Jason: "Melissa, can you use a vibrator to stimulate yourself while you give me a blow job? I would love to watch that while you are giving me head!"

He said he would feel more engaged with her in this way as well, watching what she was doing.

I suggested they have oral sex in small doses throughout the week, without bringing Jason to climax. This would increase Melissa's comfort level and decrease her resentment around being made to "get him off all the time." It would also help her to relax her muscles and learn ways to give oral sex that would not hurt her jaw. Most pain during oral sex can be alleviated when the jaw is relaxed.

Melissa also liked the idea of moving her hand on his penis while the head was in her mouth. She agreed to try the vibrator while she was giving him oral sex, and said she would be happier starting in small sessions, perhaps building up to longer periods as they practiced more of the connecting exercise.

During the dialogue the couple sat across from each other, facing each other and made eye contact. Melissa relaxed, sat back in her chair, and smiled at Jason. They made physical contact several times by holding hands, and laughed together when they were feeling shy.

The following week Jason and Melissa reported an amazing difference not only in their sexual relationship, which actually had not changed all that dramatically, but also in their capacity to talk about what was happening between them.

Jason: "Hey, I figured if we could talk about blow jobs for an hour we can pretty much talk about anything now!"

Melissa said she felt heard and understood, and no longer felt resentful. She said Jason had talked to her about how important it was for him to have these new experiences with her. She was more attached to him and felt more empathetic to his needs.

EXERCISE
Bonding over Oral Sex

The following exercise illustrates ways to stay connected to your partner, and helps with some of the resistance that you may feel when your partner wants something that feels uncomfortable for you.

During oral sex, first make eye contact. Then touch the giver's hair. Use words that describe how you are feeling in every moment. Focus on the experience, or the journey, and try to stay in the moment. Focusing on bringing your partner to orgasm can take away from the feelings of connection in the present. This is not a race to the end zone; it is an experience that you are having as a couple, to be enjoyed by both of you.

Sharing Erotic Needs with Each Other

Men and women share similar erotic needs. They also have specific needs that are determined by their gender. Some of the needs that both men and women desire include safety, trust, connection, intensity, challenge, fantasy, fear, thrill, comfort, and passion. Most of us have these needs at some level.

However, men and women also have erotic needs that are specific not only to their gender, but also to them as individuals. We have erotic tendencies that are special to us as a result of the way we grew up, how we were socialized, and how our own physical anatomy works.

EXERCISE
Sharing Our Sexual Needs

This exercise is a way to get to know your partner and compare your needs. Go down the list below and number each item according to how important this need is for you, rating it from 1 (not so important) to 10 (very important).

- Safety
- Trust
- Connection
- Intensity
- Challenge
- Fantasy
- Fear
- Thrill
- Comfort
- Passion

Have your partner do the same. Now compare lists. What do you notice about yourself and your needs? How do they compare with your partner's needs?

When Gender Makes the Difference

Sometimes we assume that because we need something, our partners should have the same need. We assume that they should know what we want because, hey, don't they want the same thing? The more we experience the erotic needs of our partners as different from our own, the more we can begin to understand who they are.

Differentiation is an advanced-level skill, but one that, when mastered, allows us some space in our relationship. And it is in this space that the longing, or the desire for another, happens. We begin to crave connection when we feel separate. This draws us to our partners and creates more intensity in the sexual relationship.

If we are totally merged with our partners, thinking they are the same as us, and want the same things and think the same way, then there is no space between us and we become overly familiar with that partner. Even though most of this is what we call projection—where we attribute certain qualities to another that are really about ourselves—we are often unaware that we do it.

We still look at our partners as extensions of ourselves, and it takes work and maturity to see them as separate people with their own unique thoughts and needs. If we can begin to see our partners that way, we can begin to understand some of their fantasies and needs, but in a new way. Now perhaps they make sense to us, and perhaps we can even fulfill those fantasies if we understand that they are not about what we want, but what our partner wants.

Men's Sexual Needs

Keeping in mind that we are all unique, most men have the following erotic needs, which are explained in detail below:

1. Physical connection. Men need to have a physical connection with their partner to feel confident and secure. Sex, to men, is an important way to find emotional security. The physicality of the erotic bond helps men feel open to communicating and talking about their feelings. Having someone to hold and touch is a powerful way for men to relate.

Direct genital contact is important for men as well. Sometimes taking our time and teasing before we get to a man's penis or scrotum is wonderful, but men need to have direct contact in the places that feel the best. Their lead time is shorter than a woman's and they crave a direct, confident touch in the places that arouse them.

2. Generosity or pleasing a partner. Men generally agree on one thing: that pleasing their partner is one of their priorities. Making a woman happy in bed, giving her an orgasm, and being sure she is enjoying the erotic connection is so important to men that when they don't feel like they are pleasing their partner they can become depressed and discouraged. See the sidebar on page 172.

3. Appreciation. Because men have spent their whole lives being recognized for what they do and not for who they are, many perceive their actions to be their most important contribution to the world.

Often the question people ask a man when they first meet is "What do you do?" The implication is that what they *do* is the most important aspect of who they *are*. This is not as true for women. Girls don't necessarily have to perform to get recognition. There is certainly pressure on girls to do well in school, and there is increased competition to get into college, which provokes more ambitious and creative forces in girls. Often, however, girls are still recognized and judged for their looks, regardless of their accomplishments.

Boys, on the other hand, are recognized for how they behave: the grades they get, the sports they play, and how they act. As adults, men still focus on their accomplishments, at least until they get older and begin to doubt their whole direction in life, which is the midlife awakening so often called the "midlife crisis."

Midlife *awakening* happens when men reach a developmental age where they have experienced some success in their lives, and they begin to realize that who they *are* does not necessarily translate into what they *do*. Perhaps they have worked hard all their lives to provide for a family or to pursue monetary or social success.

He Needs You to Come

Don and June came to my office because of June's inability to have an orgasm.

"It doesn't really matter to me if I have an orgasm with Don," June said. "I can do it when I am alone and masturbating, so I know I am capable of having one. But with Don, it's fine if we just make love and I don't come. It doesn't honestly matter to me." Don looked upset, and I asked him how he felt about it.

"Well, it matters to me," he said. "I don't enjoy sex with June if I know she won't have an orgasm."

I assured June that it is certainly enjoyable to have sex with someone you care about, knowing that he is enjoying himself, and that its not always necessary for women to have an orgasm every time. It's not always necessary for men to have an orgasm every time either! Yet, even though she claimed that she didn't need to orgasm during sex with Don, it was very important for Don. She needed to work on having an orgasm with him, not for her, but for him! And the way to do that was to teach Don how she made herself come.

Teaching your partner how to give you an orgasm is not just about your own pleasure; it also allows your partner to experience your generosity. Both partners can do this, one at a time, during one session, or in two separate sessions. Each partner should go slowly so the other can watch you and see exactly what you are doing and where you are touching yourself. Show your partner how you touch yourself to reach orgasm.

If you feel up to it, describe in detail what you are doing as you masturbate. Tell your partner about your preferences. You might say something like, "I love touching my clit on the bottom softly at first and then I go around it slowly, but with more pressure, like this." After you've reached orgasm, switch with your partner and watch him masturbate as he describes exactly what he does to ejaculate.

When you are through, you may find that you feel slightly embarrassed or self-conscious. You will also feel closer and more intimate with your partner. Now is the time to have a quiet dialogue, perhaps lying next to one another.

Midlife awakening happens when men reach a developmental age that allows them to experience success in their lives, and they have come to a place in life when they realize that who they are does not necessarily translate into what they do.

By midlife, most men begin to realize and wake up to the fact that they have never truly been able to "feel," that is, they have not been encouraged to express their emotional side but have had to repress their feelings to get by in the world. By midlife they discover that they have a wealth of emotions and a new sensitivity to the world where they crave feeling. These men sometimes gravitate toward women (or cars) that make them feel something. Some men get overwhelmed by their emotions, and others become more giving and spiritual.

Many men at midlife become better lovers because they begin to grow out of the intense self-focus and pressure to perform. They seek things in life that give them deeper satisfaction and meaning. As they age, they work harder to be in the moment.

The focus on men's actions influences their erotic needs. They need to be appreciated for their actions and their accomplishments. They want to be recognized for what they do—a need they have had since early childhood.

Whether it means feeling appreciated for bringing out the garbage or for giving their partner an orgasm, they need the feedback in an appreciative way.

Anything that a woman says to a man that is about "not doing" enough will be perceived as criticism. Male sensitivity to appreciation is due to a lifelong need to earn the affirmation around how they are "doing."

Appreciation is something that both men and women need, but men complain more about not getting it. When men complain about their partners, they say things like, "No matter what I do it's never enough" or "She doesn't appreciate all the things I do for her." In their minds, they work at pleasing their partner through their actions. Sometimes those actions may not be appreciated by their partner, since women don't recognize the need to be rewarded for all that they do.

You can work on appreciating your partner by telling him three things you appreciate about him while you are in bed with him. Whisper in his ear things you like that he is doing to you, such as "I love when you tease my nipples like that" or "I love the way your penis feels inside me."

Use explicit words. Don't expect anything in return.

Tell him afterward three things you liked about how he made love to you. Top it off with a kiss. Notice how your partner responds. Tell him what you notice. It might sound like, "You are so cute when I tell you these things—you blush right down to your toes!" or "Your smile is beautiful right now."

4. Action. Because men have been socialized to act, they need to make things happen. Male energy moves things to the next level, to the conclusion, to the end zone. In our culture, sex is often about getting to the finish line, moving things to ejaculation, which is the ultimate destination.

This need to move things to the next place also explains why men take women's flirtation as a sign that the woman is interested in them and that they want to take the relationship to a sexual level. The male need for action is what makes men have a tendency to be more directive and more dominant in relationships and in bed.

5. Languages of love. We all experience love differently. Because of the way we grew up and what we learned about love, we have needs that may not be the same as those of our partners.

Some people experience being loved and giving love in the same way. In his book, *Five Love Languages*, author Gary Chapman describes different ways that we all show and receive love. The five love languages are sex, praise, acts of service, gifts, and time.

Our languages of love are important to understand when we talk about sex and erotic needs. If our partner's language of love is time, then perhaps being in bed for long stretches of time and spending time talking about sex would make that person feel loved. If your partner's language of love is gifts, then small tokens that express thoughtfulness would go a long way toward softening the relationship. Books about sex, lingerie, massage oils, candles—all of these gifts can help your partner feel loved while at the same time improving the atmosphere in your bedroom!

Acts of service include things like keeping the house clean, shopping, building bookcases, and running errands. Doing things for our partners to make their life easier is an example of the love language of acts of service. Praise includes being verbal about things you appreciate about your partner. Sex and affection can be a way to experience love and to show love.

The following case describes ways that we love each other, and how we experience differences between us.

Speaking Different Languages of Love

Tina and Tom came into therapy because they felt the distance in their relationship was growing and they had serious questions about their ability to stay married. After twenty-seven years they wanted to stay committed to each other, but both felt unappreciated and unloved.

Tina: "I stay in the kitchen until late at night, hoping Tom will come down and help me clean up. If he would just do the dishes once in a while, I would be happy to have sex with him."

Tom: "Well, at night I am upstairs in our bed waiting for her to come up and make love. If she really loved me, we would be having sex more often. But she spends all her time futzing around the kitchen and by the time she comes up I'm asleep."

Tina's language of love is acts of service. For her, what Tom does for her to help out shows her that he loves her. She grew up in a family where her father mowed the lawn, built bookshelves, and took her mother shopping. She experienced love as an expression of what people did for her. She felt loved when Tom would unpack the groceries from the car for her.

(continued on page 176)

Speaking Different Languages of Love

(continued)

Tom's language of love is sex and physical affection. He grew up without any physical contact from his parents. Spending most of his life in an orphanage, he was not adopted until he was twelve, and his adopted family was not affectionate. He never played full contact sports, nor did he have a girlfriend until he was twenty-four. He craved physical contact, and he experienced sex and affection as healing. He felt loved when Tina crawled into bed next to him and he would sleep curled up behind her like spoons in a drawer.

Once Tom and Tina understood each other's language of love, they were able to love one another in the way that each needed to be loved. They now saw how each of them had been trying to show love to the other, but in a language the other did not understand or appreciate. The gestures were lost on each of them. When they began to see how the other person experienced that as rejection and abandonment, they were able to change things in the relationship.

Several months later, Tina reported that Tom had installed a new dishwasher for her and was helping her load it every night. They would go to bed together at the same time every night, and most nights Tina would express her appreciation for Tom's efforts and snuggle up to him in bed. Many times that would turn into sex. Tom reported feeling more connected to Tina and became more willing to love her in the ways she needed. Tina understood Tom's needs and was happy to help him feel loved and secure, once she understood how to do that!

Female Sexual Needs

In contrast to men, women have different emotional, physical, and erotic needs. Their sexual needs include the following:

1. Physical affection. For women, physical affection guarantees their security in the relationship. Touch is a way of "checking in" for women. Knowing that her partner is there, and occasionally reaching out to connect in a loving way, helps the female partner feel safe. The need to be acknowledged, to feel like "he knows I am here" is a big one.

When women complain about men, they often say things like, "He doesn't even know I'm here" or "I don't feel like he's present." Feeling physical affection reaffirms for women that their partner is indeed "there" and still cares for them.

2. Long lead time. Women have different needs from men when it comes to foreplay. Women's arousal levels are different, and they need to reach several plateaus before they reach orgasm. These plateaus are the levels of physical arousal that make sex more interesting in the moment. Women also need to reach emotional and cognitive (thinking) levels before they are ready to let go and relax into eroticism.

Getting a woman to this point can take time. Sometimes it can take days! If you want to have sex with a woman on a Saturday, then you might have to start on a Wednesday! You have learned in earlier chapters some ways to make this happen. Again, what that might look like could include the following:

- Coming up behind her as she stands by the sink and kissing her neck.
- Sending her small notes through e-mail or text messages, reminding her of how much you are looking forward to sex with her on Saturday.
- Describing in detail the things you want to do to her when you have your sex date.
- Whispering in her ear before she goes to sleep how much she turns you on.
- Bringing her a small gift, perhaps a rose, to tell her how you value her and your sexual relationship.
- Having a sex date. See exercise on page 178.

These things will help the woman look forward to the sex date. Anticipation is a great aphrodisiac.

EXERCISE
Sex Date

Make a date with your partner for sex. Four days prior to the date, use small acts to create anticipation for the big night. For example, show your partner physical affection at least three times the first day. Attempt to connect on the second day by whispering in your partner's ear the things you want to do to him or her on your sex date. On the third day, bring home a surprise. This can be something like a card or small token gift. The surprise might be something you can use on your sex date.

The fourth day is the big day, so create an atmosphere in the bedroom that will remind both of you that this is a sacred, erotic space for you to play safely in together. Light candles, put fresh flowers in the room and put soft sheets and blankets on the bed. Make an extra effort to pick out music that your partner will like.

When the big night comes, keep your expectations open and reasonable. If the evening goes well, then great. If it doesn't live up to your expectations, remember that this night can be anything that works for you and makes you feel connected to your partner. Massage, communication, and sharing fantasies using the Imago dialogue can make this an important night of sensual pleasures.

3. Emotional reminders. The need to be reminded about the connection with one's partner is not unique to women, but for women to feel relaxed and comfortable and to have a deepening of their erotic connection, they need to be reminded that they are safe. The way for male partners to do this is by reminding their women that they are still loved. Women say things to men like, "Do you still love me? Are you sure you love me?" which can sometimes be annoying for their partner.

As one man said in a sex workshop, "I told her I loved her when we got married. Isn't that enough for her? Why does she need to hear it again?"

Although this is an extreme example, it illustrates the point that men sometimes assume that their partner should know how they feel based on past conversations. But women need to be reminded, and often. It's not that they forget; it's that the reassurance of hearing it repeated on a regular basis helps them to relax into the security of the relationship. Testing the boundaries of their safety is part of what helps women to relax and surrender, knowing that their relationship has strong boundaries and will contain all of their fears and needs.

4. Permission. Because of women's guilt and shame around sex, there may be times when women don't feel that they deserve to have sexual pleasure. If there is sexual abuse in their pasts, or imagined fears that prevent letting go, then having "permission" to let go can help.

Some women don't feel like they deserve pleasure of any kind. This happens when they feel overly responsible in their lives. Their partners can tell them: "You deserve this break. You work so hard, you deserve to have all the pleasure I can give you."

5. Safety to surrender. When women receive permission, they often feel safer to surrender to the erotic moment. If they know that their partner is directive and in charge, they can relax into the experience, knowing someone is going to create an atmosphere that will help them feel like they can let go. This surrender is very important for orgasm.

There does not have to be total safety to have erotic sex or passion in a relationship. A slight bit of anxiety can heighten the anticipation and create more erotic drama for women. People are sometimes addicted to this level of excitement and arousal and look for ways to create it in their lives. The drama or crisis that is created sometimes adds an element of eroticism, particularly if there is danger or a sense of the forbidden involved.

But if the drama is risking the safety of the relationship, then it becomes toxic to a passionate partnership. This level of stimulation can be created within the partnership by planning sex that is risky or slightly scary. If women feel safe then they will not only feel turned on but will also be able to totally surrender.

6. The language of love. The way to know a woman's love language is to ask her! The languages of love are the same for women as they are for men. Finding out what her love language is can help her feel loved. Knowing her needs can help you fulfill her and give her what she wants. This is an act of generosity that shows you care about her.

The Language of Love for Women

In this exercise, we'll discover and explore how to love our partners in a way that makes them feel loved. You will need a pen and paper for this exercise.

Step One

Write down five things your partner did in the beginning of the relationship that made you feel loved. Write down five things he or she does now to make you feel loved. (There may be some overlap in these things, or they may be all new.)

Step Two

Take a look at your list and see what kind of love language you have. You may be closer to understanding your own language of love now. Which category does your love language fall under? Do you appreciate time, sex, praise, acts of service, or gifts?

Share the list with your partner. Ask for one thing that you would like your partner to do that makes you feel loved. Have your partner ask the same of you.

Step Three

Commit to fulfilling that language of love behavior at least once in the coming week.

Step Four

Meet again to talk about how it felt to get that need met. Make sure you tell your partner how much you appreciated him or her for doing this for you and making you feel loved.

Different Sexual Styles

David Schnarch, author of *Passionate Marriage,* says that there are three different types of sex—trance sex, partner engagement, and role-play.

People who are into trance sex need to shut off all outside stimulation to experience their pleasure and sensation. Being engaged with your partner means feeling emotional, intimate, and connected with your partner through sex. Role-play sex is about acting out and talking during sex. The following case illustrates how we can have different sexual styles and how at times these styles can feel confusing because they are different than our own needs. Learning more about how our partner operates sexually will help increase our understanding of what he or she needs in bed.

Dawn and Damien came into my office because of their difficulty pleasing each other during sex.

Damien: "When Dawn has sex, she doesn't want any outside stimulation. She wants to close her eyes, she doesn't want noise or talking, and sometimes she puts a pillow over her eyes or hides her face in her arm."

Dawn: "Well, I don't like it when Damien talks all the time. He is into this role-play thing and wants to talk during sex, and he wants me to talk to him."

Damien: "If she would just go along sometimes with what I want, I would love it. But she gets all embarrassed and the mood is shot. I just don't even want to try anymore."

I asked them what they had done in the past to work on their sex life.

Damien: "I bought Dawn an outfit, I have brought home porn movies, and I have tried to have sex with her in unusual places, like that time in the parking lot at my office."

Damien was a "role-play" type of sexual person. He wanted to talk during sex and was turned on when Dawn talked to him. He didn't need her to become something she wasn't, but he wanted a more active type of sex that included imagination, sex games, and playing roles during sex.

Dawn, on the other hand, was a "trance" type of sexual person. She needed to block out all outside stimulation so that she could totally focus on the sensations in her body. She was only able to orgasm if she could get lost in the experience and feel every nuance of their lovemaking.

The need for "partner engagement" includes a need to gaze into a partner's eyes during sex. When Damien asked Dawn to keep her eyes open, she would lose interest in the sex. She would pull away and they would both be angry and hurt. Neither of these preferences is wrong. However, not knowing the other's style in bed had created an atmosphere where neither had a fulfilling experience.

For couples to enjoy each other and create passion in their partnership they have to understand each other's style. At times each partner needs to push his or her edge (or limits) to try the other's style of sex. To maintain desire, both partners have to experience the other as someone who is willing and able to come to their side of the bed, and to act out their erotic fantasies. Being willing to try sex in other ways is what makes passion possible.

Use Sexual Anatomy Knowledge to Improve Your Sex Life

8

Most of the sex education handouts in our grade school health classes are of internal reproductive organs. That education is very necessary, but so is the more specific education about our sexual organs and their unique responses to stimulation and desire.

Sexual desire, and what to do about it, is not taught in school. Girls are not taught what to do when they feel an attraction to the boy sitting next to them in math class. Boys are not taught what to do with their intense sexual urges that peak in adolescence. Both boys and girls, as they reach adolescence, begin a stumbling around process that signifies the beginning of their experimentation with sex. The "backseat fumble," the reach under the T-shirt, the furtive kisses behind the ice cream shop: all of these experiences are the beginning of a journey toward erotic partnership.

To empower girls to make choices based on self-respect and integrity, they must be taught how to recognize their desires so that they can be expressed when the time feels right. Girls also need to learn about boys' sexuality. For boys to feel in control of their sexuality and to move into relationships without guilt and shame, they need education in mutual sexual desire.

Many of us are not taught about desire or what to do when we feel like acting out our feelings. Many women are confused about their body's sexual signals, which makes it hard for them to communicate their sexual needs. If women don't recognize their own erotic desires, they begin to split off from their sexuality, become dissociated during sex, and feel frustrated and dissatisfied. Men can be confused about when and how to act on their desires, and not understand a woman's sometimes confusing signals.

Test Your Knowledge

The following quiz will help you begin to identify what you know about your own sexual anatomy and that of your partner. As you take the quiz and answer the questions, notice what you are curious about. Then, after reading the rest of the chapter, take the quiz again and see how much you have learned!

Knowing about your sexual anatomy and how your body works can help you discover the endless wonders of your own sexuality. Learning about your partner's sexual anatomy and how his or her body works can help you have the sex you have always wanted.

In Imago therapy, we learn that our growth lies in what we bring *to* the relationship, not what we get *out* of it. When we give our partners what they really want, we grow into fully realized individuals.

EXERCISE
Sexual Anatomy Quiz

Answer the following questions together with your partner or separately and see how well you each score. Then, take the quiz again after reading this chapter and compare your scores. Remember, you will be testing yourselves to see how much you have learned from reading this chapter.

1. How long do women take to achieve orgasm after direct clitoral stimulation?

   3 to 5 minutes? 8 to 10 minutes? 7 to 20 minutes?
   15 to 30 minutes?

2. Where is the perineum located on women?

3. Where is the perineum located on men?

4. Where is the G-spot on women located?

5. The G-spot is actually the root of what part of the body?

6. Where is the male prostate gland located?

7. The male prostate gland is similar in nerve structure to which part of the female anatomy?

8. What is more stimulating, labia massage or clitoral massage?

9. Out of what orifice does a woman urinate?

10. Can a man orgasm without ejaculating?

11. Can a woman ejaculate while having an orgasm?

12. Are there pleasure centers in the anus?

13. What are clitoral roots?

The Ways We Become Aroused

One of the first things we need to know about sexual anatomy is that there are similarities and differences in how men and women become sexually stimulated.

Men and women both get aroused by these types of stimulation:

- **Visual.** If we are stimulated visually, then we are aroused by what we see. We will be stimulated by what our partners look like. We will get turned on by watching them. It will stimulate us to watch them having sex. We may also get aroused by watching pornography or seeing erotic photos.

- **Touch or kinesthetic.** The feel of things on our bodies is arousing. If we are kinesthetic, then touch engages us sexually more than our other senses do. Touching our partners, feeling their skin, and being held will be important to us for experiencing pleasure. Massage, feathers, feather dusters, ice cubes, and any other stimulation that creates a kinesthetic response will make us feel passionate and alive.

- **Auditory.** If we are auditory, then the sounds of lovemaking will get us excited. Listening to the soft sounds of our partner's pleasure or hearing them scream with passion will send us over the edge. Sexy music, poetry read out loud, and hearing our partners "talk dirty" will turn us on.

- **Thought or cognitive.** The stimulation of our imagination can also be arousing. Having fantasies in our minds will get us hot. Thinking about our partners and imagining them in different positions or having erotic fantasies about them will stimulate the cognitive mind.

The difference between men and women is primarily seen in their responses to arousal. Men have one level of arousal, and usually want to be touched immediately and can get an erection with little prompting. Men can go from feeling aroused to orgasm in a relatively short time. They peak, and they begin to come down almost immediately, which is why men often fall asleep after their orgasm.

For women, plateaus of arousal take longer, and there are more of them. While arousal may take a while, women can stay at higher levels of arousal for longer periods of time, allowing for multiple orgasms and a more gradual descent back to normal. This is why women need foreplay and why they stay in a sexually aroused place for a long period of time after an orgasm.

We will talk later about ways for men to stay in the higher plateaus of arousal, going from plateau to plateau and staying erect without reaching orgasm.

What We Do When We're Aroused

You may feel physical responses when you feel desire, but you do not have to act on any of them. You have a choice about what to do with your desires. When you feel sexually aroused, you have several options:

- You can act out with another person
- You can self-stimulate
- You can fantasize
- You can sublimate
- You can avoid your feelings

Acting out with another person means engaging in sex. Self-stimulation refers to masturbation and self-pleasure. Fantasizing is anything in your mind that brings erotic imagery. To sublimate your arousal means to work it out through some other positive behavior, like creating artwork or playing music.

Avoiding your feelings is perhaps the most risky option, since it implies that your feelings *can* be avoided. Feelings need to be expressed and can come out at a later time when we least expect it.

EXERCISE
Learning about Stimulation

For this exercise, find some quiet time to answer the following questions. Both men and women should take this quiz, as it applies to both sexes. You will need some time afterward to process your answers with your partner in an Imago dialogue, using mirroring, validation, and empathy.

Answer "true" or "false" to each of the following questions and share your answers with your partner:

- If I felt more comfortable in my body I think I would have sex more often.
- I recognize when my body is responding to stimulation, either visual, physical, or in my thoughts.
- I am a visually stimulated person.
- I am primarily stimulated by physical touch.
- I use my imagination to stimulate myself sexually.
- I often feel my body's signals for sexual desire.
- I would like to feel my body's signals for sexual desire.
- I like the feel of garments and materials around me, such as scarves, sweaters, etc.
- I like to have nice sheets and blankets on my bed.
- I love to take bubble baths and wear perfumes and scented creams on my body.
- I get manicures and pedicures often.
- I let people massage me and enjoy healthy nonsexual touch.

Looking at your answers, what did you notice about yourself? Share your answers with your partner, reading out loud the question and whether you answered "true" or "false." Have your partner mirror back what you say. Then your partner will validate by responding, "It makes sense you would like X because I know you like to feel X." Then your partner empathizes by guessing at one feeling he or she thinks this gives you. For example, "I imagine you feel very relaxed and sexy when you take a hot bubble bath." Then share anything you learned about your partner after hearing his or her answers.

The Avenue to Anal Stimulation

The anus has similar responses to the vagina during sex. It contracts during an orgasm in the same way the vagina does. There are lots of nerve endings in the anus, so that receiving anal stimulation can feel great if done with lots of lubricant and communication with your partner.

Be aware that receiving anal stimulation can be both pleasurable and painful. The internal and external sphincter muscles tighten and relax, controlling the passage to the anus. These muscles must be relaxed for something to enter externally.

To create the possibility of anal sex, your partner needs to work with you to help you relax. Exploring this sensitive area can include a combination of massage, lubrication, and relaxation techniques including deep breathing. Sex toys that are narrower than a finger can be used at first to test the anus's response to insertion. Make sure the anal toy is wider at the base, to prevent it from going too far into the rectum. The anus will suck things into it when it tightens, and these things may not come out. Be careful that anything you insert into the anus and rectum will be easy to retrieve.

Using good communication, couples can talk to each other during this experience to explore what feels good and what is uncomfortable. Stopping immediately when the discomfort gets too dramatic is an important thing to agree on prior to any anal play. Knowing your partner is sensitive to your body and what feels good will increase the trust between you.

Getting to Know Our Bodies

Having an orgasm for women is sometimes complicated. When they are out of touch with their bodies, women can have a hard time figuring out what gives them pleasure.

Some women at midlife have never had an orgasm, although many have faked one. And faking orgasm is confusing to men, since they don't know which signals to trust or how to create sensations for women that will lead to a real orgasm!

Even as adults, women can be ignorant of how their bodies work. Lots of women think they urinate from their vaginas. Most women have never looked at their genitals in a mirror.

Without embarrassment, can you tell your partner, with the most direct and graphic language possible, the location of your different body parts? Can you give him or her an anatomy lesson? Perhaps you will tell your partner things he or she already knows, or you may explain your body in a way that makes it a new discovery for your partner.

Try to explain to your partner what you need to achieve an orgasm and then ask your partner what kind of stimulation he or she needs to have an orgasm. Share what feels good to each of you.

This next exercise should help you teach your partner about your body and what gives you pleasure.

EXERCISE
Playing Doctor

As a passionate partner, learning about sexual anatomy, (what is where and how to use it), is an important part of being a fully present and empathetic lover. Understanding each other's anatomy leads to new journeys of exploration and connection.

For this exercise, you will need at least sixty minutes of uninterrupted time together. Make sure the room is warm and comfortable. Put on soft music and low lights, but with enough illumination to really see and appreciate your partner's body.

(continued on page 190)

(continued)

Remember, as you verbalize this information with your partner, you will use the Imago dialogue method of mirroring, so that everything your partner shares with you becomes an opportunity to help him or her feel heard and seen.

Step One

Choose who will be the sender and who will be the receiver. Senders should ask their partners (receivers) to show them all the parts of their body. Receivers should explain how these parts work and what they feel like. Senders mirror back what their partners say. Ask questions as if you were seeing these parts for the first time. Mirror back the answers.

Step Two

Senders should ask their partners what happens in specific places in their body during arousal and orgasm. Senders mirror back what they hear. Ask them how their body parts feel when they are aroused, which parts of their anatomy feel the best when caressed, and how they like to be touched in those places. Senders should mirror what they hear.

Step Three

Switch, and senders now explain to the receivers all their parts, showing and pointing to the more hidden locations so that their partners can see clearly what is happening in the sender's body.

Senders should tell receivers what stimulation their body parts need to become aroused. Receivers should mirror what they hear. Senders should explain what type of touch feels the best on what part, what happens as they get closer to orgasm, and where they feel their orgasm. Receivers should mirror what they hear.

Step Four

Thank your partner for sharing this very intimate experience with you! Share with each other what you appreciated about this exercise, mirroring back what you hear. Move into sexual play, pleasure, or intercourse if that feels right for you both in this moment. Otherwise, enjoy the appreciations and new knowledge of each other's body!

Anatomy 101: Female Genitalia

For most of us, women's genitals are a mystery—even for women! The majority of women never look at their genitals with a mirror. And since most women don't normally see other women's genitals, their own anatomy can remain a mystery.

We see men's genitals all the time. They are on statues and in fine art everywhere. Like the female breast, the penis has been immortalized in stone and in paint for centuries. But the female equivalent, the vulva, is not a popular subject of artwork. Just by virtue of the fact that the female genitalia remain hidden anatomically, women don't get a chance to see what other vulvas look like. We don't see women's vulvas in the locker room. Not all vaginas are alike. They differ as widely as penis shapes do.

Here's a rundown of what you should know about female genitalia, including the famed G-spot.

The **vulva** consists of two sets of **labia**, or lips. The word *labia* is derived from the Latin word meaning "lips." The outer lips, *labia majora*, are what we see if a woman is shaved or has no hair on her vulva. The inner lips, the inner labia or *labia minora*, are smaller and thinner, protect the opening of the vagina, and are extremely sensitive. Labia or lips are folds of skin that vary in size and elasticity. Not all labia look alike! They are as unique to the individual as any other part of a woman's body. The labia swell when aroused. Sometimes the inner labia hang outside the outer labia and sometimes they are covered. Both are normal.

Looking at a woman directly while she is lying on her back, the vulva is slightly pear-shaped, with the narrower part on top and the wider parts at the bottom. Or it can be narrow at both ends and wider in the middle. Inside the inner labia the **clitoris** (klit-er-iss) is at the top. The opening to the vagina is in the wider part of the vulva. In between the clitoris and the vagina is the **urethra**. The urethra is the opening where women urinate. Women do not urinate from their vagina, even during orgasm.

The **clitoris** is a small projection, approximately the size of a pea, situated above the vagina, at the top of the vulva. The clitoris can project out from between the labia minora or be hidden in the folds of the labia. Women's clitoral size varies. It can be anywhere from the size of the tip of a pinky finger to two inches long.

The **anus** is below the vagina, and the **perineum** is the area in between the bottom of the vagina and the anus.

When touching a vulva, always have clean hands. Go slowly at first, and be gentle. Touching the sensitive parts of the vulva using dry fingers can catch and drag the skin and feel uncomfortable, so use a water-based lubricant.

The urethra is sensitive to bacteria, and nothing should be dragged or rubbed over this area that might have bacteria from the anus or dirt from fingers or hands. Lubricants with scents or heating effects can cause urinary tract or yeast infections. Any chemical that comes into contact with this area can cause burning, discomfort, and infection.

The **frenulum** of the clitoris is the skin that attaches it to the body. Like a penis, the clitoris becomes erect when it is aroused. There is a "hood" or **prepuce** over the clitoris, which is skin that covers and hugs the clitoris and pulls back as the clitoris becomes erect. When erect, the clitoris is very sensitive and cannot normally be rubbed directly.

Like the penis for men, the clitoris is the center of sexual arousal for women. It has the highest concentration of nerve endings in the body, and is the seat of pleasure on a woman's body. Stimulating the clitoris is the secret to pleasing a woman and giving her an orgasm.

The clitoris extends upward and to the back, before splitting into two parts called the **crura**, or clitoral *roots*. It can extend its shaft up inside the body and can be as long as five inches internally. The roots extend around and into the interior of the labia. These two bundles of nerves and tissue can extend deep into the vaginal walls, or they can be connected closer to the surface of the labia. It is possible that the clitoris has its primary root or origin in the G-spot, which is anatomically behind the clitoris and located in the vagina.

The clitoral roots actually extend internally all the way down and around both sides of the vagina, into the perineum, and down to the anus. These roots can be stimulated and enhance sensations leading to orgasm.

The inner and outer sections of the clitoris, and its extensions or roots down around the vagina, make the clitoris similar in structure to the penis, with the clitoris mirroring the sensitive head of the male penis.

The G-Spot

Famed German gynecologist Ernst Grafenberg "found" the **G-spot** in 1950, and it was aptly named after him for his discovery. Grafenberg described this area as a possible "second internal clitoris." Many refuted the idea, questioning the existence of the G-spot at all. Others have claimed that it is the "back side" of the clitoris, while current research is trying to prove that the G-spot is probably home to the ultimate roots of the clitoris.

The G-spot is an area two inches inside the front wall of the vagina, behind the pubic bone. When stimulated through the vagina, the G-spot expands or swells upon arousal. The G-spot has a different texture than the rest of the vagina. It can feel smoother or rougher than the vaginal walls. It can also feel like a spongy area, and be anywhere from the size of a pea to the size of a half-dollar coin. The G-spot can be stimulated to create heightened levels of arousal and, for many women, vaginal orgasm.

One way to know that you have found the G-spot is when pressure on the area creates a pressure to urinate. The G-spot is located just above the bladder and can press on the urethra. If this feeling can be tolerated, the area will continue to respond and more intense pressure can be applied.

Stimulating the G-Spot

G-spot orgasm can be intense and actually trigger strong emotional responses, like crying. Doing G-spot massage and concentrating on this area should be done with respect and sensitivity, so that any and all feelings can become part of the experience.

The good news about G-spot orgasms is that women can have one before, during, or after a clitoral orgasm. Before women recover from a clitoral orgasm, stimulation to her G-spot can trigger another orgasm.

The good news about

G-spot orgasms is that women can have one before, during, or after a clitoral orgasm.

The stimulation can feel intense when a woman is already engorged and throbbing from the clitoral response. Women can have multiple orgasms in this way, or go up close to the point of orgasm and come back down again, riding the wave to the ultimate climax. This experience not only triggers strong emotions but can also induce an almost trancelike state, similar to meditation but more blissful.

G-spot orgasms can be explosive. Some women emit a vaginal fluid that can actually squirt out of the vagina at the time of orgasm. Some women will experience this female ejaculation during a G-spot orgasm. Female ejaculate is a clear fluid and is not urine. It is not created in the bladder, but emanates from the vaginal walls themselves.

A G-spot orgasm can take longer than a clitoral orgasm. Vaginal climax only happens when the clitoris is aroused simultaneously, either directly or indirectly. This can happen when the clitoris is stimulated by direct touching, by rubbing the clitoral roots in the labia and opening to the vagina, or by stimulating the clitoris through the G-spot.

The G-spot is engorged when it is aroused. It can't be found unless the woman is already turned on. Trying to rub or caress the G-spot before a woman is totally stimulated can sometimes cause discomfort or pain.

Vaginal and clitoral orgasms feel different. During a vaginal orgasm, there is a pushing down sensation in the vagina and cervix, and the contractions push out. Women might even push out their lover's penis or fingers! When women have a clitoral orgasm, there is a suction effect created by the contractions, and the pulsing of the muscles will squeeze from inside.

The partner stimulating the G-spot needs to know that this is a wonderful experience and should be honored. However, a vaginal orgasm is not always possible. Partners will need to use more pressure and time to stimulate the vagina or G-spot to orgasm, compared to the stimulation needed for a clitoral orgasm. For most women, stimulating the vagina alone is like stimulating only the scrotum on a man. It feels nice, but is not likely to get them off.

How to Stimulate the Clitoris

Because the clitoris is so sensitive, it must be approached with tenderness and sensitivity. Some women can tolerate stronger and deeper pressure as they become more aroused. A good rule of thumb for partners is to start by applying well-lubricated pressure in a circular motion around the clitoris.

When the clitoris is aroused it will become engorged, erect, and more visible. Just prior to orgasm it actually rises up so that it may look like it is disappearing back into the folds of skin above and around it. This is an indication that orgasm is approaching.

Using the clock exercise in chapter 7, partners should try sliding their fingers around the clitoris in a circle, starting at twelve o'clock. Determine where the clitoris is the most responsive.

Experiment with gentle light flicking or pulling, kissing or soft biting, squeezing and pinching as the clitoris becomes more and more stimulated. Working with your partner, communicate exactly what is happening in your body, and tell your partner what you are feeling.

Use this next exercise to teach both partners where your clitoris is most sensitive and responsive to stimulation.

EXERCISE
Clitoris Play

For this exercise (an extension of "Clitoral Clock"), you'll need a warm room, and a bed, couch, or pillows on which to lie. Women should lie back, open their legs to their partner to receive soft stimulation, and keep their eyes open to gaze at their lover. The sender should apply water-based lubrication to his or her fingers.

For the partner stimulating the clitoris, start with gentle strokes on the inside of the thighs. Move closer to the vulva, lightly stroking the outer labia. Using deeper strokes, begin massaging the labia, sliding your well-lubricated fingers over the

(continued on page 196)

(continued)

inner and outer labia and getting into the outer area or threshold of the vagina. This will stimulate the area and you may feel the labia swelling or becoming engorged. The vagina may become naturally wet and lubricated, or a finger can be used to smooth lubricant into the outer opening of the vagina.

Begin pinching the labia between the palms of your hands, using longer strokes to stretch toward and gently stroke the clitoris. Come back to the vagina and down to the anal area, stimulating the perineum and the whole vulva area. Move up again to the clitoris, creating a teasing and a buildup of sensation. Insert a finger into the vagina occasionally, using a "come hither" motion to swipe the G-spot area, and come back to the clitoris. Wind around the clitoris with your finger using the clock motion. Ask your partner to make a noise or use words to describe when you are hitting supersensitive spots that feel great.

For many women, touching the top-left quadrant of the clitoris feels great. Try it, moving your fingers in tighter and tighter circles around the clitoris, leaning your palm on the vaginal area or using your other hand to stimulate the G-spot area inside the vagina.

Continue the clitoral stimulation for at least ten to fifteen minutes. Try a windshield wiper movement with two fingers over the clitoris, waving them back and forth, as your other hand is inserting a finger into the vagina and stimulating the G-spot.

Know that each of you can move around and adjust if you are getting cramps or feel uncomfortable. But keep coming back to the clitoral area, watching for signs that she is ready to orgasm.

Ask her now to tell you exactly what to do to bring her to orgasm. Have her use words or put her hand on yours to show you the exact move that will bring her over the edge. As she is coming, keep up the stimulation, although move softly on or around the clitoris. Stimulation at this point will feel very intense and can be uncomfortable.

Stopping too soon and discontinuing can also feel disconcerting. Some women like pressure or a finger inside their vagina as they come down from their orgasmic plateau.

Orgasm

The word orgasm is from the Greek word "orga," which means explosion. This makes sense because orgasm can feel like an explosion of pleasure and bliss. It is not uncommon for women to cry during or after orgasm, as the experience liberates stress and withheld emotions.

Women can orgasm for as long as twenty seconds. The intensity of the orgasm can vary, depending on G-spot, vaginal or clitoral stimulation.

Interestingly, a study from the Netherlands found that the area of the brain that controlled fear and anxiety was switched off during orgasm. This may indicate that letting go and surrendering is the easiest way to bring yourself to orgasm. The result is that feelings of fear and anxiety decrease.

Each woman will have her own wealth of knowledge regarding her body and what she needs to orgasm. No matter what the studies say, each woman is her own orgasm expert, the one who knows best what kind of stimulation and situations lead her to climax.

Anatomy 101: Male Genitalia

The **penis** is a highly sensitive area, with several parts—the **shaft**, the **glans** (or **head**), and the **scrotum**.

The glans of the penis is the most sensitive area, with the ridge surrounding the helmet shape being the most sensitive. The urethra is the opening at the head of the penis, and men can urinate when soft or erect. Men do not urinate and ejaculate at the same time.

The shaft is rigid during erection and soft when not erect. An uncircumcised penis has skin that reaches up and over the head of the penis. When the penis is erect, the foreskin, or skin covering the head, pulls back and the head is exposed.

The foreskin is removed at the time of circumcision. Both circumcised and uncircumcised penises are stimulated in the same way.

The scrotum is a soft, sensitive sack that holds the testicles. The scrotum has many nerve endings that can feel very pleasurable when stimulated. The testicles are kept warm and fertile in this sack, allowing an environment for sperm to thrive.

Men become erect during stimulation, and also involuntarily at times during REM sleep. Most stimulation feels good on a man's penis, and yet communicating about what feels the best can lead to a more positive experience for couples.

Try the following exercise as a way of finding out what kind of stimulation works best on your partner's penis.

EXERCISE
The Penis as a Work of Art

Take at least forty-five minutes for this exercise. Find a quiet, comfortable place where you will not be interrupted. For this exercise you will need markers (water-based) or different colored foods.

Men should take washable, water-based markers—scented ones are fine, too—and choose colors that represent sensation. You'll use these colors on your penis to show your partner which areas are the most sensitive to touch. For example, red can indicate the most sensitive area, green can show areas that feel good when touched, and yellow might show areas where you are the least sensitive.

Stimulate your penis to erection, using masturbation or your partner's manual manipulation. Using lubricant or saliva at this point will make it difficult to see the markers and decrease their efficacy. You will color small areas, about half an inch, directly on your penis.

Use different colors to show your partner the areas that feel the most sensitive and where you want to be touched. Do this exercise with your partner, drawing on these areas while your partner watches, or have your partner draw with the markers where you indicate.

Notice the beautiful work of art you both have created as your penis becomes a canvas of pleasure. If you have scented or flavored markers, your partner can lick off the colors, starting with the least sensitive areas and moving to the red hot zones. You can use food for this exercise as well, such as chocolate or strawberry sauce, whipped cream, or jelly.

Note: Make sure you wash off the marker before penetration to prevent possible infection.

The Prostate and Ancestors of Anal Beads

The prostate is a gland located internally in men. The prostate gland or "P-spot" is above the perineum and inside the anal wall. This area has as many nerve endings as the woman's G-spot and is many times equivalent in sensitivity.

The prostate secretes fluid into semen prior to ejaculation and controls the mobility of sperm. This fluid helps the sperm swim up the vagina and into the cervix, and keeps them viable long enough to connect with the egg in a woman's uterus. As men age or if there is prostate dysfunction, this fluid can decrease, and ejaculate amounts will also decrease. This does not influence the amount of sperm, but it can reduce their life span.

The prostate, when stimulated, enhances pleasure for men and can cause orgasm and ejaculation. Seventeenth-century sailors discovered this secret from the courtesans and prostitutes on the Orient shores where they landed. Sailors would request the ships that made runs to the Orient, because they knew that these women could stimulate them to ejaculation quickly and get them back on the ships before they left port.

These women developed a technique where they tied knots in silk scarves and inserted the scarf into a sailor's anus, then pulled it out slowly, stimulating their prostate. During orgasm, the knots would pull past their prostate and out of their anal sphincter muscles, creating intense waves of orgasmic pleasure. These scarves are the ancestors of plastic anal beads available today in sex toy stores and catalogs. The toys serve the same purpose, to stimulate the prostate as well as the anus itself.

The prostate has as many
nerve endings as the woman's G-spot
and is many times equivalent in sensitivity.

There are two ways to stimulate the prostate. One is to insert a well-lubricated finger into the anus and reach up about two inches, feeling for a round ball approximately the size of a golf ball. The prostate can be smaller or larger, depending on health and heredity.

Before inserting a finger into the anus, make sure you have lots of water-based lubricant on your finger and around the anal area. Go slowly, and only with permission.

Some men are hesitant about letting themselves feel the powerful sensations of prostate pleasure if they equate anal pleasure with homosexuality. Some men have shame and embarrassment about anal stimulation, although most men, if it is done correctly, will enjoy the sensations.

The second way to stimulate the prostate is through prostate massage. Because the prostate sits on the perineum, the area between the scrotum and the anus, outer massage can be done without going through the anus. Using lubricant, so the skin will not become irritated, massage with firm pressure. You may feel the shape of the prostate and you can massage to the depth that feels comfortable. With the right stimulation, this can be a very pleasurable experience for a man. Try this next exercise to stimulate the prostate.

EXERCISE
Prostate Massage

For this exercise you need at least sixty minutes of uninterrupted, safe time together. Make sure you will not have distractions or worries about children or responsibilities at this time.

Create a setting that reflects the mood you would like to have for this exercise. Soft rock, jazz, or classical music can be played in the background. Lower the lights, but not enough so you can't see one another.

Step One

Have the male partner lie on his back, knees bent. Ask him whether you may put your finger in the opening of his anus. Insert a well-lubricated finger into his anus and slide your finger slowly inside, feeling for the round shape of the prostate about two inches inside. Move your fingers in a "come hither" motion along the wall of the rectum that faces the front of his body.

Step Two

Stimulate his penis by rubbing it with your other hand, which should also be well lubricated, up and down, paying special attention to the head. As you slowly maneuver your finger deeper into his anus, if so, continue the "come hither" motion. Use your finger to gently massage the prostate.

Step Three

Ask him whether these motions feel good. Try several different strokes and pressures, asking him which feels better. Try squeezing his scrotum gently. Give him choices, such as "does this feel better, or this?"

Step Four

Put his penis in your mouth and keep massaging his prostate with your finger. Ask him to tell you when he is ready to come. Have him take a deep breath when you feel he is getting ready. If his penis is making jerking motions up toward his body or if he swells to a hard erection, he is getting ready to climax. Tell him to bear down on your finger, pushing your finger out of his anus. The combination of sensations will drive him crazy with pleasure.

Sexual Massage for Him and Her

All kinds of massage can be used to relax and awaken erotic feelings. The beginning of reexperiencing positive and generous touching can start with back rubs and body massage and move to massage of specific sexual parts.

These next three exercises will show you how to massage, stimulate, and pleasure your partner. These are direct contact exercises, where you will need lots of privacy and water-based lubricant. Make sure the room is warm and lit with candles or other soft light. You want adequate time to focus on pleasing your partner and uninterrupted space to feel relaxed and fully present for these erotic encounters.

For Her: Labia Massage

Using lots of water-based lubricant, explore your partner's labia, both the inner and outer lips, using different techniques and strokes.

Put your palms together and slide the vulva between your hands. Smooth the vulva down and then back up with the palm of your hand. Using your fingertips, gently push into the area, massaging each side separately. Massage with your fingers slowly from the crease in the leg to the vagina, and go back out again. Combine labia massage strokes with strokes over and around the clitoris, vagina, and anus. Be careful to keep any fingers that touch the anus away from the rest of the vulva.

Massage the clitoris and vaginal area to orgasm, or just use this massage experience as a way to give and receive pleasure and sensation. Massage can be a wonderful way to connect with your partner, and it does not need to lead to the "finish line." Sometimes pleasuring each other can be the goal.

EXERCISE
For Him: Scrotum Licking

For men, scrotum licking can be an intense experience that brings joy and pleasure.

Using your tongue, bathe the scrotum in saliva, tasting each area of the scrotum from the inner leg to the perineum and back to the base of the penis. Play with the sack and testicles inside of it gently. Take one testicle in your mouth at a time and suck it gently, lubricating it with your saliva and your tongue. Lick all around the scrotum and then slide to the penis with your mouth.

Now using lubricant, massage the whole area from the base of the penis to the perineum. Make sure that you use a firm grip, at times gently pulling or rolling the scrotum sack. Never yank or pull too hard.

EXERCISE
For Both: Perineum Massage

The perineum is the area from the vagina to the anus on women and the area from the scrotum to the anus on men. These areas can be massaged and bring prostate stimulation to men and possibly some clitoral stimulation for women.

Start with lots of lubricant and experiment with different pressures, from a light scratch or tickle with your fingertips to harder movements and strokes. Try rubbing and pressing with your palm, and ask your partner what he or she would like more of.

This can be a wonderful way to connect your partner to his or her root, the base of the perineum, where there is a lot of power and energy. That energy can be drawn up into the genitals, the belly, and the heart. In the next chapter we will talk more about sex and spirituality and how to combine the anatomical moves with breathing and meditation.

Women's Struggle with Body Image

For women, sex with a passionate partner can be the beginning of waking up and reexperiencing being totally present in the body. As women become more open about their need for sex, they may be faced with feelings about their own bodies.

Most women today are concerned with their appearance and worry about how they look naked. Only 5 percent of women fit the standard ideal for models in this country—the average woman is 140 pounds, 5'4", and a size 14. The modeling industry is made up of women whose average height is 5'10" and an average weight of 107 pounds. Feeling the pressure of our culture, our media, and the fashion industry, women find it difficult accepting and loving the body they are in.

There are new standards in the fashion industry, particularly in Spain and other parts of Europe, where models are required to have a healthy percentage of body fat on their frames before they can become fashion models. As these standards trigger change all over the world, women may feel less pressure to conform to an unrealistic standard.

The pressure to stay youthful in our society also makes women feel anxious to be in top physical shape and to fight aging through liposuction, Botox injections, and plastic surgery.

Most women polled say that if they felt more comfortable in their bodies they would have sex more often. Women can learn from this, by pushing their edge and trying to have sex even when they feel uncomfortable about their physical selves. (Notice how you feel after a wonderful lovemaking session. Are you less insecure about your body parts?)

Working on body image is an important part of a relationship, because being physically confident helps you bring your whole self to the relationship. Performing the following exercise when you have negative thoughts about your self-image can help you feel more accepting of your body.

EXERCISE
Accepting Your Body

Look in the mirror and repeat this affirmation ten times a day for two weeks: "I love and accept myself exactly as I am." You may notice that when you have a negative body thought, this phrase begins to come up instead. And over time you may actually come to believe it.

Every time a negative thought or self-doubt comes up, repeat the affirmation until it drives out the negative thought from your mind. Every time you have a less than complimentary thought about your looks, repeat the affirmation to yourself. This exercise will help replace negative thoughts with self-acceptance.

It is only through acceptance that you will learn to love your body. Good sex means being totally present and open without the need to hide any part of yourself.

Men's Struggle with Body Image

The need for sex is normal and natural for women and is important for body image recovery as well as healthy eating patterns. Many men have body image issues as well.

While women worry that they are not small enough, sometimes men feel insecure about not being big enough. Men feel pressure to appear muscular, particularly as they get older. As they lose their hair or gain weight around their waists, men can have a negative body image as well.

Men worry about how their bodies compare to those of other men. They have fears about whether or not they can satisfy their female partners. Mostly, they worry about their penis size. When men are asked what they would most like to change about their bodies, they say "hair, stomach, and a larger penis."

For men, having sex makes them more comfortable in their bodies. When men feel that their partner loves and appreciates their penis, it helps them to relax in their sexuality. Comparing their penis size to actors in porn movies makes men feel insecure. Male genitals in pornography are many times larger than the average-sized penis. Men can feel competitive over the size of their penis, and they need to know that their size and shape are perfect for you.

Letting your partner know the things you really like about his body can help. Praise him for the way he moves in his skin, for the way he uses his hands, for how good his hard chest feels against your soft body. Use your auditory skills to tell him how much you love his penis.

A way for both men and women to become more comfortable and appreciate their bodies in all their wonders is to learn how the body responds in its skin. Discovering what feels good sensually helps you value your body and feel connected to its sensual desires. The following exercise will help you begin to appreciate that your body is not just a clothing size or a number on the scale, but is a receptor for sensual delights.

EXERCISE
Getting in Touch with the Sensual World

Create sensuality for your body and your senses by trying some of these exercises:

- Wear soft clothes that feel sensual against your skin.
- Use soft sheets with a higher thread count and blankets that have a sensual touch, as well as soft pillows and comforters on your bed.
- Place soft throw pillows and blankets around you in your home.
- Light scented candles and add fresh flowers to your bedroom.
- Take a hot soapy bath with fragrant bath soaps and salts.
- Start massaging you body with scented lotions and creams.
- Add a manicure and pedicure to your weekly routine (men can get manicures and pedicures with a nail buff instead of polish).
- Brush your hair 100 times, just to feel the sensation on your scalp.
- Get a massage using scented and slippery massage oils.
- Try appreciating all of your physical sensual self.

A Lifetime of Passion

When you "wake up" a relationship and allow each partner to be present to the gifts of each other's fantasy life, you create a stronger, more committed partnership. To have this long-term passion, there needs to be healthy communication about sexual needs, including a way to deal with anger and resentment, such as channeling it into the sexual relationship.

Anger can be dysfunctional when it interferes with healthy sexuality. But it can also be channeled into a passionate sex life.

If there is anger in a relationship, there is energy. It means that the relationship is alive and awake. In a partnership, being "awake" includes a mutual sexual appreciation of each other, where you both feel seen and desired. When signs of "drowsiness" appear, the sexual energy in a relationship can be awakened using Imago therapy techniques.

In our society we like to say, "Never go to bed angry." The problem is that if we can't bring our anger into the bedroom in a constructive way, we put off a chance for two loving partners to resolve conflict.

Channeling resentment into your sexual relationship can be scary, but it solves several dilemmas. One, it allows relief from the stress of the conflict and it helps us trust that our partners are being honest about their feelings. If we can be connected to our partners even when they are angry, then there is less fear that anger will cause a permanent disconnection. If we withdraw from our partners when we are angry, we never resolve the problem, and we grow farther and farther apart.

Knowing that anger is okay takes some of the pressure off of the partnership. It is unrealistic to think that you will never be angry at your partner. Understanding what to do about anger and how to work through it is a way to build a permanent connection.

Being honest about your anger and expressing it in healthy, nonviolent ways can help you connect with your partner. (Note: Anger is healthy but violence is not. Make sure you get help if you are experiencing a violent relationship, either as the one inflicting violence or the one receiving it.)

Chemical Romance

When we are angry, we get a surge of the brain chemical adrenalin, which signals conflict to our bodies. But we don't have to wait until we work through our conflict to engage in sex. Other brain chemicals like oxytocin, dopamine, and serotonin are all released when we have sex, which makes us feel calmer and more attached to our partner.

When we first meet, we are attracted to a potential partner because of the serotonin levels that are triggered in our system. We feel a rush of good feelings and some obsessiveness, too. That is why we think about our new love all of the time. Longer-term attraction is created by higher levels of oxytocin, the feel-good chemical that is released after sex.

If the initial physical "serotonin attraction" wears off, it would seem you need more oxytocin in the relationship, which leads to long-term satisfaction. And because oxytocin is released in the body during and after sex, wouldn't it make sense that the more sex you have the more attracted to your partner you are for longer periods of time?

The more sex you have, the more of these "love hormones" you release. When you stop having sex, your body naturally lowers its estrogen and testosterone levels. So, having sex makes you want more sex. Sex is the ultimate aphrodisiac.

Maximizing versus Minimizing Anger

Without safety in a relationship there can be no true intimacy, either physical or emotional. Yet, stuffing your anger does not help your partner feel safe. Anger has a way of coming out sideways when we don't express it directly.

Passive-aggressive anger is resentment that is not direct, but is acted out in more subtle ways, such as coming home late, ignoring our partner, or withholding sex as a punishment. Withholding sex as a way to express resentment can be toxic to a good partnership.

This doesn't mean we shouldn't get angry—anger is a normal and natural response to frustration. What we do with our anger is the important issue. Most of us have conflict in our relationship at some time. When there is conflict, we react by **maximizing** or **minimizing** it. "Maximizers" have a tendency to create drama when they don't feel heard. This is their way of testing the bond of the partnership. They blow things out of proportion and dramatize their feelings. This can be a sign that what the maximizer is really craving is safety, not an argument! Maximizers test the walls of the box to make sure they are strong.

"Minimizers," on the other hand, are people who avoid conflict. They would rather withdraw from the problem and spend time alone to figure out an answer. They retreat into their emotional cave, fleeing the conflict or danger.

When a maximizer's partner retreats, the maximizer feels abandoned and pursues the minimizer, forcing this person deeper and farther into the cave. The more the maximizer pursues the minimizer, the more the minimizer persists in his or her pattern of responding—the fight escalates and both partners feel misunderstood.

Changing this pattern of defensive responses in your relationship can go a long way toward resolving conflict. For example, the best thing to do for minimizers is to give them space. For maximizers, this might be very difficult. If they can give minimizing partners a little time to process the conflict, they will come out on their own when they feel safe.

A minimizer can help a maximizer feel safe by staying present for the conflict for a little while longer than feels comfortable. Minimizers might want to retreat and hide out until the conflict passes, but if they can try something different and stay present for just a few extra moments, they can begin to change the pattern.

Responding to a Maximizer and a Minimizer

Learning how to have a "dialogue" instead of a conversation can go a long way toward helping maximizers feel safe. A dialogue helps maximizers feel that they are being heard. The maximizer feels dismissed when the minimizer says things like, "Why are we fighting over this? It's no big deal." A maximizer will react by saying things like, "You don't care how I feel."

How we respond is important. Instead of retreating during an argument, let the maximizer know, "Look, I am here, everything is good, you are safe. I can handle this. I am not going anywhere." This reassuring language can make a potential flare-up fizzle out.

When minimizers are angry they may withdraw, becoming uncommunicative and silently resentful. They don't want to be pursued and usually don't want to talk about the conflict. Minimizers aren't sure how to express their anger in healthy ways and many times would rather avoid it altogether. As stated above, giving minimizers space and time can help them gather their thoughts. And then it is important to let them know that anger can be talked about and that it is safe to come out of the cave!

We all act as minimizers and maximizers, depending on the issue, and this happens in all relationships. How we recognize this and respond to it is more important than trying to stop it. Try the next exercise as a way to step out of old fighting patterns.

EXERCISE

Containing Your Reactivity

Consider how you react when you are angry at your partner. What do you want to do? Walk away? Fight? Hide?

Whatever your reactivity is, your behavior when you are upset or angry at your partner is the behavior that scares him or her the most. It's hard to keep our reactive behavior in check. When we are scared or hurt we go into reactive, defensive behavior. Many times this looks like anger.

If you are a maximizer, you may find it challenging to hold back your reactivity, especially when you are angry. Minimizers may find it difficult to stay fully present when they feel anger.

Decide where your growth edge lies. Your growth edge is the area where you need to change your behavior. Knowing how you need to change and actually making those changes is how you grow. If you are unsure where your growth edge is, check with your partner. He or she usually knows where your growth lies.

Challenging your personal growth edge means pushing yourself into a new behavior, a new way of reacting when your partner gets angry. This may feel uncomfortable at first, especially in the middle of feeling the anger.

For this exercise, you will need to practice it when you are in a conflict. Next time you feel your reactive behavior kick in during a conflict, use a container exercise. This means pushing your edge of comfort, and staying uncomfortable for a few more moments than is normal for you. For instance, if your reactive behavior is to walk away during a conflict, engage your partner, talk, touch, and contain your feelings for one or more moments longer than you feel comfortable. Then walk away if you have to.

Do the same thing if you typically argue when you are angry—breathe, hold the feeling, talk, touch, and contain.

Each time you do this exercise you will be growing out of your usual behavior pattern. This will reassure your partner—and yourself—that the cycle of resentment and anger can change.

How Understanding Differences Can Lead to Trust

As discussed earlier, we all have both male and female "energy," which is simply a way to describe how men have what are considered female qualities and women have what are perceived as male qualities.

Male energy is very directed. Male energy wants to get to the next destination; it wants to reach the final climax, whether in bed, in an argument, or in a career. Male energy is what gets us to the next level. These traits are a great way to get things done, but they can sometimes be perceived as insensitive to feelings.

Women want men to take charge.
This makes women feel safe. This, however, does not mean women want to be controlled.

Feminine energy is "in the moment." Sometimes female energy is experienced as a force that digs in and will not let go. Female energy is in the present and experiences all of the senses. Female energy is the sensual and creative force behind our relationships.

Male energy wants to solve problems; female energy wants to experience the emotions until there is a relief of tension. This can lead to stress between partners, misunderstandings, and anger. If a woman is upset, she will want to talk about it until the energy is spent. If a man is upset, he will devise a way to "fix" the problem. For men, listening to women talk endlessly about their feelings can be frustrating. If a woman continues to talk about the problem after the man has offered his advice, he may become resentful, feeling like she did not appreciate the solution he came up with for her. A woman will experience this as a shutdown of her feelings. She will resent his trying to "fix" her and feel like he is not listening to her when she wants to talk. Understanding these differences can lead to greater trust and less need to act out anger and resentment.

For example, one of the sexiest things a male partner can do is to be directive. Women want men to take charge. This makes women feel safe. This does not mean women want to be controlled, and it is important for anyone in a relationship to feel he or she has a voice. But there is something about a man taking charge in bed that appeals to feminine sexuality. Many couples are intrigued by the capacity to channel their anger and resentment into sexuality in a healthy way.

On the other hand, couples who build resentment between them have a tendency to withdraw from each other, and move farther apart. What if that resentment could be verbalized, perhaps through a healthy dialogue, and then channeled into a strong and passionate sex life? What if, instead of withdrawing into our cave, we could integrate it into our sexual partnerships? What would that look like?

Think about the romantic paperback novels where the man throws the woman on the bed and they make mad, passionate love. There is sometimes a sexiness that comes from having sex that is a little "rougher." Not all women can play this game. They need to feel comfortable and secure before lovemaking, but if they can surrender to the passion and the power, the sex can be even better than "make up" sex. It can be "work through it before the argument" sex!

Surrendering to the Moment— and to Our Partner

The more we trust our partners and let them in, the more confident they will feel. The more we can surrender, or let go, the more our partners can please us. Receiving love in the form of sensual pleasure can be more of a challenge than giving love and sensual pleasure. We need the safety of healthy boundaries to surrender to the moment. If we trust that anger can be managed and worked through, then this will allow us to relax and receive.

One way to redirect the angry energy is to reawaken the inner adult. The inner adult is different from the inner child. We all have an inner child—a youngster that lives in us from our childhood. Don't we all act like six-year-olds in our relationships sometimes?

We tend to behave at our lowest possible functional level at home and with those we love and feel safest with. Remember having a good day at school, and then getting off the bus and acting cranky with Mom? You were tired and stressed, and when you were home with loved ones you could express your frustration. We sometimes act like six-year-olds as adults, too.

Recognize in an argument that you don't want to be six years old. You want to be an adult. You want to recognize that when you feel like your inner six-year-old, it's because something is happening that reminds you of your childhood. Then tell your partner how you feel, using the Imago dialogue. It might sound like:

"When you say that to me it makes me feel X and that reminds me of when I was a kid and Y."

Partners should simply mirror back what you are saying, if they are able to. Or, if they are very angry, ask them whether they can validate your feelings for you.

One way to redirect the angry energy is to reawaken the inner adult.

Invite your adult self to the conflict. How does it want to act? Think about responding intentionally instead of being reactive to what your partner triggers in you.

For example, if we want to be our inner adult in our relationship, we need to communicate as an adult partner. Being direct and honest and not withholding feelings can all lead to a new connection. If you can't resolve all of your issues in one sitting, don't be afraid to go to bed! Your erotic life can help work out your issues for you, just like the couple in the following case.

Working Out Anger in Bed

Average husband closes his book and reaches over to turn off his bedside lamp. Typical wife rolls over away from him in her sleep, pulling all the covers onto her side of the bed. He lies awake on his back, feeling the distance between them. The resentment that has been between them for years has been creating distance and friction in the relationship.

He is afraid that if he wakes her up to have sex, she will be angry and complain about having to get up in the morning. This makes him feel like he is being criticized by one of his parents. He feels a moment of pain and frustration and tenses his body, not sure if he should roll over and give her the cold shoulder or wake her up to argue with her.

Typical wife, half asleep, feels the distance between them. She wonders whether he wants to make love. Part of her wishes he would just try; this would confirm for her that he still finds her attractive even though she has gained weight since the kids were born. She wants him to affirm his love and attraction for her, but she doesn't know how to ask for this. Sometimes she feels abandoned and alone.

Average husband waits and wonders whether she will pursue him. His low self-esteem has been triggered over and over through the lack of sexuality in their relationship. He wonders whether he can really honor his commitment to her and stay married. Why is it called "settling down" anyway? He doesn't feel like he settled for his wife. He knows he was attracted to her for a reason, and wants the relationship to stay erotic and connected.

Typical wife wonders whether her partner still finds her sexually attractive, since he hasn't initiated sex in a while. She used to have such great erotic energy, she thinks. She remembers every fantasy she has ever had, and she wonders about his.

The moment comes when they both take a deep breath, and decide to push their edge, just like in yoga class that morning when the instructor asked them to push through the discomfort of a pose just slightly, finding a new edge, without forcing. She tries to reach out her hand toward him to see if he will respond. He rolls toward her. They both breathe. They lie facing each other, and with eyes open, begin to focus on making eye contact. He reaches out and pulls her closer to him.

"I love you," he says.

"You love me?" she asks.

"Yes, I love you," he says.

"I love you, too," she says, "even though I am so angry at you all the time."

He responds, "So you love me even though you are angry at me all the time?"

"Yes," she says, smiling. They breathe together, slowing down their breath. He begins to stroke her back as he exhales, and she relaxes.

They are on their way to a new connection, and a new erotic and passionate partnership.

The Spiritual and the Physical

Spirituality and sex are intimately and irrevocably linked. Our bodies, minds, and souls unite during sex and connect us to the Divine in a way that no other spiritual work can. Most of the spiritual practices today focus on taking us out of our bodies and away from the physical. Other practices, such as yoga, psychotherapy, and bodywork (in our Westernized versions) eliminate the sexual connection and often skip over the sensual altogether. Incorporating sexuality into a spiritual practice helps us connect to each other and to the spirit of our partners through a deep appreciation of sexuality.

Energy is raised when there is arousal, the observation of time slows down, and sex goes in slow motion. The more aroused we are, the slower and more sensual the dance, and the more spiritually connected we feel.

This next exercise links the spiritual and the sensual so that you and your partner can feel connected on another level. Take your time, enjoy the moment, and appreciate the closeness.

EXERCISE

Spiritual and Sensual Closeness

For this exercise, you will need at least sixty minutes of uninterrupted time. Make sure the children are taken care of, the phone is off, and you have no obligations. Find a quiet, warm space where you and your partner can be together. Lie down facing one another. Find a comfortable position to be as close as possible to each other.

Step One

Breathe deeply into your lower abdomen and exhale longer than you inhale. Try to make your breath an exercise in letting go. Breathe deeply into your pubic area and the root of your spine. Try to match your breath with your partner's. Don't hold your breath. Relax all of your muscles. Gaze into your partner's left eye, the receptive eye. Use your mouth to exhale, making any noises that feel comfortable to express. Continue to breathe until you feel a rise of energy in your genital area.

Step Two

Rock gently back and forth in your pelvis and hips. Move together without penetration, feeling the experience mesh with your breath. See whether you can feel your partner at a different level as you gaze into his or her soul. Get a sense of who he or she is in spirit.

Step Three

Take turns saying something to each other that you would not normally think of. For example, what is it that you truly want from your partner? Perhaps you have never expressed this before. What is it you long for from him or her?

Have your partner mirror back what you ask. Take longer breaths, breathing into your genitals.

Step Four

Rock back and forth from your hips. When you both become aroused, shift into gentle massage. Stroke your partner on the exhalation only. Take turns. Slowly sweep your hands along your partner's back. Stop and inhale. Take your time. You can move to your partner's chest and eventually the genitals. Massage on the exhalation.

(continued)

Step Five

Use penetration to focus on your rhythm and exhale as you penetrate. Tighten and release your perineum muscles, then relax. Keep the gaze on each other's eyes.

If you feel that you are coming close to orgasm, stop and breathe and gaze into your partner's eyes. Focus on your perineum muscles, tightening and releasing.

Encourage your partner to breathe deeply into the abdomen if his or her breath gets shallow or rapid. Help your partner by slowing down your own breath and continuing eye contact. Do this "pause" several times as you come close to orgasm, pulling back and reconnecting with your partner.

Step Six

When and if you are ready to orgasm, see whether you can breathe deeply and push down while you come. Try to relax, breathing deeply, bearing down, and tightening only your perineum area. Relax into the orgasm. Stay in this position as you come down from orgasm, moving as little as possible and continuing to gaze into your partner's left eye.

Continue to breathe together. Keep eye contact, kiss, and stroke as you both come down.

If you want to, you can begin again.

Tolerating Joy

As is often the case, we become comfortable with our habits. The things we do, the words we say, and even the thoughts we entertain and invite into our minds are patterns that get stronger the more we practice them.

We always get more of what we focus on, whether it's positive or negative. For instance, if we are focused on what we don't like in our relationships, then we may notice that those things seem to increase. If we focus on what brings us joy in our relationship, we feel it more often. For some of us, joy can be almost uncomfortable when we have gotten used to being miserable. Sometimes the moments of true joy in our relationships can feel fleeting. Could it be that when we feel joy we push it away?

Joy is a state of mind and a state of spirit. If we are focused on the joy in our partnerships and learn to sit in that feeling for longer periods of time, we find that more joy comes in and stays around.

The journey toward having a more passionate partnership can be a joy-filled journey! Having a more passionate partnership begins by communicating your erotic needs. The increased sexual connection and passion that result can be used as a foundation to work through all issues in the relationship, creating safe mirroring and decreasing fear and anxiety for the future.

Focusing on the joy of the journey, rather than the final destination, means we can be fully present in our relationship.

EXERCISE
Positive Sexy Flooding

For this exercise, you will need uninterrupted quiet time together. Make sure the kids are taken care of. Set up the room with a romantic atmosphere. Turn the lights down low, light candles, and put out fresh flowers or incense.

The first step of the exercise will be writing down a list of all the things you appreciate about your partner sexually. The second part of the exercise will be taking turns flooding each other with these positive sexual statements. Receiving can be harder than giving. Let yourself be filled up when your partner floods you.

Step One
Find a comfortable place to make a list. Write down all of the things you love and appreciate about your partner sexually. This may include a list that describes how your partner makes you feel, how he or she looks, how your partner touches you, and so on. Anything else you appreciate about your partner sexually should go on this list. Use a few words to describe each appreciation.

Step Two
Decide who will be the sender and who will be the receiver. Receivers should sit in a chair in the center of the room. Senders should walk slowly around their partner, list in hand, and read everything they appreciate, whispering loudly enough in their partner's ear to be heard and leaning down to get as close as possible.

Senders should tell their partners specifically how they appreciate the things they do in bed and how they appreciate each part of their body. They should tell them the things they love to do to them and why, all the while whispering and walking around them. Flood them with sexual appreciation.

(continued)

Step Three

The sender's voice can be louder than a whisper now. Senders should notice how the receiver responds. Senders can say the appreciations in their most sexy voice, letting their partners know with their hands that they love to touch them. They should repeat the appreciations that cause the most reaction.

Step Four

Now switch. Senders become receivers and the new senders send over their list of sexual appreciations.

Step Five

When you are both done and feeling flooded with positive appreciation, move directly into lovemaking if you wish. Or you can take a few moments and share one thing you appreciated about this exercise with your partner. Make sure you mirror your appreciations now in this closing piece. You may feel overwhelmed with positive feelings. You may even feel joy. Allow yourself to have this moment of joy. Before you separate and break your connection with your partner by getting up and moving, let yourself experience the joy for a little longer than you can tolerate.

One of the greatest gifts we can bring to our relationship is to acknowledge the moments of joy, focusing on what it feels like to be truly connected and in our Eros energy. Our creative life force makes us feel passion. Passion makes us feel connected. Being connected brings joy.

In this next exercise, be with your partner in a moment of joy. Find the feelings that make you happy, content, and connected. Tolerate the joy for one more moment than you might normally experience. You deserve it, and so does your partner.

Our creative life force makes us feel passion. Passion makes us feel connected. Being connected brings joy.

Feel the Joy

Find some time where you can focus on your partnership and the passion that you crave. Make sure the kids are taken care of, the phone is turned off, and you have uninterrupted time to be together. Set up the room for romance and passion. Light candles, turn off the lights, spread rose petals on the bed, and use pillows and blankets that feel sensual on your body. Have lubricant and massage oil handy.

Prepare yourself by taking a warm bath or a hot shower. Shave, moisturize, and take the time to get ready for lovemaking with your partner. Put on sexy lingerie or let yourself be comfortably naked. Anticipate the joy of connection with your partner.

Step One

Make love to an orgasm. You might use one or more of the methods discussed in this book. Take your time. Don't rush to the finish line. Appreciate the journey of getting there together. Let yourself experience with all of your senses what it feels like to be in the moment, making love with your partner.

Step Two

After making love and experiencing an orgasm, kiss your partner but do not speak. Lie together and do not move your body. Let yourself feel the energy that has been created by your lovemaking. Feel the stillness in the room and around you. Let yourself feel the air on your skin. Feel the joy that comes with orgasm and pleasure.

Try to remain still, maintaining the connection with your partner. Touch your partner, but let yourself be still. Appreciate the feeling that spreads out from your genitals to the tips of your fingers and toes. Feel the energy circulate throughout your internal system. Feel the joyful energy of touching another person, physically and spiritually. Feel the joy of being totally in your body and yet out of it at the same time. Notice how far your energy radiates around your body.

Step Three

With your eyes closed, visualize the joy-filled energy as it dissipates, floating into the air around you. Let go of the energy; do not try to hold on to it. Feel the power of the journey.

Step Four

When you are completely back to earth, embrace your partner and settle in for sleep or feel the energy created that will allow you both to move back into the world, energized, alive, and living your most passionate partnership!

ACKNOWLEDGMENTS

I would like to thank my children, Tyler and Emma, for their tireless patience and for being such great people. Thanks to my sister Melanie Barnum for her support. And thanks to Will Kiester at Fair Winds Press, for believing in the potential of this book, and to Cara Connors, for gently guiding my thoughts. Thanks to all my Imago teachers, including Harville Hendrix, Jette Simon, and all of my colleagues and friends who have been there for me and encouraged me to write the book.

Special thanks to all of the couples who have come to me for help and taught me so much. You know who you are.

And thanks, Mom, I feel you smiling down on me.

ABOUT THE AUTHOR

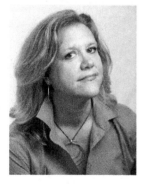

Tammy Nelson, Ph.D., is a licensed psychotherapist and world-renowned expert in sexuality and relationships, with over twenty-five years of experience working with individuals and couples. She is a Certified Imago Therapist, a board certified sexologist, and an international speaker.

She has been a featured expert in *Glamour, Cosmopolitan, Redbook, MSNBC, Healthy Life Magazine, Shape, Men's Health, Women's Health, Men's Health UK, Twist Magazine,* and as a source in *Time* magazine. She writes for the *Huffington Post* and YourTango.com; is the founder of the Institute for Sexuality and Human Development; and trains professionals in the field of psychotherapy, sexuality, and human development worldwide. Tammy gives workshops and intensives for couples, and trains psychotherapists around the world on global relational change.

To connect with Dr. Tammy Nelson or find more info, go to www.drtammynelson.com.

The Yale Law School
Guide to Research in
American Legal History

JOHN B. NANN and MORRIS L. COHEN

Yale UNIVERSITY PRESS

New Haven and London

Published with support from the Lillian Goldman Law Library, Yale Law School.

Yale University Press books may be purchased in quantity for educational, business, or promotional use. For information, please e-mail sales.press@yale.edu (U.S. office) or sales@yaleup.co.uk (U.K. office).

Set in Minion type by IDS Infotech Limited
Printed in the United States of America.

Library of Congress Control Number: 2017956187
ISBN 978-0-300-11853-7 (paperback: alk. paper)

A catalogue record for this book is available from the British Library.

This paper meets the requirements of ANSI/NISO Z39.48–1992 (Permanence of Paper).

10 9 8 7 6 5 4 3 2 1

To Morris, an exemplary person and librarian

Contents

Acknowledgments

My colleagues at the Yale Law Library, especially Fred Shapiro, provided support throughout the process. My students in the Research Methods in American Legal History class over the years have made the class a joy, and they have all provided me with great opportunities to learn; that is our purpose. Morris Cohen deserves all of my thanks; it was an honor working and teaching with him: he truly is a librarian and a person to emulate. Bryn Williams provided great help as both a student and a Research Assistant. The professionals at Yale University Press have provided me with great support. Janet Blake, with kindness and great skill, tried to make my writing as active as possible. I hope that researchers in American legal history find this useful and that this work, in some small way, contributes to better history in the law. Most important, my wife, Marléna Soble, and daughters, Jordan and Micayla, who inspire me daily, have made this book possible through their support and assistance. Thank you.

The Yale Law School
Guide to Research in
American Legal History

Introduction

I am quite convinced that political societies are not what their laws make them, but what sentiments, beliefs, ideas, habits of the heart, and the spirit of the men who form them, prepare them to be, as well as what nature and education have made them.

—*Alexis de Tocqueville,* Selected Letters on Politics and Society

Historians and scholars often have to consult legal information, while attorneys often consult historical sources. Users of legal information must keep in mind that legal material is part of a specialized world that employs its own language and norms. The world of law and legal information is not static; the materials, language, and norms that serve a researcher today may be inadequate when applied to the law of the past. For example, terms used to describe the employment relationship in 1820 differ from the terms used today.

Terminology also differs between the research worlds of the historian and attorney. To an attorney, a "primary source" is or was the law. Any regulation or statute that has the effect of law is a primary source, whether or not that law is still in force, but a congressional report or proposed regulation is never a primary source. To a historian, contemporary material—whether a newspaper, letter, diary, restaurant menu, or flyer—is a primary source.

An attorney might conduct legal history research if the law at question in a legal dispute is very old: the U.S. Constitution and the Bill of Rights are well over two hundred years old. Even the most recent constitutional amendments were passed decades ago. Many statutes, rules, and regulations that remain law are also quite old. One of the most important theories of legal interpretation, originalism, requires that the law be interpreted as it was originally intended. The "original" meaning can be found only through historical research.

The U.S. legal system is a common law system, which means that cases can make, interpret, and define the law. Even when statutory or regulatory law governs an issue, cases define the statute. A legal researcher must find all relevant cases from the past to determine how a statute or regulation will be applied in a particular case.

Historical research also comes into play when the question at issue is what the law was at a certain time in the past. Since ex post facto laws are unconstitutional, people are held to adhere to the law in place at the time of their actions or when the cause of action arose. Whether certain behavior breaches a contract will generally be judged according to the law that existed when the behavior occurred.

Historical legal sources also serve other purposes. Since many important historical figures were lawyers, familiarity with legal material grounds the understanding of their work. For example, President William Howard Taft was also chief justice of the U.S. Supreme Court. The educator Horace Mann studied law at the Litchfield Law School. Researchers who want to understand these men will need to know the law that colored their views of the world.

Law plays an important part in the political and social history of the United States. For example, the history of women in the United States could be written through the various laws that affected women differently from men. The laws of coverture, inheritance, and citizenship all play a role above and beyond voting and equal rights. Researchers interested in almost every aspect of American life will have occasion to use legal materials.

Among the questions that lawyers using historical materials and historians using legal materials must consider are the following:

- What are the "proper" ways to use legal materials?
- How should they be used and who can and should best use them?
- Does a lawyer have sufficient historical background to understand the past?
- Does a historian have enough legal background to understand how the laws of the past would have looked and worked for members of the legal fraternity at the time?
- Is either group equipped to do this research? Are both?
- Is there a special sensitivity that a lawyer needs to bring to the examination of the past or that a historian needs to bring to legal materials?

The research necessary to answer these questions will be a blend of legal and historical research. Some of the insights and tools that modern legal researchers are familiar with will be useful, although the nature of the sources makes working with versions from long ago different. Not only will the sources be different, but researchers will also want to begin to develop a historian's relationship with the past. Similarly, as historians work through legal materials, they will find that the structure of the information is designed to aid in the law and the information may not make sense without first developing an understanding of why lawyers, judges, and legislators were making law as they were and why printers and publishers who supplied them created what they did.

Several classes of research guides may be helpful to someone new to legal history research. The first are current guides and textbooks designed to teach modern students how to conduct legal research. These are geared to current sources and techniques, but since much of the law from the past is still relevant today, these current tools and strategies should be a part of the legal history researcher's arsenal. A subcategory of this class is the specialized guide. While the list of guides below is necessarily incomplete, this problem is especially acute with specialized guides, for at least two reasons: there are many of these guides, and they can take a number of forms. It is our hope that the searching skills and catalog sources described in the next chapter will allow readers to locate specialized guides that we do not mention.

Another class of research guides is the guides and textbooks written for students and researchers in the past. A research text from the 1930s can be the best source to teach a researcher how to find the law from the 1930s. Another class is modern guides, collections, bibliographies, and checklists of historical resources.

State-specific research guides, which have been written for each state, deserve special mention. However, their quality and depth vary. Perhaps the best is William H. Manz's *Gibson's New York Legal Research Guide*. This extensive guide (the fourth edition is more than seven hundred pages long) provides researchers with in-depth information about the sources and process of research in New York State and New York City. It also covers current and historical research. A catalog search for legal research ("[state name]") will direct researchers to the guides for any particular state. *Prestatehood Legal Materials* contains brief guides to legal research for each state's law from before statehood.

From the standpoint of the historian, legal history is fragmented along many axes, some that are reflected in the sources and some that are more theoretical. In this book, we have elected to take an American realist view of the terrain. We include English material insofar as it *is* American, as the colonial material is, and we do not delve deeply into the legal past of any place much before it became part of the United States. As for the theoretical axes, we discuss the sources central to the creation and promulgation of law within the various governments in the United States. We briefly touch on some sources slightly beyond this core, but researchers interested in approaching the material from directions different from those a lawyer or traditional practiced legal researcher at the time may have taken will need to start with what we have here and expand their reading into the core materials of the direction chosen.

Almost every profession and area of scholarship has a language and a culture. In the United States, when attorneys write or speak, especially for each other, they make certain assumptions about language and culture. The further researchers proceed into the literature of an area, the more of the specialized language and culture they must understand. Rather than jumping into the language armed with a legal dictionary, as we discuss in chapter 11, researchers new to the law may be more comfortable spending time with an introductory legal research text geared toward novices. Such texts traditionally set the scene by describing some of the assumptions that are a part of the culture. They also introduce the most basic specialized language.

As we have seen, historians and attorneys have different definitions of the term "primary source." The remainder of this chapter describes how primary sources, as lawyers define the term, have been published or otherwise made available over time. It also describes the general classes of research tools that readers will encounter in the following chapters. However, before delving into the sources of law or the publication of law, researchers must understand context. In the law, the most important context is legal authority: what law is effective in a particular place and at a particular time, and what law prevails when laws conflict.

The U.S. Legal System and Legal Authority

This discussion of lawmaking and legal authority concentrates on the federal government, while noting that the structure of the federal government is substantially similar to the parallel systems of lawmaking in each state. The following description of the American legal system is necessarily overly simplified. For more details, see the books included at the end of this introduction or William N. Eskridge Jr., Philip P. Frickey, and Elizabeth Garrett's *Legislation and Statutory Interpretation* (2006) or Peter Hay's *The Law of the United States: An Introduction* (2017).

Government in the United States has changed over time; as researchers focus on a particular period, they will want to determine what the lawmaking bodies, especially the courts, looked like at that time. Since chronology roughly forms the organizing principle here, our discussion of important periods of change will also cover the resources that explain the structure of a government at a given time.

In the field of law, a primary source is the law, and three factors must be in place to make law. First, a body capable of making law must make a statement; second, that body must be acting according to the required methods; and, third, it must have the intent to make law. Lawmaking bodies work with or produce a lot of material that is not law. This additional material can be useful when interpreting the law, but unless the three factors are present, it is not the law.

A lawmaker's capability to make law can be limited in a number of ways. The Constitution empowers the federal government to make law in specified topical areas, with the remaining areas left to the states. Lawmakers are also limited geographically. In most cases a state's law is effective only in that state. An opinion by a state's supreme court on the meaning of a statute has the force of law only in that state or with regard to that statute.

Each method of lawmaking has a process associated with it. It may be straightforward or complex, but the process must be followed. A federal legislative law requires approval by both houses of Congress and signature by the president. A federal court opinion requires that a controversy exist between parties, that the court has personal and subject-matter jurisdiction over the controversy, and that the part of the opinion that constitutes the law is necessary to reach the opinion. Finally, the body must intend to make law.

In the United States, two constitutions may play a role in an event. The U.S. Constitution is the fundamental law for all Americans and all U.S. governments (although there are some complications relating to whether and how much the Bill of Rights may apply to the states); and each state also has its own constitution that controls the state government and may offer protections to people in the state.

In considering a hierarchy of law from the most powerful to the weakest or from the most difficult to change to the easiest, the Constitution sits at the top. No law made by any other lawmaking body may violate the Constitution. The next most powerful law is that made by Congress. In the United States the lawmaking power comes from the people, and Congress represents the people. Executive branch law, regulations, executive orders, and other items are the next level of law. They are closely related to statutes. The power that the executive has to make law comes from two sources: from the powers granted expressly by or implied in the Constitution, and from statutes. Congress often passes statutes to give agencies, either independent agencies or those that are a part of the executive branch, power to make law in a limited area. The Constitution also grants power to the president to make law as the commander in chief and also as the chief executive with the responsibility to ensure that the laws are faithfully carried out.

To make law, Congress must pass a statute, which might be referred to by a number of terms depending on the circumstances: laws, public laws, session laws, and so on. An identical bill must pass both houses of Congress, and the bill must be signed by the president. If the president vetoes, or "pocket vetoes," the law, the veto must be overridden. *The American Congress,* by Steven S. Smith, Jason M. Roberts, and Ryan J. Vander Wielen, presents a more complete description of congressional lawmaking.

The executive branch has made law since the nation's founding, though the early output was a trickle compared with the amount of today's lawmaking. Since the late nineteenth century, the executive branch has enjoyed expanded lawmaking privileges. Executive organs, whether agencies created by Congress or other bodies, have increasingly been allowed to promulgate rules and regulations, adjudicate disputes, and otherwise act as lawmaking bodies. While some of the executive's lawmaking power derives from the Constitution and therefore is limited only by the Constitution, a great deal of its lawmaking power derives from Congress, so its scope is dependent on Congress.

The judicial branch spends most of its time interpreting existing law, whether the Constitution, statutes, or rules and regulations. When no other law exists that will solve a dispute, the judiciary can make law; however, a later statute can supersede any judge-made law or interpretation. Although judge-made law is susceptible to invalidation by the act of one of the other branches of government, which might make judge-made law look weaker than the law from the other branches, remember that judges have the power of interpretation and can invalidate unconstitutional actions by the other branches. Cases decided by judges give life and meaning to the statutes and regulations flowing from the other branches.

Federal courts are open to two kinds of cases: those that deal with federal law, and those between citizens of different states as long as the requested damages are over a certain amount. If a suit does not meet either criteria, the litigants use state courts. If the litigants want, they can have issues of federal law decided in state courts. Therefore, it is common for a state court to interpret federal law and for a federal court to interpret state law. There are also many instances, whether by "choice of law" rules, or contract, or otherwise, in which a court will interpret the law of another state. This subject can quickly become very complex, and readers are directed to *Choice of Law* by Symeon C. Symeonides.

At present, federal courts and the courts in most states have three levels. There are trial courts of either limited or general jurisdiction. Most systems have courts that specialize in certain areas, such as small claims courts, land courts, or probate courts. All systems have a trial court of "general juris-diction," which is open to the cases not sent to the courts of limited jurisdiction. Above the trial courts, there is almost always an intermediate appellate court, and above the intermediate appellate court is a supreme court. In most instances, a party that loses at trial can bring complaints about trial court errors of law to the intermediate appellate court. Generally, appeals to a supreme court are by leave of the court: a request is made to the court, which it may grant or deny.

Attorneys use the term "case" to mean two very different things. It can refer to the entirety of a dispute between parties, including the filing, all of the pretrial work, the trial, and so on. In legal research, however, the word refers to the written opinion from an appellate court. This is important to an attorney because it is a statement of the law that can be used to show another court what the law is. Materials associated with cases of the first type are generally very difficult to locate and often require archival work. The written appellate decision is much easier to locate.

It is important to understand what these appellate opin-ions look like before discussing some of the issues related to the legal authority that certain courts' decisions have. When an appeal is made, the litigants can raise only issues of law. The appellate court cannot change the findings of fact; all it can examine is how the law was applied and interpreted at the trial. The appellants must raise all possible errors in their appeal. If they do not raise them, they are lost. The appellate court will get briefs and hear arguments, and then consider all of the alleged errors and make a decision. Often, the appellate court will give an opinion with no reasoning; the opinion could be as short as "affirmed." If the court does write an opinion, it will treat all of the significant issues raised. Therefore, most appellate opinions deal with several different areas of law.

The loser at the intermediate appellate court can usually petition the supreme court and ask it to hear the case. If the supreme court agrees, the litigants will submit briefs and offer oral arguments. If the supreme court hears a case, it will almost always make and deliver a reasoned decision. While court opinions of all types are increasingly available, only a small percentage of trial or even intermediate court opinions are reasoned written opinions.

Not all court opinions are equal. The opinion of a higher court can compel a lower court to decide a case in a certain way. In fact, when attorneys do legal research, they often seek cases that will compel the court to decide the case their way. Of course, the art of lawyering is persuading the court that such a case is more relevant than the opponent's case.

While state court systems are generally simpler than the federal system, the latter will serve here to describe judicial authority. The federal courts are divided into three levels, with one Supreme Court, thirteen appellate courts (first through eleventh circuits, the District of Columbia Circuit Court, and the Federal Circuit Court), and ninety-four federal judicial districts, each with at least one district and one bankruptcy court.

The Supreme Court's authority is nationwide. The numbered circuits each cover several states or territories. The District of Columbia Circuit Court acts like the numbered circuits; it is an appeals court of general jurisdiction that covers the District of Columbia. The Court of Appeals for the Federal Circuit, on the other hand, is a limited jurisdiction court of appeals: it hears patent and other specialized appeals. The district courts have jurisdiction over a state or a part of a state. Each state has at least one federal judicial district.

The decisions of the U.S. Supreme Court act as mandatory authority on all courts that fall below it. The Supreme Court is not the final arbiter of a state constitution or a state law, except when considering whether either violates the U.S. Constitution. However, since the Supreme Court can decide which cases to hear, it hears cases in its area of authority. When the Supreme Court has not decided on an issue, the court of appeals can interpret the law. The court of appeals decisions about U.S. constitutional issues and federal statutes are mandatory authority on the district courts within its circuit. However, when the courts of appeal from different circuits disagree about a law, a court's opinion will have the force of law only in its geographical region. For example, the Court of Appeals for the Second Circuit is the intermediate federal court that covers Connecticut (and other states, including New York). A decision from this court is the law in Connecticut. Massachusetts is in the First Circuit, so the law there may be different. Decisions from courts above the court in question and from the same path of appeal must be followed; however, convincing and well-reasoned decisions, no matter where they are from, can be used in an argument. Court decisions that are not considered mandatory authority are said to have persuasive authority. Thus, a case from another state interpreting a similar law, or from another circuit interpreting the same law, would be considered persuasive by a court. The court decides how persuasive a case is; it is not compelled to follow a persuasive case. A similar situation occurs when a court is confronted by one of its own opinions. A court has the power to reverse itself, but this power is circumscribed by the doctrine of stare decisis, which holds that a court should reverse itself only when there is compelling reason to do so. The theory is that people expect the law to remain constant and only change through legislation, by constitutional revision or amendment, or under dire circumstances.

Interpretation of Law and Originalism

One of the main jobs of a court is to interpret law that was written in the past, often far in the past. When conducting legal research, researchers also try to interpret the law and will use a variety of tools and doctrines to try to determine what the law means or what a court may decide that it means.

There are established doctrines of interpretation that should serve as the starting point for any work in this area. Two good places to start are William Eskridge's recent treatise *Interpreting Law: A Primer on How to Read Statutes and the Constitution* and Lief Carter and Thomas Burke's *Reason in Law*. A search of a library catalog or the online union catalog WorldCat using the subject heading "law United States interpretation and construction" will result in books and other materials about the interpretation of law generally. A more focused set of results can be found by adding terms to the search that describe the type of law, such as "statutory," or the type of interpretation, such as "originalism." Presently, since originalism is a relatively new term in the law and has one primary meaning, a search for the word originalism alone can be useful.

A special case of interpretation is constitutional originalism, an interpretive doctrine that has developed since the late twentieth century. Initially, constitutional originalism assumed that the interpretation of the Constitution must adhere to the original intentions and understandings of the drafters and therefore focused on using conventional historical methods to determine what the framers thought when drafting or ratifying the Constitution or its amendments. The method of constitutional originalism changed, however, after criticism pointed out that determining the distilled intent of many people is difficult and after the historical method exercised by lawyers was criticized (see Jack N. Rakove and Edwin Meese, *Interpreting the Constitution: The Debate over Original Intent*). More recently, the method has moved from a historical examination of the context of the law to the development of an understanding of what the words used in the law would have meant to ordinary readers at the time of enactment. For more, see Lawrence Solum, "What Is Originalism? The Evolution of Contemporary Originalist Theory," in Grant Huscroft and Bradley W. Miller, eds., *The Challenge of Originalism: Theories of Constitutional Interpretation*. Also see the materials mentioned at the end of this chapter under "Originalism" and materials indexed in Legal Source (see chapter 6) under the descriptor "Originalism (Constitutional Interpretation)" and materials cataloged in WorldCat or other catalogs (see chapter 1 for more information about catalogs and catalog searching and consider searching a catalog under the subject "Constitutional Law United States Interpretation and Construction" or under the keyword "Originalism.")

The early methods used by constitutional originalists required that researchers develop an understanding of the context and intent of the historical actors, while the current form of constitutional originalism requires that researchers examine the definitions of terms at the time of enactment. The current form can be accomplished with the dictionaries and other legal literature mentioned in the following chapters.

The doctrine of originalism and its development have generated a significant literature. Two books that offer a good starting point are Jack M. Balkin, *Living Originalism,* and Antonin Scalia and Bryan A. Garner, *Reading Law.* Two historical takes on originalism are Jack N. Rakove, *Original Meanings: Politics and Ideas in the Making of the Constitution,* and Edward A. Purcell, *Originalism, Federalism, and the American Constitutional Enterprise: A Historical Inquiry.*

The tools necessary for undertaking an originalist's reading of the law are described elsewhere in this volume. When trying to determine meaning at the time a law was made, researchers will, of course, use contemporary dictionaries and dictionaries like the *Oxford English Dictionary* that track the development of and change in the use and meaning of words. Researchers will also consult contemporary literature that will provide insight into the context of the making of the law and into how the terminology that appears in the law was used in the wider legal and popular conversation at the time. Monographs, justice of the peace manuals, news and periodical articles, cases, statutes, reports, floor debates, and other examples of the language being used in the law will provide insight into its meaning.

Publication of Law

Over the past two centuries, attorneys and legal publishers have worked to develop tools to overcome the difficulty of finding the law about a particular topic. Several factors make this a challenge, and understanding this challenge helps researchers understand how and why the resources work. The first obstacle is the lack of early legal publishing in the United States. Once the law was published, it was done so chronologically.

As we will see in chapter 5, case reporting has developed dramatically over the past two centuries. In 1800 most courts gave their opinions orally. There was no system for capturing a court's opinion or making it available to lawyers. In the late eighteenth century, some lawyers began to publish their notes of courts' opinions, and by the early nineteenth century, many opinions from appellate courts were being noted and published. During the nineteenth century the courts took more control over opinions. Judges began to write their opinions and to provide a written opinion to the court reporter. Soon the courts hired someone to gather the decisions and publish them on the court's behalf. At this point, judges could control which opinions were published and which were not. Until very recently, the only court opinions generally available were those released, as useful statements of law, by the court for publication. By the middle of the nineteenth century, important cases, which could include several legal issues, were published roughly chronologically. The next issue was to find a way to discover the parts of cases relevant to a particular topic.

When a legislature passes a law, it is published in a chronological set. The *United States Statutes at Large* contains the full text of all federal laws in the order they were passed. But just as court opinions can cover a variety of subjects, federal legislation can include many subjects; at the federal level it is relatively easy to insert unrelated law within another law and pass the whole thing. One example of this is the Hyde Amendment, a rider that prevents federal funds from being used to fund abortions, which has been attached to appropriations bills annually since 1976. Another is COBRA, which is a part of, and gets its name from, the Consolidated Omnibus Budget Reconciliation Act of 1985 and allows some employees to retain health insurance for a period of time after leaving an employer. For researchers, the challenge is to create a system to provide topical access to legislation. This same pattern holds true for regulations. Regulations are promulgated by agencies and published immediately in the chronological daily *Federal Register*.

The same solution to the problem of looking for topical material in a chronological set of law was used for statutes and regulations: codification. The statutes and regulations are separated into topical parts and organized into a topical structure. The good news about researching statutes or regulations in a code is that each code title covers one subject; however, the subjects are often broad. As the statutes are organized into a topical arrangement in the United States Code, the regulations are organized into a topical arrangement in the *Code of Federal Regulations.*

The problem of searching chronological publications containing multiple topics was resolved differently for the different kinds of law, but it remains as important a research issue today as it was in 1800. In the early twentieth century, the federal government sanctioned and partially adopted a statutory code and a regulatory code—topically organized versions of the laws or regulations currently in effect. The problem of case research has been attacked from several angles; structured outlines of parts of cases and online searches are the most important case research tools. To research the law effectively, researchers should understand not only how the law is made, but how the law is published.

Citations and Abbreviations

In the United States, most law communication uses the citation form described in *The Bluebook: A Uniform System of Citation.* The *Bluebook* is also a valuable research tool. For instance, Table T1 of the *Bluebook* lists, for all U.S. jurisdictions, all of the courts and court reports (with dates of coverage), as well as the current statutory compilation, administrative compilation, and administrative register. Often, researchers will encounter a legal citation that they do not recognize. *Prince's Bieber Dictionary of Legal Abbreviations,* available in print and as part of the electronic database Lexis as *Bieber's Dictionary of Legal Abbreviations,* is the first place they should turn to. If the abbreviation is not included in *Bieber's*, they may check the Cardiff Index to Legal Abbreviations (http://www.legalabbrevs.cardiff.ac.uk/).

Change

All research guides, including this one, represent a snapshot in time. The law changes, publishers change, databases change, publications change. We have tried to deemphasize particulars about too many resources and databases and instead emphasize the aspects of the research tools that will be most long-lasting. While the look and feel of the databases change frequently, the data included, the structure of the data, and the methods for locating the data change far more slowly. We hope that this book will help provide readers with a view of what to expect from historical American legal literature. What exists now or may exists in the future? How might that be described? Who might be the players in the print and online literature? What are the challenges that providers of legal information must struggle with, and what are their likely solutions? By developing an understanding of these issues, researchers will be able to identify new resources and will be better placed to track and understand developments with the existing resources.

Major Legal Databases

Many research sources are important in legal research, but today, three general legal research databases are the most important: Bloomberg Law, Lexis, and Westlaw. These database systems share many similarities: they contain the full text of most reported state and federal cases, current state and federal codes (and archival versions back to the 1980s or 1990s), state and federal administrative codes, many secondary research sources such as looseleaf services, legal treatises, and law review articles; and they provide an extensive citator that provides reference to later materials that cite an earlier document. Each also supplies access to news, some foreign and international legal and business materials, and many other sources of information. The systems often contain material from their own collection of publishers so that one system may have the classic treatise in one area while another system may have the classic treatise in another area. They offer Boolean and natural language searching, though the details of each are different. As is true with every database, it is important to spend time becoming familiar with the details of the system's operations. The systems provide help in various formats. Researchers should be aware that the systems are extremely expensive, and access to a large proportion of the database is often available only at law schools and law firms. However, both Lexis and Westlaw offer systems for universities that offer access to case law, codes, citators, and some secondary sources.

Another database that is of special importance to researchers in U.S. legal history is HeinOnline. HeinOnline contains collections of many law reviews back to their first issue, session laws, historical codes, legal treatises not covered by copyright, and a great number of other important resources. We will mention when important classes of material discussed later are available at HeinOnline. One drawback to HeinOnline is its searching capability. The database supports Boolean searching, though researchers should consult the help section before attempting more than a very basic search. Also, while the scanning and OCR is generally adequate, a large proportion of the text has not been proofread. Titles and authors have been proofread, so searches in those areas should be accurate, but searches in much of the material will likely miss relevant items.

Most of these databases and many resources cost a great deal of money. There are some good free resources, and we include some in this book, but most free solutions available today do not have the coverage that the for-fee databases offer. We are hopeful that this will change soon and that less expensive or free databases will provide more complete access to the law, but sometimes a for-fee resource is so much better than a free one that researchers should seek access to that version. It is possible to do good historical research without access to the for-fee resources, but it is much more time-consuming and difficult. Also, some avenues of inquiry are reasonable to undertake only with a database. This book does not provide a comprehensive guide to every possible tool researchers may want; we concentrate on the better resources that are more widely available. Most of the resources mentioned are available at good university libraries, law school libraries, or excellent public libraries.

Databases change along with everything else. The resources discussed in this book are those available at the time of publication, and the means of access are the means most supported at the same time. Databases will change names, interfaces, and contents, so the steps researchers take to access information will also change. But the basic structure of the information, the type of information, and the actual legal information created in the past do not change. Sometimes, databases are simply digitized versions of materials that a nineteenth-century researcher would recognize. At other times, the online systems provide new access and visualizations, but the underlying material will not change. Just as a nineteenth-century researcher would recognize the material underlying today's databases, future researchers will find that this book can help them understand the materials underlying the new information resources, however they look.

Coordinating Historical Legal Research:
A Six-Step Approach

No one style of research will work in every instance: each research problem is unique. Here we offer six points to consider in approaching a research project. Remembering that legal research is recursive, the researcher must remain open to new ideas to consider, new collections of cases to examine, or new statutes to integrate into an understanding of the law as useful information is unearthed. As a research project unfolds, consider the following steps:

1. Analyze facts and tentatively frame a research question.
   - A scholar or researcher will look to prove or disprove a thesis; a practicing lawyer will look to argue for or against a proposition.
   - Do the facts of the inquiry suggest time or jurisdiction limitations that may shape the research?
   - Framing the research question should not be absolute; it should be a continuous process. A research question can be refined or even revised as the research reveals new insights or new dimensions to the problem.
2. Develop an overview of the subject area.
   - What types of laws are required? Is it a federal or state problem? Are colonial sources likely to be relevant? Does a constitutional issue appear to be involved? Is it the sort of dispute that will likely become the subject of litigation? Is it an area regulated by statute?
   - A treatise from the relevant jurisdiction and period may define the types of authority to be researched. If the subject area is unfamiliar, whether factual or legal,

look for a useful introduction in a history or legal monograph related to the time and place involved. For example, each of the following situations requires a different sort of factual and legal investigation: a maritime problem involving British seizure of U.S. shipping in the Caribbean in 1810; Indian treaty violations in upper New York State in 1790; free black seamen being arrested as runaway slaves in Southern ports.

- Use appropriate dictionaries or texts to understand the meanings or usage of unfamiliar words or phrases.
- Begin developing a sense of what sources of authority are likely to be relevant. If the issue is litigation-based, a researcher should determine where the precedents can be found and what sources might help determine the procedural situation.

3. Make an in-depth search for legal authorities.
   - Consider both online and traditional sources.
   - Work from a known case or statute.
4. Read and evaluate the primary and secondary authorities.
   - A list of research sources will undoubtedly expand in the process as references to sources not previously encountered are found. Keeping notes (with full citations) of everything, whether relevant or useful or not, will avoid the aggravating waste of time involved in rechecking materials.
5. Bring historical research up to date.
   - Recent publications (periodical indexes, dissertation abstracts) may shed additional light on the research subject.
6. Pay attention to when the research will be considered complete.

- If the research has produced a sufficient body of material to support or negate the thesis, it is time to stop. (Some cynics would interpret this as "when one runs out of time.")
- For the practicing lawyer, research should stop when the cost exceeds the expected benefit for the client.
- When a search for primary sources turns up the same material again and again, research is complete.

The following chapters describe the research tools available to an attorney of the past as well as the tools that a researcher of today will use to find the law of the past. The development of legal publications and research tools during the past three hundred years serves as a framework in which to examine the resources. At the end of each chapter, we present a research example to show how the resources might be used to find information. In addition, each chapter is followed by a brief list of sources that may be of interest to readers and a list of the more important sources mentioned or discussed in the chapter. The latter list is divided into print resources and databases. Please note that we will not list Lexis, Westlaw, Bloomberg, or HeinOnline in the list of databases following a chapter; assume that they would follow every chapter. Some of the readings provide context, and others are sources for further research.

Further Reading

Amar, Akhil Reed. "Intratextualism." *Harvard Law Review* 112, no. 4 (1999): 748–827.

Barnett, Randy E. "The Gravitational Force of Originalism." *Fordham Law Review* 82, no. 2 (2013): 411–32.

————. "An Originalism for Nonoriginalists." *Loyola Law Review* 45, no. 4 (1999): 611–54. Baude, William. "Is Originalism Our Law?" *Columbia Law Review* 115, no. 8 (2015): 2349–2408.

Cornell, Saul. "Originalism on Trial: The Use and Abuse of History in District of Columbia v. Heller." *Colloquium: District of Columbia v. Heller* 69, no. 4 (2008): 625–40.

Dworkin, Ronald. "Comment." In Antonin Scalia, *A Matter of Interpretation: Federal Courts and the Law,* edited by Amy Gutmann, 115–27. Princeton, NJ: Princeton University Press, 1997.

Flaherty, Martin S. "Historians and the New Originalism: Contextualism, Historicism, and Constitutional Meaning." *Fordham Law Review* 84, no. 3 (2015): 905–14.

Gordon, Robert W. "Historicism in Legal Scholarship." *Yale Law Journal* 90 (1980): 1017–56.

Lichter, Brian A., and David P. Baltmanis. "Foreword: Original Ideas on Originalism." *Symposium: Original Ideas on Originalism. Northwestern University Law Review.* 103, no. 2 (2009): 491–94.

Scalia, Antonin. "Common-Law Courts in a Civil-Law System: The Role of the Federal Courts in Interpreting the Constitution and the Laws." In Antonin Scalia, *A Matter of Interpretation: Federal Courts and the Law,* edited by Amy Gutmann, 3–47. Princeton, NJ: Princeton University Press, 1997.

Solum, Lawrence B. "Faith and Fidelity: Originalism and the Possibility of Constitutional Redemption." *Texas Law Review* 91, no. 1 (2012): 147–73.

————. "Originalism and Constitutional Construction." *Fordham Law Review* 82, no. 2 (2013): 453–537.

Whittington, Keith E. "Originalism: A Critical Introduction." *Fordham Law Review* 82, no. 2 (2013): 375–409.

Important Sources Mentioned in This Chapter

Carter, Lief H., and Thomas Frederick Burke. *Reason in Law.* 9th ed. Chicago: University of Chicago Press, 2016.

Eskridge, William N., Philip P. Frickey, and Elizabeth Garrett. *Legislation and Statutory Interpretation.* 2nd ed. Concepts and Insights Series. New York: Foundation, 2006.

————, eds. *Statutory Interpretation Stories.* New York: Foundation, 2011.

Eskridge, William N., and John Paul Stevens. *Interpreting Law: A Primer on How to Read Statutes and the Constitution.* University Treatise Series. St Paul: Foundation, 2016.

Force, Peter. *American Archives: Consisting of a Collection of Authentick Records, State Papers, Debates, and Letters and Other Notices of Publick Affairs, the Whole Forming a Documentary History of the Origin and Progress of the North American Colonies; of the Causes and Accomplishment of the American Revolution; and of the Constitution of Government for the United States, to the Final Ratification Thereof.* Washington, DC: M. St. Clair Clarke and Peter Force, 1837–1853.

Hay, Peter. *The Law of the United States: An Introduction.* New York: Routledge, 2017.

Smith, Steven S., Jason M. Roberts, and Ryan J. Vander Wielen. *The American Congress.* 4th ed. New York: Cambridge University Press, 2006.

Symeonides, Symeon. *Choice of Law.* Oxford Commentaries on American Law. New York: Oxford University Press, 2016.

Originalism

Arthur, John. *Words That Bind: Judicial Review and the Grounds of Modern Constitutional Theory.* Boulder, CO: Westview, 1995.

Balkin, J. M. *Living Originalism.* Cambridge, MA: Belknap, 2011.

Bennett, Robert W., and Lawrence Solum. *Constitutional Originalism: A Debate.* Ithaca, NY: Cornell University Press, 2011.

Calabresi, Steven G., ed. *Originalism: A Quarter-Century of Debate.* Washington, DC: Regnery, 2007.

Charles, Patrick J. *Historicism, Originalism, and the Constitution: The Use and Abuse of the Past in American Jurisprudence.* Jefferson, NC: McFarland, 2014.

Cross, Frank B. *The Failed Promise of Originalism.* Stanford, CA: Stanford Law Books, 2013.

Dworkin, Ronald. *Justice in Robes.* Cambridge, MA: Belknap, 2006.

Huscroft, Grant, and Bradley W. Miller, eds. *The Challenge of Originalism: Theories of Constitutional Interpretation.* New York: Cambridge University Press, 2011.

McGinnis, John O., and Michael B. Rappaport. *Originalism and the Good Constitution.* Cambridge, MA: Harvard University Press, 2013.

O'Brien, David M., ed. *Judges on Judging: Views from the Bench.* 4th ed. Thousand Oaks, CA: CQ, 2013.

O'Neill, Johnathan G. "Challenging Modern Judicial Power: The Emergence of 'Originalism' in American Constitutional Theory, 1954–1987." PhD diss., 2000. Available through ProQuest Dissertations & Theses Global. https://www.proquest.com/products-services/pqdtglobal.html.

Purcell, Edward A. *Originalism, Federalism, and the American Constitutional Enterprise: A Historical Inquiry.* New Haven, CT: Yale University Press, 2007.

Rakove, Jack N. *Original Meanings: Politics and Ideas in the Making of the Constitution.* New York: A. A. Knopf, 1996.

Rakove, Jack N., and Edwin Meese. *Interpreting the Constitution: The Debate over Original Intent.* Boston: Northeastern University Press, 1990.

Scalia, Antonin, and Bryan A. Garner. *Reading Law: The Interpretation of Legal Texts.* St. Paul: Thomson/West, 2012.

Citation Manuals and Abbreviations Dictionaries

Harvard Law Review Association. *The Bluebook: A Uniform System of Citation.* Cambridge, MA: Harvard Law Review Association, 2012.

Prince, Mary Miles, and Doris M. Bieber. *Prince's Bieber Dictionary of Legal Abbreviations: A Reference Guide for Attorneys, Legal Secretaries, Paralegals, and Law Students.* Buffalo, NY: W. S. Hein, 2009.

Current General American Legal Research Texts

Armstrong, J. D. S. *Where the Law Is: An Introduction to Advanced Legal Research.* 4th ed. Edited by Christopher A. Knott. St. Paul, MN: West, 2013.

Barkan, Steven M. *Fundamentals of Legal Research.* 10th ed. Edited by Barbara Bintliff and Mary Whisner. St. Paul: Foundation, 2015.

Berring, Robert C. *Finding the Law.* 10th ed. Edited Morris L. Cohen. St. Paul: West, 1995.

Brostoff, Teresa, and Ann Sinsheimer. *United States Legal Language and Culture: An Introduction to the U.S. Common Law System.* 3rd ed. New York: Oceana/Oxford University Press, 2013.

Cohen, Morris L. *How to Find the Law.* 9th ed. Edited by Robert C. Berring and Kent C. Olson. St. Paul: West, 1989.

———. *Legal Research in a Nutshell.* 11th ed. Edited by Kent C. Olson. St. Paul: West, 2013.

Doyle, Francis R. *Searching the Law.* Ardsley, NY: Transnational, 2005.

Healey, Paul D. *Legal Reference for Librarians: How and Where to Find the Answers.* Chicago: American Library Association, 2014.

Kunz, Christina L. *The Process of Legal Research: Authorities and Options.* 8th ed. New York: Wolters Kluwer, 2012.

Manz, William H. *Gibson's New York Legal Research Guide*. 4th ed. Buffalo, NY: William S. Hein, 2014.

Nedzel, Nadia E. *Legal Reasoning, Research, and Writing for International Graduate Students*. 4th ed. Aspen Coursebook Series. New York: Wolters Kluwer, 2017.

Olson, Kent C. *Legal Information: How to Find It, How to Use It*. Phoenix: Oryx, 1999.

———. *Principles of Legal Research*. 2nd ed. St. Paul: West, 2015.

Sloan, Amy E. *Basic Legal Research: Tools and Strategies*. 6th ed. Aspen Coursebook Series. New York: Wolters Kluwer, 2015.

Older American Legal Research Texts

Ames, Charles Lesley. *Reference Book: A Companion Book Illustrating the Third Edition of Brief Making and the Use of Law Books*. St. Paul: West, 1914.

Bogert, George Gleason. *How to Find the Law*. Chicago: Blackstone Institute, 1916.

Eldean, Fred August. *How to Find the Law: A Legal Reference Handbook, Including Chapters on Brief Making*. St. Paul: West, 1931.

Foster, George N. *Lawyers Legal Search: Rules and Problems of Search Illustrated by Diagrams or Geometric Charts*. Rochester, NY: Lawyers Cooperative, 1920.

Hicks, Frederick C. *Materials and Methods of Legal Research*. Rochester, NY: Lawyers Cooperative, 1942.

Kiser, Donald J. *Principles and Practice of Legal Research*. Brooklyn, NY: American Law Book, 1924.

Law Books and Their Use: A Manual of Legal Bibliography, Legal Research and Brief Making for Lawyers and Students. Rochester, NY: Lawyers Cooperative, 1925.

Notz, Rebecca Laurens Love. *Legal Bibliography and Legal Research*. Chicago: Callaghan, 1952.

Pollack, Ervin H. *Fundamentals of Legal Research*. Brooklyn, NY: Foundation, 1956.

Price, Miles O., and Harry Bitner. *Effective Legal Research: A Practical Manual of Law Books and Their Use*. New York: Prentice-Hall, 1953.

Townes, John Charles. *Law Books and How to Use Them*. Austin, TX: Austin Print, 1909.

Bibliographies and Guides to Historical Legal Sources

Chiorazzi, Michael G., and Marguerite Most, eds. *Prestatehood Legal Materials: A Fifty-State Research Guide, Including New York City and the District of Columbia.* New York: Haworth Information, 2005.

Cohen, Morris L. *Bibliography of Early American Law.* Buffalo, NY: William S. Hein, 1998.

Databases

Bloomberg LP. Bloomberg Law. https://www.bna.com/bloomberglaw/.

Hathi Trust. Hathi Trust Digital Library. https://www.hathitrust.org/.

Internet Archive. Internet Archive. http://archive.org.

LexisNexis. Lexis Advance. https://www.lexisnexis.com/en-us/products/lexis-advance.page.

———. LexisNexis Academic. https://www.lexisnexis.com/en-us/products/lexisnexis-academic.page.

ProQuest. *ProQuest Dissertations & Theses Global.* https://www.proquest.com/products-services/pqdtglobal.html.

Thomson Reuters. *Campus Research.* http://legalsolutions.thomsonreuters.com/law-products/westlaw-legal-research/campus-research.

———. Westlaw. http://legalsolutions.thomsonreuters.com/law-products/westlaw-legal-research/.

University of Wales. *Cardiff Index to Legal Abbreviations.* http://www.legalabbrevs.cardiff.ac.uk.

William S. Hein and Co. HeinOnline. http://www.heinonline.org/.

———. *Spinelli's Law Librarian's Reference Shelf.* https://heinonline.org/.

Wolters Kluwer Law and Business. IntelliConnect. http://www.wolterskluwerlb.com/intelliconnect/.

1
General Bibliographic Sources

Before we delve into how to conduct research, a brief introduction to the landscape of print and online publishing may be useful for an understanding of what researchers will encounter. The early twenty-first century is an interesting vantage point from which to examine legal resources. A great deal of the past has been digitized, but it has been digitized by different organizations for different purposes. While underlying vendors and their needs may seem unimportant, their needs dictated the final product. Understanding what they are trying to accomplish can help researchers learn to work with the resources.

Some material is digitized by large for-profit vendors. These vendors create large, and often very expensive, databases of materials designed for particular markets. In the 1970s, Lexis was one of the first full-text online databases. Lexis was developed for practicing lawyers and that is still its primary market. This leads Lexis, and its competitors in that market, including Bloomberg Law and Westlaw, to make content and other decisions based on the needs of practicing lawyers. One area where this benefits legal history researchers is case law.

Since very old cases may be relevant to current legal disputes, Lexis, Westlaw, and Bloomberg Law have developed databases that contain the full text of most published appellate decisions promulgated in the United States. However, since lawyers do not generally need very old statutory codes, Lexis, Westlaw, and Bloomberg Law do not supply them. Their coverage is only from the later twentieth century.

Some material is digitized by large for-profit vendors for sale mainly to large academic libraries. These databases must be general enough to draw interest from enough departments in a university and from enough universities to make the database profitable. A number of these databases specifically contain legal materials, for example the several components of Gale's *Making of Modern Law,* and a number of larger general collections of materials happen to contain a lot of law. Readex's *Early American Imprints, Series 1: Evans, 1639–1800* (http://www.readex.com/content/early-american-imprints) is a collection of digitized versions of the books listed in the great bibliography by Charles Evans. Among these are many colonial statutes, justice of the peace manuals, and other legal sources.

Some niche publishers create databases of legal materials that may not have the same market as those digitized by larger vendors. The advantages of these databases is that researchers can get access to many items that may not otherwise be available to them. But there is a trade-off. The searching capabilities and interface to these systems are often less robust and user-friendly than what researchers may be used to.

Many other groups are also digitizing and making material available to researchers. Aside from explicitly governmental groups, which will be discussed below, these organizations run the gamut from quasi-governmental to universities to cooperative projects and even private citizens. The quality of these databases varies widely, and some are tremendously useful. It is important, however, for researchers to understand who is funding the effort and why.

Governments are large publishers and have digitized a lot of their materials. Governments publish materials because it is their duty to do so, they want explain what they do, or they want to ensure that necessary information is available. For example, the U.S. government publishes a lot of the law, but not all of it. The Government Printing Office (GPO) publishes the *United States Reports,* the case reporter that covers the U.S. Supreme Court, but it does not publish the opinions of the federal courts of appeal or district courts. Those are published, in print, by West Publishing Company. The federal government has been slow to publish case law and, to a slightly lesser extent, statutory law online; however, it has done much more with administrative law. For a variety of reasons, funding being not the least, the government can also be very slow to publish. In many areas of law, private publishers have been stepping in since the beginning to fill the gaps or speed up the process.

Of course, the terrain and players will both change, but it seems likely that the main classes of players—large corporations, small corporations, universities, and other nonprofits—and the government will continue to play important roles in the dissemination of legal information. A major part of the research process is determining what materials are available to researchers and in what format the materials are available. Some sources will not be available to all researchers. Some of the materials we describe will be available to researchers in other formats or databases that may be more widely available. Other materials will be accessible only through expensive databases generally available at large academic or specialized libraries. Savvy researchers will consider alternative sources of materials or find more useful versions of materials that might not be available to them through the vendors mentioned below.

Another important aspect of research is understanding how the material came to be and that the identity of the creator of the material or the organization making the material available affects content and access. Much of the remainder of this book covers these issues, but a few general observations are in order. Much of the material reflects how the law is made. For example, cases are decided one after another, and a prior case may have little in common legally with a subsequent case. This fact leads to chronologically organized case reports with legal topics scattered throughout the collection. Research tools were created to overcome this problem, but the value and use of such tools make little sense unless the user knows about the reports.

Legal materials were originally created in ways that made sense when one considers how the law was made. When the law was digitized, this print understanding of the way that the law is made and researched was ported directly into an online environment. The print structure of legal materials is still readily apparent in online systems. Indeed, all online vendors need to know where pages break in print volumes that the user may never use. Legal research today is just beginning to consider how to think about information apart from print. The legacy of print will be important to researchers for years to come.

The print orientation of online databases in not limited to the law. Among the great databases is the digital version of Charles Evans's bibliography, which maintains much of what makes the print bibliography useful—the entry points and controlled vocabulary—while adding full-text searching and ready access to the texts. However, the database is still clearly an electronic version of the print tool. Other databases have taken large collections of print items, digitized them, and provided basic access. An example of this is the collection of law journals available at HeinOnline. Hein has made available scanned, searchable versions of many law journals, as if a law library's journal collection were scanned and placed online. Hein offers the researcher access via citation and searching. Authors, article titles, and journal names can be designated as search fields, and the material in those fields has been proofread. However, the remainder of the content, while searchable, is not broken down or proofed. In addition, no additional entry points, such as subject headings, are added.

Once researchers understand the terrain, they can begin to contemplate the search. In developing a search strategy, an awareness of general bibliographic tools and online searching strategies and procedures is useful.

Beginning the Search

When starting a research project, researchers must define, as specifically as possible, the question at hand. A well-defined query leads researchers to a vision of the type of material required. From that vision they can identify not only the most useful resources, but also the terminology needed to describe the material.

The strategies needed to plan a research project are the same whether one is using print or online materials. Consider the following: the nature of the material sought; the nature of the resources in which the material might be found, including format and coverage; whether the material might be indexed; whether the material might be searchable; and whether the full text might be available.

Early on, researchers will need to master the specialized language used both in the era researched and in the subculture examined. They will want to develop lists of likely terms to use when consulting a print index or an online database. The recursive nature of research will quickly become apparent; a found source will likely raise a new term or idea or suggest a new perspective on an issue. They should then return to the resources previously consulted with the new term or idea in hand and see what these new searches might add.

In developing a search strategy, researchers must strike a balance between comprehensiveness and accuracy. They can construct a search strategy that will return only, or almost only, relevant items. But such a search, by its nature, will miss some pertinent information. On the other hand, a search designed to not miss any possible relevant items will, by its nature, contain a great deal of irrelevant information. Researchers must consider whether they want an accurate search or a comprehensive search as well as what sources they will consult.

Almost every database supports searching using the "and," "or," and "not" logical connectors. So-called Boolean searching allows researchers to construct a logic statement and have every item that meets the requirements of the statement returned in their results. The Boolean "and" connector narrows the results because the terms on either side of the "and" must be present in order to meet the requirements of the search statement. The "or" connector broadens the search by allowing for alternative terms. The "not" connector will return every item that meets the requirements outlined in the search statement preceding the "not," but if the term(s) following the "not" are in the found item, it will be discarded. The basic Boolean connectors can allow for quite complex logic statements, and most databases support Boolean searching.

Many databases take Boolean searching further by introducing signals that allow researchers to specify that terms appear within a certain number of words of each other or appear within certain parts of a document. Most databases also allow researchers to replace certain characters in a word with a "wildcard" or to "truncate" search terms. Both of these are very useful to historical researchers. Truncation can easily save a great deal of typing. Consider employment. Almost every word beginning with "employ" will be relevant to most searches. Rather than having to think of and type all of them, researchers can retrieve them all by simply using the truncation character after the letter "y." As regards wildcards, anyone who has spent any time reading materials printed much before 1800 is familiar with the "long s." To modern eyes, this character looks like an "f," and many optical character-recognition (OCR) readers do not know what to do with it. By replacing the "long s" with a wildcard character, researchers will get far better and more complete results. For instance, a search in *Early American Imprints* for the word "manuscript" returns 255 items. Replacing the "s" with the wildcard operator, in this case the "?," and searching for "manu?cript" yields 1,129 items. Many databases support these extensions. However, while the Boolean "and," "or," and "not" are represented much the same in many databases, the "proximity" connectors and "field" descriptors vary from database to database. But all databases will have a help section that describes the search capabilities of the database.

As we describe the data contained in the books and databases that historical legal researchers use, it is important to note what the data look like: full text of a book or a case or a magazine article? An annotated code, in which case each document can be several thousand pages long? Or a bibliographic record similar to what a researcher finds with a library catalog search? With the latter, the entire document might be less than fifty words long. The size of the document may encourage the use of the "and" connector or, in a larger document, perhaps a "proximity" connector. Also, the researcher will want to note whether the documents that make up the database are broken into fields that may allow more exact searching. Frequently, the date of issue of a case or newspaper or other material is important in locating the item. If the date can be searched, and it almost always can be, locating the item is much easier. Another important type of field is the "descriptor" or "subject" field. This type of metadata is often added to books, articles, and other items to assist researchers. The cataloger or indexer selects terms that describe the book or article from a limited list of terms. When researchers determine the terms that are used, they can easily find all of the relevant documents.

In addition to Boolean searching, many databases support some sort of algorithmic search—that is, a search, as with Google, in which the researcher enters terms that tend to describe the result wanted; then the database determines, by means of an algorithm, the best results. There are times when researchers will want to use a search algorithm, and times when they will want to construct a Boolean search. While experience is the best guide, the legal research texts mentioned at the end of the introduction or other research texts are also useful references for helping to determine the optimal search strategy.

Just as each book is indexed and organized differently, each online database works differently. The method of searching, the existence of subject headings, and the type and quality of the underlying data can differ. These differences factor into the development of search strategies. For example, some of the full-text databases were constructed by scanning or keying in print originals, and some were constructed using a microform copy of the print original. In the second instance, the digital copy is an additional generation removed from the original item. Once a digitized copy is created, special OCR software creates a text-based copy of the items. Searches are constructed on the text-based copy. Unless extensive proofreading is performed on the text copy, many errors will remain in the text. In some instances, the software will misread a letter, and in other cases, a word may break at the end of a line or page and the complete word may not be found in a search. The quality of the scanning and proofreading is not always made clear by the database description; however, by paying close attention to search results and by examining text snippets when they are made available, careful researchers can develop a sense of the quality of the material being searched. In most cases, careful researchers will get positive results and can be assured that they have found a portion, even a significant portion, of the relevant material in a database. Unless the database has undergone excellent proofreading, no careful researcher can claim to have found every relevant item.

Catalogs

Almost any research project will employ library catalogs and bibliographies. Library catalogs may include the collection of a single library or of many libraries, and bibliographies range widely in scope and size.

Catalogs, the main tools used to find items held by libraries, give bibliographic details of books (and occasionally other material). WorldCat, the largest catalog, contains the bibliographic records of Online Computer Library Center (OCLC) member libraries. By the middle of 2017, it held almost 400 million records provided from libraries around the world (http://www.oclc.org/en/worldcat/inside-worldcat.html). The documents or records are brief, containing author, title, publisher and publication information, and notes, which may include a table of contents and subject headings. WorldCat is available via subscription or, in a slightly limited form, for free. The subscription version offers additional searching and sorting functions.

Most of the items cataloged by WorldCat are monographs. Journals are also included, but since few libraries catalog journal articles, WorldCat is not a reliable tool for identifying them. WorldCat also includes archival materials, such as personal or institutional papers, some sound recordings, some images, some pamphlets, and the like. WorldCat does not include every book ever published, but it does describe more monographs than other catalogs, making it an important tool for identifying and locating books. It can also serve as a secondary or tertiary resource for identifying and locating other types of material. Since WorldCat contains so much material, search results can be overwhelming, although large result sets can provide good information about how a subject has been treated.

The advanced searching capacity on the subscription version of WorldCat allows complex Boolean search expressions, including truncation and wildcards; it also allows researchers to limit results through a variety of factors, including date, language, the number of libraries that hold the item, format, whether the item is meant for a juvenile audience, and whether it is a work of fiction or nonfiction. Researchers can even limit a search to a specified library. The advanced search at WorldCat.org allows most of the same search capabilities as well as the ability to create and share lists of resources.

Catalogs of single library collections can also be important research tools. A search in a large database will often return too many items, whereas a focused, limited catalog search will return fewer false positives and may provide faster and easier access to the material needed.

Some catalogs cover only one library, others cover many libraries, and others fall in the middle and include a few specific libraries. Such catalogs can be very useful, especially if a focus on a group of libraries aligns with a researcher's needs. The University of Manchester's Copac (copac.ac.uk), an example of this type of catalog, provides free access to the online catalogs of many major university, specialist, and national libraries in the United Kingdom and Ireland, including the British Library.

Many catalogs that a researcher in U.S. legal history will find interesting are available for free on the Internet. When a researcher is dealing with archival material, as we will see in chapter 8, these catalogs often cannot substitute for the kind of collection descriptions that archivists create, but they can be useful for locating archival collections.

Bibliographies

Bibliographies offer descriptions of books or other items that are related in some way: by time or nation of publication, author, or subject. Many bibliographies seek to be comprehensive.

National bibliographies are an important research resource, and those that cover discrete periods of time are often very useful. Among the most helpful national bibliographies for researchers working in U.S. legal history are the following (see also more complete information at the end of this chapter):

- Evans, *American Bibliography* (1941), supplemented with Shaw and Shoemaker, *American Bibliography* (1958), and Shoemaker, Cooper, and Shaw, *A Checklist of American Imprints* (1964). Online from 1639 to 1819 in Readex's *Early American Imprints.*

- Sabin, Joseph, Wilberforce Eames, and R. W. G. Vail. *Bibliotheca Americana. A Dictionary of Books Relating to America, From Its Discovery to the Present Time.* New York, 1868–1936. This bibliography describes books, pamphlets, and periodicals printed in the United States or related to the United States from 1639 (the date of the first printing in what was to become the United States), no matter where printed; early newspapers are not included, nor broadsides printed after 1800. The original edition covered through the mid-nineteenth century, but later work brought it into the twentieth. Online at Gale, *Sabin Americana, 1500–1926.*

- Wing, Donald Goddard, *Short-Title Catalogue of Books Printed in England, Scotland, Ireland, Wales, and British America, and of English Books Printed in Other Countries, 1641–1700,* and online as the English Short Title Catalogue (1473–1800) (ESTC). Note that this is not a full-text database.

- The Library of Congress, *National Union Catalog* (1956). This appeared in several series; the pre-1956 imprints, a set of more than seven hundred volumes, contains the catalog records of major U.S. and Canadian libraries. This massive set is available in major libraries.

Many of the older bibliographies have been digitized and are available through Google Books and the digital library HathiTrust. In addition, Sabin, *Bibliotheca Americana: A Dictionary of Books Relating to America,* has been digitized by the American Council of Learned Societies (ACLS) and is available through the ACLS Humanities E-Book project at http://www. humanitiesebook.org/default.html and through HeinOnline. Members of the associated societies have access to the ACLS version, and individual access to that version is not very expensive; but the searching is not very sophisticated, and only the bibliographic records, not the full text of the underlying books, are searchable.

Researchers of U.S. legal history will also consider subscription databases of historical law books that contain treatises published after 1800. The major databases are not comprehensive but together contain the most important legal treatises published between 1800 and 1926. Gale's *The Making of Modern Law: Legal Treatises* contains the most important British and U.S. legal treatises published between 1800 and 1926. The material can be searched by bibliographic reference or by full text. The complete books are available in a page-image format. Thomson/West's *Rise of American Law* is a similar database available on Westlaw. It is also full-text searchable and provides access to the complete text in page-image format. One additional benefit of *Rise of American Law* is that the coverage extends beyond 1926 into the 1950s, with some titles into the 1990s. HeinOnline also provides many legal treatises; the *Legal Classics* library contains more than forty-five hundred important legal treatises that can be identified by author, title, broad subject, or full-text search. Searching HeinOnline is a little more complex than many other databases, but by using these databases, researchers can conduct full-text searches of the important legal treatises published from the time that the printing press appeared in England until at least the 1920s.

The *Making of Modern Law: Legal Treatises* and *Rise of American Law* are examples of topical bibliographies. The best way to locate others is to search WorldCat or a large library catalog using "bibliography" or "checklist" as a term in the title or to search for "bibliography" as a subject. Since many bibliographic records note when a book contains a bibliography, no matter how small, a broader search that allows "bibliography" to appear anywhere in the record will return a lot of books that are not bibliographies.

The most important subject bibliography for researchers interested in U.S. legal history is Morris Cohen's *Bibliography of Early American Law*. It covers monographs and trial materials published in the United States from the beginning of the colonial period through 1860. Indexes include author, title, subject, jurisdiction, party, place and publisher, language, and a chronology. It is available in print at major libraries and at HeinOnline. Another bibliography, Betty W. Taylor and Robert John Munro's *American Law Publishing, 1860–1900,* provides bibliographic records for the remainder of the nineteenth century.

Some examples of book-length bibliographies that may be of interest to legal historians include Paul Finkelman, *Slavery in the Courtroom* (1985), and William Hamilton Bryson, *A Bibliography of Virginia Legal History Before 1900* (1979). In many legal research projects, a bibliography covering a seemingly unrelated field can also be useful. For example, Evald Rink's *Technical Americana* (1981) refers to a great deal of material on the relationship between the law and industrial development during the first half of the nineteenth century. For instance, it includes references to many items related to *Gibbons v. Ogden* (22 U.S. 1 [1824]), the U.S. Supreme Court Commerce Clause case that specifically dealt with the steamship trade on the Hudson River.

Websites

Many publishers, historical societies, scholars, libraries, and individuals have created websites that contain material of interest to legal researchers. When considering such sites, researchers should think about how to locate them, how reliable they are, whether they will exist in the future, and how they can be used.

Always keep in mind the ultimate purpose of any research. For instance, if page images are important for citation or other reasons, then sites that do not provide page images will not be very helpful.

Judging the reliability of a website requires understanding the purpose, prejudices, and mission of its author and determining whether sufficient checks on the content make the site acceptable. Recognize that the problems of mission and prejudice arise with all materials, whether printed or online, whether created by a scholar or by a layperson. Websites with specific agendas can still be extremely useful; indeed, several of the sites mentioned in the following chapters have specific political, social, or other purposes, but the material can be useful if researchers factor in the agenda of the provider when deciding when and whether to use the material.

There are several ways to find websites useful for historical legal research. One is to consider authorship: what organization might have unique access to the material being sought? Many archives are making parts of their collections available, and many legislative libraries are making legislative materials available. As the only location for their holdings, these are logical places to look. For example, one of the best places to find out about what is happening in Congress is at its website, https://www.congress.gov.

Another method is to consider what groups or organizations might make use of the materials in question. For instance, Liberty Fund publishers, which have a particularly libertarian bent, might focus on political or philosophical purposes. Alternatively, a law faculty might develop a site as a new kind of publishing, to cultivate a scholarly reputation, or to advance knowledge. Finally, money-making ventures will provide access to materials that are more widely sought.

Research Example

We will search for books about witchcraft and the law as an example of how to use a basic word search in an online catalog to gather terms that will enable us to both expand and focus our search as we begin to learn about the subject. For this example, we will use WorldCat for our searches although the same processes will work for almost any catalog.

If we enter the search "witchcraft AND law AND trial" in www.worldcat.org, we get almost nine hundred items. The first relevant looking item is a book by Peter Alan Morton and Barbara Dähms, *The Trial of Tempel Anneke: Records of a Witchcraft Trial in Brunswick, Germany, 1663* (2006). While interesting, it's a little far afield if we are researching American law; but it gives us some clues. One of the subject headings is "trials (witchcraft)," to which geographical limits are attached.

If we now conduct an advanced search for the subject "trials (witchcraft)," we get almost three thousand items, but the results look more relevant. We can now use the facets on the left to limit the results. By limiting myself to "books," "nonfiction," and "nonjuvenile" with the topic "law," we get about three hundred items. One of the first is Katherine Richardson, *The Salem Witchcraft Trials* (1994), published by the Peabody Essex Museum in Salem, Massachusetts; still on the first page is Emerson W. Baker, *A Storm of Witchcraft: The Salem Trials and the American Experience* (2016), published by Oxford University Press; and another near the top is Peter Charles Hoffer, *The Devil's Disciples: Makers of the Salem Witchcraft Trials* (1998), published by Johns Hopkins University Press.

When we look at the subject headings, we don't get much help as they are almost all using "trials (witchcraft)" as the relevant heading. We are getting material mainly about trials; if we want to expand the search to include other legal issues, we might consider an advanced search for the subject "witchcraft" and the subject "law" limited to nonjuvenile, nonfiction books with the topic "law." This returns eighty-one books that look at the law of witchcraft a little more broadly in scope and geography. For example, one of the first is Jo Bath and John Newton, *Witchcraft and the Act of 1604* (2008), and another is John Hund, *Witchcraft, Violence and the Law in South Africa* (2003).

By starting with searches using terms that we think are most relevant, we identify a collection of material. Close examination of that collection will inform us of the controlled terms that are used to describe the ideas that interest us. By understanding the nature of those terms and by conducting additional searches based on those terms, we will begin to get a sense of how the topic has been addressed and will identify the most relevant items.

Early American Imprints uses the same subjects as World-Cat; however, since there are far fewer items in *Early American Imprints* than in WorldCat, we might want to try a less restrictive search. Searching *Early American Imprints* for the word "witchcraft" and requiring that it appear in the subject heading yields only sixteen items. If we require the term "law" to also appear in the subject headings, we get nothing. But by loosening the search a little and requiring that the word "witchcraft" appear as a subject and that the word "law" appear anywhere in the description, we find the act of the Massachusetts legislature in 1713 that reversed the attainders of George Burroughs and others for witchcraft. We can then look at a digital copy of the actual document. We could further loosen the search by allowing the words to appear within a particular number of words of each other in the text of the documents or anywhere in the text of the documents. But we should remember that as we loosen the search restrictions, we allow more irrelevant material into the results.

The data being searched in some of the databases in this example and in many to follow is not static. If you conduct the searches mentioned above in WorldCat today, your results will be different from mine since more books are added to the database every day. However, the underlying concepts described in the examples will remain valid.

Further Reading

Berring, Robert C. "Full-Text Databases and Legal Research: Backing into the Future." *High Technology Law Journal* 1 (1986): 27–60.

Gordon, Robert W. "Historicism in Legal Scholarship." *Yale Law Journal* 90 (1980): 1017–56.

Musson, Anthony, and Chantal Stebbings. *Making Legal History: Approaches and Methodologies.* Cambridge: Cambridge University Press, 2012.

Presser, Stephen B. "Legal History or the History of Law: A Primer on Bringing the Law's Past into the Present." *Vanderbilt Law Review* 35 (1982): 849–90.

Important Sources Mentioned in This Chapter

Cohen, Morris L. *Bibliography of Early American Law.* Buffalo, NY: W. S. Hein, 1998.

Evans, Charles. *American Bibliography: A Chronological Dictionary of All Books, Pamphlets, and Periodical Publications Printed in the United States of America from the Genesis of Printing in 1639 Down to and Including the Year 1820.* New York: P. Smith, 1941.

Sabin, Joseph, Wilberforce Eames, and R. W. G. Vail. *Bibliotheca Americana. A Dictionary of Books Relating to America, from Its Discovery to the Present Time.* New York, 1868–1936.

Databases

Gale. *The Making of Modern Law.* http://www.gale.com/primary-sources/the-making-of-modern-law.

———. *Sabin Americana.* http://www.gale.com/c/sabin-americana–1500–1926.

OCLC (Online Computer Library Center). WorldCat. https://www.worldcat.org/.

Readex. *Early American Imprints, Series I: Evans, 1639–1800,* and *Early American Imprints, Series II, Shaw-Shoemaker, 1801–1819.* http://www.readex.com/content/early-american-imprints.

Thomson Reuters. *Rise of American Law.* Westlaw. http://legalsolutions.thomsonreuters.com/law-products/westlaw-legal-research/.

2

English Foundations of American Law, 1500s–1776

In the early seventeenth century, most of the colonists in the eastern part of North America saw themselves as English subjects bound by English laws. As Justice Joseph Story noted in *Commentaries on the Constitution of the United States,* "the colonists, continuing as much subjects in the new establishment, where they had freely placed themselves . . . as they had been in the old, carried with them their birthright, the laws of their country; because the customs of a free people are a part of their liberty" and "the jurisprudence of England became that of the colonies, so far as it was applicable to the situation" (Boston: Hilliard, Gray, 1833, p. 138). Although colonial charters, legislation, and court decisions adapted to different conditions made the law a little different, at base, the laws of the colonies were the laws of England.

Research in the laws of the colonial era requires an understanding of both the legal regime and institutions of the colony in question and the legal regime and institutions of England. This chapter describes current sources and techniques useful for finding seventeenth- and eighteenth-century laws of England and introduces some methods an attorney in England in the seventeenth and eighteenth centuries might have used.

Sources of Law

Before researchers can find the law, they must know what was considered to be the source of law in the period being investigated. The common law system was developed in England during the Middle Ages, and under it, the law is "found" by the application of reason and precedent to particular matters. Common law was imposed in North America and elsewhere during colonization and has largely been retained in former colonies. Later attorneys can discern the law by pulling together various applications of law appearing in relevant cases. Therefore, reporting, publishing, and finding cases has been important in English law for centuries.

The English legal system was not unchanging. In the fifteenth and sixteenth centuries, the increasing availability of case law affected the development of precedent, and the adoption of Protestantism and the departure of the Roman Catholic Church's courts from England affected the way that the courts of chancery and equity developed. During the seventeenth century, a major conflict concerned the place of Parliament, which expanded its lawmaking function mainly at the expense of the monarch. A result of a more active Parliament is that fewer legal issues have to be developed by courts alone. The work of common law courts has changed so that they spend more time interpreting legislation than finding law.

While the legal system of most of Great Britain and its former colonies is based on the common law, today most of the rest of the world uses a civil law system. There are many differences

between the common law and civil law systems, including the role
of judges and the education of lawyers. The most important difference is in the source of law. Civil law countries look to codes
of laws that are, at their root, based on codes going back to ancient
Rome and the rationalization of the law undertaken in the sixth
century under the auspices of Emperor Justinian and published
in the *Corpus Juris Civilis*. Questions of interpretation are solved
by reference to ancient explanations included in the *Institutes* and
Digests, collected by the creators of the *Corpus Juris Civilis*, as well
as to scholarly treatments of the subject.

The common law has always been made up of more than
cases. Today, we would say that legislation and administrative
rules and decisions and municipal enactments are the major
sources of law. In the United States, the written federal and state
constitutions are also obvious sources of law. But what would
an attorney in the seventeenth century look to as law? In 1628,
Lord Coke, former chief justice of the Common Pleas and of
the King's Bench, included a list of the sources of law:

> *En la Ley.* There be divers Lawes within the Realme
> of England. As First,
>
>   (a) *Lex Coronæ*, the Law of the Crowne.
>
>   (b) Lex & consuetudo parliamenti. Ista lex est
> ab omnibus quaerenda, à multis ignorata, à paucis
> cognita.
>
>   (c) *Lex naturæ*, the Law of nature.
>
>   (d) *Communis lex Angliæ*, the common law of
> England sometime called *Lex terræ*, intended by
> our Author in this and like places.
>
>   (e) Statute Law, Lawes established by authori-
> tie of Parliament.
>
>   (f) *Consuetudines*, Customes reasonable.

(g) *Jus belli*, The Law of Armes, Warre, and Chivalrie, *in republica maximè conseruanda sunt jura belli.*

(h) *Ecclesiasticall or Canon Law* in Courts in certaine Cases.

(i) *Civill Law* in certaine cases not only in Courts Ecclesiasticall, but in the Courts of the Constable and Marshall, and of the Admiraltie, in which Court of the Admiraltie is observed the *ley Olyron, anno 5.* of *Richard* the first, so called, because it was published in the Isle of Olyron.

(k) *Lex forestæ*, forest Law.

(l) The law of Marque, or reprisall.

(m) *Lex mercatoria*, Merchant, &c.

(n) *The Lawes* and Customes of the *Isles of Jersey, Gernesey, and Man.*

(o) *The Law* and priviledge *of the Stanneries.*

(p) *The Lawes of the East, West, and middle Marches which are now abrogated. (The First Part of the Institutes of the Lawes of England,* ch. 1, pt. 1, sec. 3)

Among the sources that Coke lists are the law of the crown, the law and custom of Parliament, the laws of nature, the common law, statutory law, and customary law. Of these, the most important sources of law in the colonies, and those focused on here, are the statutes of Parliament and the common law. Some of the resources, especially those that enable law-finding by topic, and some treatises may refer a researcher to other sources of law. This chapter discusses the sources that were available to a seventeenth- or eighteenth-century attorney as well as resources that have been developed since that allow modern researchers to locate law from that time.

It is important to understand how seventeenth- or eighteenth-century lawyers were educated and what sort of law was familiar to the educated layperson. Legal education in England was undertaken at one of the Inns of Court in central London. The Inns started as boarding houses and clubs for lawyers practicing in London but quickly took on responsibility for educating the profession; indeed, their educational activities predate the sixteenth century. But education in civil law was more widely available; it was the law taught in the universities. Until the 1860s and 1870s, Cambridge and Oxford universities did not offer a degree in English common law. A university-educated person who had studied law was trained in the civil law. Until Henry VIII's break with Rome, a fully functioning civil law system, parallel to the common law system, was operating in the ecclesiastical courts in England. Many eighteenth-century Americans were familiar with civil law and read widely about political philosophy and the law. Early American lawyers were either immigrants who has been educated at the Inns of Court or they apprenticed in the law or had been associated with the Inns of Court. However, as we will see, their libraries reflect a sophisticated understanding of both civil and common law.

The story of the development of law, legal writing, and publishing up to 1800 as well as many of the details of English practice after 1800 are fascinating and beyond the scope of this work. Several good guides point to sources of English law that could be found during the American colonial period and the tools that lawyers would have used to find the law. One is the chapter on legal literature in J. H. Baker's *An Introduction to English Legal History;* another is the chapter on historical sources by W. W. S. Breem in Elizabeth M. Moys's *Manual of Law Librarianship: The Use and Organization of Legal Literature.*

Legislation

The early colonial period, from the reign of James I to William and Mary, saw a diminution of royal power and a concurrent increase in parliamentary power. While seventeenth-century parliamentary legislation was not as important, or even often of the same nature, as nineteenth-century legislation, parliamentary enactments during the colonial period play an important part in the framework surrounding any particular legal issue.

The *Public Acts of Parliament* have been published regularly, when Parliament is in session, since the late fifteenth century; and except for the Interregnum, publication continued throughout the colonial era to today. The acts are available fairly widely; however, two problems can arise in conducting research in them. First, they are generally published chronologically, making a finding aid necessary to locate the legislation that covers a particular issue. Second, many of the online sources and easily available finding aids cover only acts that are presently "in force." Although much of the law from the American colonial period is still in force in Great Britain, a great deal is not.

Official versions of parliamentary acts can be found in the "parliament roll" for the session in which it passed. The public laws of Parliament continued to be published on a manuscript roll until the mid-nineteenth century, and the official versions are still printed on parchment and stored in the Public Records Office and at Parliament in Victoria Tower. The parliamentary rolls from the reign of Edward I through the reign of Henry VII were published starting in the eighteenth century under the name *Rotuli Parliamentorum*, many volumes of which have been digitized and are available online through Google Books. These rolls are also available through *The Parliament Rolls of Medieval England, 1275–1504,* a subscription database. The rolls from 1327 forward are available for inspection at the National Archives at Kew. The only exception is the parliamentary enactments from the Interregnum. These can be found in *Acts and Ordinances of the Interregnum, 1642–1660*, a print and online source edited by C. H. Firth and Robert S. Rait. Although the rolls are the most official source, they are rarely consulted; various printed versions of parliamentary legislation were used in the eighteenth century and are still used today.

Since the nineteenth century, a main source for acts passed before the death of Queen Anne in 1714 is the *Statutes of the Realm.* It includes acts passed by the Parliament of England to 1707 and the Parliament of Great Britain from 1708 to 1714. It has recently been reprinted and is widely available in print and through HeinOnline; some volumes are available online through Google Books and the Internet Archive. Researchers should note that while the *Statutes of the Realm* contains statutes through the early eighteenth century, it wasn't published until the early nineteenth century. Most acts since 1235 were collected and published in sets generally known as *Statutes at Large.* Attorneys of the American colonial period would have consulted these volumes. Researchers of today will also use these sources to find laws passed between 1713 and 1797. After 1797, *Public Acts* should be consulted. *Statutes at Large* is fairly widely available in print; a researcher can locate and search those published in the eighteenth century in the Eighteenth Century Collections Online database. One drawback to the *Statutes at Large* is that it usually contained only the laws in force at the time of printing. If a lag occurred between the passage of a law and its printing, which often happened during this period, and if the law was repealed in the interim, the printed source often would not contain the text of the law. In these instances, a researcher might consult additional versions of the *Statutes* or other sources.

The Justis Publishing database provides the most complete online source for finding acts of Parliament. It contains all acts, both those that have been repealed and those that are still in force from 1235. Acts can be found by full-text searches and by searches in a variety of fields, including title of the act, year or range of years, section number, and whether or not it has been repealed. Lexis and Westlaw contain full-text searchable acts currently in force from the thirteenth century, and the National Archives has made some legislation available at www. legislation.gov.uk. While this website does contain legislation as far back as the thirteenth century, complete coverage doesn't begin until 1988. Researchers should know that in addition to the lack of complete coverage of pre-1988 acts, the Parliaments of England (acts from 1267 to 1706), Great Britain (acts from 1707 to 1800), and the United Kingdom (acts from 1800 on) are housed in three different collections.

The acts contain the law as passed by Parliament. Later acts may amend or supplement earlier ones. Often, a legal researcher seeks not a specific act but rather the law on a particular topic. To find acts on a certain issue, several tools are available today.

If the acts are still in force, *Halsbury's Statutes of England,* available in print in many libraries as well as online from Lexis UK, is the best first tool. Within each category, this topical arrangement of parliamentary acts chronologically lists the parts of acts that are still in force. It offers a good index, and each edition is updated with annual supplements until the publication of the next edition. A researcher can browse *Halsbury's Statutes* as an encyclopedia or consult the index. Online, of course, full-text searching is available. In print, *Halsbury's*

Statutes is now in its fourth edition. Its contents were originally contained in a legal encyclopedia, *Halsbury's Laws,* which
started in 1907. In the late 1920s, *Halsbury's Statutes* was spun
off from *Halsbury's Laws.* If the act in question was in force at
almost any time during the twentieth century, a researcher can
turn to *Halsbury's.*

  If the law is no longer in force, several alternatives exist.
One is to conduct online searches within the databases mentioned above. If researchers know roughly when Parliament
acted, they can look through the chronological list of acts at the
front of the volumes that cover the years in question. Or if they
know the subject, they can consult the indexes in the *Statutes
of the Realm* or the *Statutes at Large* that cover the relevant years.

  Once researchers have located an act of interest, they will
want to discern whether the act was repealed or amended during the selected time period. Here, a statutory citator will help.
The easiest online tool to use is the citator JustCite, from Justis
Publishing. When searching for a statute using JustCite, or just
pulling up a statute on Justis, the service offers information
about the current status of an entire act (or section if only a
section was amended), any amendments to earlier acts made
by the selected act or section, any cases interpreting the act or
section, and any amendments to the act by later acts. In print,
the best source is the *Chronological Table of the Statutes,* which
lists every act that Parliament has passed. For each, it also indicates any later act that amended or repealed any section.
Various publishers have put out this style of resource for years;
Halsbury's version is probably the most widely available. The
current volume should have what any researcher needs. The
full set of *Halsbury's Statutes* will provide repeal and amending
information as long as the initial act was in force during the
publication history of *Halsbury's,* since 1907.

Throughout the American colonial period, topically organized versions of statutes were published, usually in abridged
versions. One example, Edmund Wingate's *An Exact Abridgment
of All Statutes in Force and Use from the Beginning of Magna
Charta* (1700), went through several editions. Several others,
including John Cay's *An Abridgment of the Publick Statutes in Force
and Use, from "Magna Charta," in the Ninth Year of King Henry
III, to the Eleventh Year of His Present Majesty King George II*
(1739), followed. Many abridgments have been recently reprinted
and may be found in libraries; otherwise, they are available at
Eighteenth Century Collections Online or Early English Books
Online.

Case Law

English law is built on a foundation of common law, which is
built on case law. Finding cases that relate to a particular topic
is critical in research. However, until the nineteenth century,
case reporting, although becoming more organized, was haphazard, and the reports varied widely in quality. During this
era, case finding—that is, finding all relevant material on
a topic—was unheard of; rather, several collections of cases
carried weight, and lawyers were on the lookout for new material. Later work has imparted some rationality on the cases
reported during this era, but it is still possible to uncover previously unknown reports of cases. The development of a rational-
ized case-reporting and case-finding system proceeded with
stops and starts and reversals and jumps forward from at least
the eighteenth century forward.

Although the eighteenth and nineteenth centuries wit-
nessed the most important developments that led to a rational
case-publishing and case-finding system, case reporting and

discovery had been developing slowly from before the advent of the printing press. There have been several important periods of case reporting in English history. From even the earliest times, basic records exist. These records were kept in "plea rolls" and are available from at least the turn of the fourteenth century; forty volumes of the plea rolls have been published. Because the rolls were created to ensure that the king collected money due or properly exacted punishment, they did not include much useful information about the development of the law. The legal reasoning used to arrive at a decision was generally not included; rather, the rolls include the fact of the verdict, perhaps the charge, and the punishment or amount due. A complete set of the plea rolls is held at the National Archives of the United Kingdom in several series, including E13 (Exchequer) and CP40 (Common Pleas). A search for the phrase "plea rolls" at the National Archives website can help locate the series reference.

Some of the plea rolls have been published by the Selden Society, a society of legal historians. These materials are available at many libraries as well as at HeinOnline. The Public Records Office published a calendar of the plea rolls, *List of Plea Rolls of Various Courts, Preserved in the Public Record Office,* in the late nineteenth century and again in the early twentieth century. These have also been reprinted and are available in many academic libraries, and some editions can be found online through HathiTrust and Google Books.

Beginning around the time of Edward II, notes of cases organized by court term began to appear. These collections, later termed "Year Books," are anonymously written and outline the reasoning of cases. The Year Books date from around 1270 and continue into the sixteenth century. Many were later collected and published. The most important collection for seventeenth- and eighteenth-century lawyers was the Vulgate edition of the Year Books that was printed by George Sawbridge between 1678 and 1680; this has been reprinted by the Selden Society in the Year Books Series.

Within its collection of annual publications, the Selden Society has published thirty-four volumes of Year Books that cover cases from 1307, the first year of Edward II's reign, to cases from the early sixteenth century. The reports in the Year Books are by no means complete records. While the origin and purpose of the Year Books remain unclear, they may have originally been designed as learning aids for or by the apprentice lawyers at the Inns of Court. The Year Books were organized by judicial terms; however, there are many terms and reigns with no cases, and some are mistakenly assigned to the wrong time.

In the sixteenth century collections of case reports, much like those included in the Year Books, ascribed to named authors begin to appear. These, the so-called Nominative or Nominate Reports, slowly became better and more useful for aspiring lawyers and researchers. The highly regarded *Les Commentaries, ou Les Reportes de Edmunde Plowden* in the sixteenth century and *Les Reports de Edward Coke ... de Diuers Resolutions & Judgemens Donnes* in the seventeenth century are good examples. From the seventeenth to the mid-eighteenth centuries, case reporting continued to grow in volume though modern commentators consider most of these reports to be lacking in quality. John William Wallace's *The Reporters, Chronologically Arranged with Occasional Remarks upon their Respective Merits* (1845), a review of the reports and the reporters, is useful for determining the value of various accounts. *The Reporters* is available at many libraries and online through Google Books.

Nominative Reports were compiled using a variety of methods. Some are the reorganized notebooks of a presiding judge, published after his retirement or death; some are reports by lawyers or other spectators outlining the proceedings. During the nineteenth century, judges began to take a greater interest in the accurate reporting of their reasoning, and the position of reporter became more professionalized. As hundreds of Nominative Reports were published in small print runs during the seventeenth and eighteenth centuries, gaining access to the various writings was difficult.

In the late eighteenth century the relations between the courts and certain reporters had become closer, and some of the reporters developed standards. While judges always had opinions about the quality of the reports, they began to favor some of them, to the extent that some judges shared their notes with the reporters. During that period, the idea of an "authorized" report developed (similar to what became designated as an "official" report in the United States). By the late nineteenth century in the United States, the government printed case reports containing the cases released by a court for publication. In the United Kingdom, private organizations printed authorized reports that contained the cases the publishers deemed important; however, these reports were given priority as the preferred version for citation and the version used by the courts. The most important, the *Law Reports*, published by the Incorporated Council of Law Reporting, has been published since 1865.

By the mid-nineteenth century it had become clear that some sort of collection of reports would make research more efficient for attorneys. One of the first collections was the 149-volume *Revised Reports; Being a Republication of Such Cases in the English Courts of Common Law and Equity, from the Year 1785, as Are Still of Practical Utility*, published in 1891 by Sweet and Maxwell. This collection reprinted the cases from law and equity from 1785 that were still of practical utility in the mid-nineteenth century. The *Revised Reports* are available in print at larger law libraries and at HeinOnline.

During the twentieth century, new series of law reports developed in the United Kingdom. The *English Reports, Full Reprint,* published in the early twentieth century, runs to 176 volumes and contains the full text of almost one hundred thousand cases decided between 1220 and 1867. The set is organized by court and includes citation to the Nominative Reports and the page breaks in the Nominative Reports. The bulk of the cases come from the late fifteenth century on. Of course, as a collection of the reports that happened to get written and happened to have been included, the *English Reports* should not be confused with a comprehensive reporter. The idea of comprehensively reporting the work of a particular court is another nineteenth-century development.

The print version of the *English Reports* is difficult to use. There are only two print finding aids: a table of cases (by name) and a table that converts Nominative Reports citations to *English Reports* citations. Therefore, online access to this set is very useful. The *English Reports* can be found online and searched at Justis, Westlaw, HeinOnline, and, for free, the Commonwealth Legal Information Institute (CommonLII, at www.Commonlii. org). All versions are backed up by PDF page images. The versions at HeinOnline and CommonLII are more difficult to search than those at Justis and Westlaw, but the data are available in all four databases.

In the 1930s, the *Law Journal* began a set of reports designed to compete with the Incorporated Council of Law Reporting's *Law Reports.* The *All England Law Reports* was begun in 1936 and covers the main courts of the United Kingdom. In the 1970s, the *All England Law Reports,* then owned by Butterworth and now a part of Lexis, published the *All England*

Law Reports Reprint. This set printed about six thousand important cases decided between 1558 and 1936.

Finally, the database of the British and Irish Legal Information Institute (BAILII, at www.bailii.org), while mainly known for more recent cases, does include some cases from the past (for example, a chancery case from 1595). This site is not nearly as comprehensive as other resources, but it is free and easy to use.

The reports of state trials are often of particular interest to historians since these volumes contain treason trials and other trials relating to offenses against the state. Several collections of state trials were published throughout the eighteenth and nineteenth centuries. The largest set, *Cobbett's Complete Collection of State Trials and Proceedings for High Treason and Other Crimes and Misdemeanors from the Earliest Period to the Present Time . . . from the Ninth Year of the Reign of King Henry, the Second, A.D. 1163, to . . . George IV, A.D. 1820,* published in the early nineteenth century, fills thirty-four volumes and includes a name and topical index. This set is available in print at many libraries (there was a 2007 reprint) and at HeinOnline. An earlier set originally collected by Thomas Salmon was first published in the early eighteenth century. It appeared in six volumes, was soon supplemented with a seventh, and reached eleven volumes by 1781. This version covers from 1388 through 1777. It is available in print at some libraries but apparently has not had a modern reprinting although Hein has made the 1720, 1737, and 1744 editions available online.

Several databases provide online access to historical cases. As previously mentioned, CommonLII has the *English Reports, Full Reprint;* HeinOnline has the *English Reports, State Trials,* the publications of the Selden Society, and some additional Year Book cases; Justis has the *English Reports, Full Reprint* as well as the *State Trials* set; Westlaw has the *English Reports, Full Reprint,* the *All England Law Reports Reprint,* and the publications of the Selden Society, which contain many Year Book cases; and Lexis provides access to the *All England Law Reports Reprint.*

The cases that can be found in the reporters mentioned above are usually cases that dealt with the application of the law to new or difficult legal or factual questions. Often, a historian would like to know how the law affected real people day to day. One website, The Proceedings of the Old Bailey (https://www.oldbaileyonline.org/), provides access to information about all cases that took place at the central criminal court in London from the seventeenth century to the twentieth. This free resource provides as much information as possible, including transcriptions of testimony, and can be searched by keyword, various name fields, offense, verdict, punishment, and time period.

Case Finding

A twenty-first-century researcher has more options than one from the seventeenth century for finding a case that deals with a specific legal topic. A modern researcher can conduct full-text online searches using Boolean logic through most cases that are available for the period up to American independence using the databases of Westlaw, Justis, HeinOnline, or CommonLII. All offer full-text searching, albeit with different syntaxes.

Full-text searching, however, may not be the most efficient way to find cases that treat a specific type of legal issue. Problems of language, such as shifts in word meanings and spellings over the centuries, and inconsistent terminology used to describe legal concepts could impede the search process. For example, taking the property of another person might be described as just that, or depending on the facts of the case, a more technical term such as "larceny," "burglary," or "embezzlement" might be used.

Sometimes a better case-finding option is a digest of cases; these have been written over the centuries, as have abridgments and treatises on particular areas of law. Each of these tools can help a researcher find cases that treat a particular legal topic. Some will also help to explain the law.

Modern researchers should also consider using the tools that lawyers of the seventeenth century used to find the law. Nicholas Statham's *Abridgment des libres annales* was first published in the late fifteenth century, but the sixteenth century saw the development of more comprehensive "grand" abridgments. These abridgements are organized alphabetically by legal topic. The law for each topic is described and cases and statutes are cited. *La Graunde Abridgement* by Anthony Fitzherbert was first published in 1514–1516. Robert Brooke's *La Graunde Abridgement,* first published in 1573 and revised in 1586, followed it. These were the most important of this genre during the first century of colonization. Three abridgments were published in the seventeenth century, but as John Baker in the chapter on legal literature in *Introduction to English Legal History* points out (4th ed.; London: Butterworths Lexis Nexis, p. 185), none was close to the standard set by Brooke. William Sheppard's *A Grand Abridgment of the Common and Statute Law of England: Alphabetically Digested Under Proper Heads and Titles . . .* (1675), William Hughes's *The Grand Abridgment of the Law Continued* (1660), and Henry Rolle's *Un Abridgment des Plusieurs Cases et Resolutions del Common Ley: Alphabeticalment Digest Desouth Severall Titles* (1668) are considered to be of mediocre to poor quality. But other than the treatises described below, these were the best material available for finding cases after Brooke. All of these abridgments of the law can be searched and browsed in the Early English Books Online database.

The mid-eighteenth century saw publication of several additional abridgments of the law. All were highly regarded and remained important tools well into the nineteenth century. *A General Abridgment of Cases in Equity Argued and Adjudged in the High Court of Chancery, &c. . . . by a Gentleman of the Middle Temple* (1734 and continued for five editions), John Comyns's *A Digest of the Laws of England* (1762), Matthew Bacon and Timothy Cunningham's *A New Abridgment of the Law* (1736), and Charles Viner's *A General Abridgment of Law and Equity: Alphabetically Digested Under Proper Titles . . .* (1742) were and remain critical to locating and understanding English law to the time of American independence. All of these abridgments can be found and their full texts can be searched through the Eighteenth Century Collections Online database. With William Blackstone's *Commentaries on the Laws of England* (1765), Viner's *General Abridgment* was one of the most important English law books in early America. In addition, some digests or abridgments brought out in the nineteenth century may be of interest. Some of these are available online through the Internet Archive, but Eighteenth Century Collections Online is the most certain resource in which to find them.

Explanations of the law also began to appear as early as the fifteenth century. The first printed book in England that tried to explain the law in a simpler form than was common in the earlier manuscript "readings" was Thomas Littleton's treatise on property law, *Tenures,* published in 1518 (written between 1450 and 1460; it was first printed in 1481). Several subsequent books written in the sixteenth century tried to describe the law and bring the expanding case law into the discussion. But the first book that we would recognize as a legal treatise was Edward

Coke's extremely important and influential *Commentary* on Littleton in 1628. This is but a part of Coke's *Institutes of the Laws of England,* the rest of which was published after his death and included a commentary on older statutes, criminal law, and the law of the crown. Coke supplied an extremely learned gloss on Littleton's text. *Coke on Littleton,* as it became known, was the principal textbook on property law in use in England into the nineteenth century.

Matthew Hale (d. 1676) was the next important legal writer. However, while Coke published his reports of cases and the first part of the *Institutes* during his lifetime, Hale directed that his writings on the law not be published. Despite that, the first to appear, the *Pleas of the Crown: or a Methodical Summary of the Principal Matters Relating to that Subject,* was published in 1678; *The History and Analysis of the Common Law of England* was published in 1713; and *The Analysis of the Law: Being a Scheme, or, Abstract, of the Several Titles and Partitions of the Law of England, Digested into Method* followed in 1713. His final book, *The Prerogatives of the King,* was not published until 1976. Some of Hale's books still remain extremely important treatments of their subjects. *Pleas of the Crown* can be found in Early English Books Online, and Hale's books published in the eighteenth century can be found and searched in Eighteenth Century Collections Online.

Blackstone's *Commentaries on the Laws of England* (1765–1769) is the most important prerevolutionary English treatise in the development of American law and also has worldwide importance (it was translated into many languages). Many editions and abridgments of Blackstone's *Commentaries* were published throughout the eighteenth and nineteenth centuries and into the twentieth. It is a readable, compact, and coherent restatement of the law of England, and it was the first source that most nineteenth-century U.S. lawyers encountered during their legal educations or when they faced a new legal problem. Reprints of the *Commentaries* are very common and should be easy to locate. It is also available free on the web through the Avalon Project of Yale Law Library and many other places, including *Early American Imprints* and Eighteenth Century Collections Online. Several editions of the complete and abridged *Commentaries* with later and U.S. cases are available at HeinOnline and the database *Making of Modern Law: Legal Treatises.*

In addition to these more complete treatises, books on more limited areas of law, for example, Samson Eure and Giles Duncombe's *Trials per Pais: Or the Law of England Concerning Juries by Nisi Prius, &c. with a Compleat Treatise of the Law of Evidence* (1718), were published throughout the seventeenth and eighteenth centuries. Others are more comprehensive, such as Geoffrey Gilbert's *The Law of Uses and Trusts: Collected and Digested in a Proper Order, from the Reports of Adjudg'd Cases, in the Courts of Law and Equity, and Other Books of Authority. Together with a Treatise of Dower* (1734). These can be found at Early English Books Online and Eighteenth Century Collections Online.

There have been several more recent digests of English case law. The most important current digest is simply titled *The Digest: Annotated British, Commonwealth, and European Cases,* first published in 1919. It provides an organized snapshot of more than five hundred thousand cases from the medieval period to today. An earlier important digest is John Mews's *Digest of English Case Law, Containing the Reported Decisions of the Superior Courts and a Selection from Those of the Scottish and Irish Courts to the End of 1924* (a later edition and supplements go forward in time, but that is beyond the scope of this chapter). In addition, more limited digests might cover a particular topic, a particular set of case reports, or a particular time period. The later nineteenth century saw publication of some digests that can shed light on eighteenth-century law, including Robert Alexander Fisher's *A Digest of the Reported Cases Determined in the House of Lords & Privy Council, and in the Courts of Common Law, Divorce, Probate, Admiralty & Bankruptcy* (1870) and Charles Petersdorff's *Practical and Elementary Abridgment of Cases in the Courts of King's Bench, Common Pleas, Exchequer, and at Nisi Prius* (1825–1830), which might be the most useful.

Over the past century some English legal encyclopedias have been published that provide a succinct statement of the law with citation to statutes or cases that express that rule. The encyclopedias are not comprehensive, but the historical researcher can still find them useful. The *Encyclopaedia of the Laws of England* was first published between 1897 and 1903. *Halsbury's Laws of England* is now in its fifth edition and has been published since the early twentieth century. The encyclopedias are organized into a logical system and also have indexes and tables of cases and statutes.

Any of these tools can be helpful, but one from the time period being researched can make the issue of whether the law later changed easier to discern. For the colonial period, the most useful source is probably John Comyn's *Digest of the Laws of England.* First published in 1762, it was owned by Thomas Jefferson, Alexander Hamilton, and Robert Treat Paine, among others. It continued to be published into the 1820s in England and the United States.

Privy Council

Among the powers that the crown retained in order to control the colonies was the right of the Privy Council to void any objectionable colonial law, the right of the colonial governor to veto legislation, and the right to appoint members of the colonial legislature's upper house in all colonies except Connecticut, Rhode Island, and Massachusetts (Massachusetts's upper house was appointed by the crown after 1774). The Privy Council also served as a court of last resort for the colonies. *Acts of the Privy Council of England: Colonial Series, 1608–1783* (London: His Majesty's Stationary Office, 1908–1912; reprint 2004), covering 1613–1783, includes an index and a table of colonial acts approved and disapproved. Joseph Henry Smith's *Appeals to the Privy Council from the American Plantations* (1950) provides detailed information about appeals to the Privy Council.

The Privy Council and increasingly over time other royal ministries were deeply involved with the workings of the colonies. The official materials that passed between the colonial governments and the royal departments were indexed in *Calendar of State Papers: Colonial Series.* Published in the nineteenth century, it covers to 1759, is chronologically arranged, and contains a brief description of an action with a citation to the document. There is also an index to the papers. Several volumes are available online through Google Books and the Internet Archive. Also, a database published by ProQuest, *Colonial State Papers,* covers the activities of the England in its various colonies from 1574 to 1759. Another version published by Gale, *State Papers Online,* covers English domestic state papers from 1509 to 1714.

Research Example

We return to the subject of witchcraft and the law, researching legislation and cases surrounding witchcraft in England from the sixteenth and seventeenth centuries as well as considering the place of law and gender in relation to claims of witchcraft in the Massachusetts Bay Colony in the late-seventeenth century. In addition to legislation and cases, we will also look for any seventeenth-century law books that might deal with witchcraft.

To find English legislation on the topic, we search the legislation database on Justis for the term "witch*," truncated using the asterisk, in the full text of the statutes passed before January 1692. This returns thirteen results from eight acts. The first, from 1511, decries the unlettered practitioners of folk medicine and requires the examination of physicians practicing within seven miles of London. The second, from 1541, makes it a felony (at the time, felonies carried the death penalty) to practice witchcraft. In 1542, an act was passed to reconcile the acts of 1511 and 1541 to ensure that herbalists could still practice. The Witchcraft Act of 1562 lessened the severity of the 1541 law by making witchcraft a felony only if another person was harmed. As we can see, the law was mainly concerned with witches as practitioners of herbal medicine. In 1580 it was made a felony to use witchcraft to attempt to determine the date upon which the queen would die. In 1603 the law was changed slightly; the second offense became a felony, and the move from ecclesiastical courts to civil courts was solidified by the requirement that a peer of the realm hear the case. Finally, in 1660 witchcraft was excluded from the general pardon act.

At the time of the Salem witch trials, under English law, the Witchcraft Act of 1603 would have been the governing statute. The statute reads: "An Act against Conjuration, Witchcraft, and dealing with evil and wicked Spirits. The Penalty for practising of Invocation or Conjuration, &c. Conjuration or Invocation, whereby any Person is killed or lamed. Declaring by Witchcraft, where any thing is hidden, Procuring unlawful Love, &c. The second Offence Felony. No Forfeiture of Dower or

Inheritance. Trial of a Peer of the Realm" (1 Ja. I, C. 12). The citation indicates that this was the twelfth law passed in the parliament that sat during the first year of the reign of James I.

Our next step is to look for cases preceding 1692 that deal with witchcraft. A search of the *English Reports* online through Justis for "(witch or witchcraft*) not slander*" returns eighty-eight cases decided between 1567 and 1688 (as well as one case from a reporter that covers a long time period, which may predate 1567). We excluded "slander" to eliminate the many cases in which the issue was not witchcraft but the slander of calling someone a witch. A search of the *English Reports* at Commonlii.org returns similar results, but while the data are the same, the search is a little more difficult to conduct. Including the term "witch*" will return the relevant cases but will also include those in which one of the parties' names starts with "witch," an unfortunately frequent occurrence. HeinOnline is a little more awkward to search. A search for "(witch OR witchcraft)" returns 340 cases before 1800, and date limits or organization by date is difficult. Limiting HeinOnline to "witchcraft" returns 141 cases, along with the same date issues.

We have now identified the English statute and a group of cases that will contain any relevant cases that, barring colonial law, would have applied to any action related to witchcraft in Massachusetts in 1692 and that did apply in Great Britain in 1692. Next we look for any contemporary treatises or other writings that can give us insight into how the law saw witchcraft in Great Britain in 1692.

The first place to turn is WorldCat. A search for the keyword "witchcraft," the Library of Congress subject heading most frequently used, and the keyword "law" further limited to material published between 1500 and 1700 brings us more than 130 bibliographic records. Several describe the same title, but we have a number of publications to turn to for a sense of the late-seventeenth-century law's treatment of witchcraft. Among the titles, we find William Drage's *A Physical Nosonomy; or, a New and True Description of the Law of God (Called Nature) in the Body of Man . . . also in the Second Part of This Book is a Practice of Physick . . . to Which is Added, a Treatise of Diseases From Witchcraft . . .* (1665), and *A Magazine of Scandall: Or, a Heape of Wickednesse of Two Infamous Ministers, Consorts, One Named Thomas Fowkes of Earle Soham in Suffolk, Convicted by Law for Killing a Man, and the Other Named John Lowes of Brandeston, Who Hath Beene Arrainged for Witchcraft* (1642).

A search in Early English Books Online for the keywords "witchcraft and law," further limited to materials published to 1700, returns more than two thousand items because the keyword search is broader than a subject search. Among the items is *A Question Deeply Concerning Married Persons and Such as Intend to Marry Propounded and Resolved According to the Scriptures, by A.L.* (1653), which instructs a woman to be obedient because "rebellion is as the sin of witchcraft." By requiring that the concept of witchcraft appear as a subject, we find Thomas Ady's *A Candle in the Dark Shewing the Divine Cause of the Distractions of the Whole Nation of England and of the Christian World* (1655). On the title page, Mr. Ady writes, "This Book is profitable to bee read by all Iudges of Assizes, before they pass the sentence of Condemnation against poor People, who are accused for Witchcraft; It is also profitable for all sorts of people to read who desire Knowledge."

Other databases, such as Gale's *17th and 18th Century Burney Newspapers Collection* or its *British Newspapers, 1600–1950* might also contain valuable material. As we move further from the law, more general historical resources come into play. A brief introduction to some of these resources appears in chapter 11.

Further Reading

Baker, J. H. *An Introduction to English Legal History.* London: Butterworth, 1997.

Baker, John H. *The Oxford History of the Laws of England.* Vol. 6. New York: Oxford University Press, 2003.

Barnard, John, and D. F. McKenzie. *The Cambridge History of the Book in Britain.* Vol. 4. Cambridge: Cambridge University Press, 2002.

Hellinga, Lotte, and J. B. Trapp. *The Cambridge History of the Book in Britain.* Vol. 3. Cambridge: Cambridge University Press, 1999.

Holdsworth, William Searle, Arthur L. Goodhart, Harold Greville Hanbury, and John McDonald Burke. *A History of English Law.* London: Methuen, 1903.

Moys, Elizabeth M. *Manual of Law Librarianship: The Use and Organization of Legal Literature.* Boulder, CO: Westview, 1976.

Important Sources Mentioned in This Chapter

Blackstone, William. *Commentaries on the Laws of England . . . By William Blackstone, Esq. Vinerian Professor of Law, and Solicitor General to Her Majesty.* Oxford, Clarendon, 1765.

Brooke, Robert. *La Graunde Abridgement, Collect & escrie per le Iudge tresreuerend Syr Robert Brooke, Chiualier.* London: In aedibus Richardi Tottell, 1573.

Cay, John. *An Abridgement of the Publick Statutes in Force and Use, from "Magna Charta," in the Ninth Year of King Henry III, to the Eleventh Year of His Present Majesty King George II, Inclusive, by John Cay . . .* London: R. Gosling, 1739.

Comyns, John. *A Digest of the Laws of England: By the Right Honourable Sir John Comyns.* London, 1762.

Fitzherbert, Anthony. *La Graunde Abridgement.* London: John Rastell and Richard Pynson, 1514.

Great Britain. "The Statutes at Large, of England and of Great-Britain from Magna Carta to the Union of the Kingdoms of Great Britain and Ireland." Printed by George Eyre and Andrew Strahan, 1811.

Great Britain, Privy Council. *Acts of the Privy Council of England: Colonial Series . . . A.D. 1613–[1783].* London: His Majesty's Stationary Office, 1908–1912.

Great Britain and Hardinge Stanley Giffard Halsbury. *The Complete Statutes of England: Classified and Annotated, in Continuation of Halsbury's*

Laws of England; And, for Ready Reference, Entitled "Halsbury's Statutes of England." Vols. 1–40. London: Butterworth, 1929.

Great Britain and Record Commission. *The Statutes of the Realm, Printed by Command of His Majesty King George the Third, in Pursuance of an Address of the House of Commons of Great Britain, from Original Records and Authentic Manuscripts [1101–1713].* London: Record Commission, 1810.

Halsbury, Hardinge Stanley Giffard. *The Laws of England: Being a Complete Statement of the Whole Law of England.* London: Butterworth, 1901.

Howell, Thomas Bayly, Thomas Jones Howell, and William Cobbett. *A Complete Collection of State Trials and Proceedings for High Treason and Other Crimes and Misdemeanors from the Earliest Period to the Year 1783: With Notes and Other Illustrations.* London, 1809.

Smith, Joseph Henry, Columbia University, and Foundation for Research in Legal History. *Appeals to the Privy Council from the American Plantations.* New York: Octagon, 1965.

Viner, Charles. *A General Abridgment of Law and Equity Alphabetically Digested under Proper Titles with Notes and References to the Whole.* London, 1742.

Databases

Gale. *Eighteenth Century Collections Online* (ECCO). http://www.gale.com/primary-sources/eighteenth-century-collections-online.

HathiTrust. Hathi Trust Digital Library. https://www.hathitrust.org/.

Justis Publishing. *English Reports, Full Reprint.* http://www.commonlii.org/uk/cases/EngR/.

———. Justis. http://www.justis.com.

Old Bailey Proceedings Online Project. *The Proceedings of the Old Bailey, London's Central Criminal Court, 1674 to 1913.* http://www.oldbaileyonline.org/.

ProQuest. *Colonial State Papers.* https://www.proquest.com/products-services/Colonial_State_Paper.html.

———. *Early English Books Online.* https://www.proquest.com/products-services/databases/eebo.html.

3
Colonial Law, 1600s–1770s

The North American colonies changed dramatically over time. From the beginning of the seventeenth century when the English possessions were merely small outposts, to the late eighteenth century when Philadelphia, Boston, and New York played important roles in the British economic system, the relationship between the colonies and London also changed. As the colonies grew from small self-governing or corporate-governed groups to complex societies with sophisticated lawyers and political thinkers, the ideas of law and government also grew. Researchers examining the resources used to find colonial-era law must keep in mind the nature of life at the time.

Each of the thirteen colonies had different fundamental laws, charters, and local legislation and courts. This chapter examines the sources and techniques useful for finding information about the legal culture and law of individual colonies. Current guides, for example, *Prestatehood Legal Materials: A Fifty-State Research Guide, Including New York City and the District of Columbia*, edited by Michael Chiorazzi and Marguerite Most, can help focus research in the states that emerged from the colonies.

A good recent history of the law in colonial America is *The Common Law in Colonial America* by William Edward Nelson. Volume 1, in a planned four-volume series, was published in 2008 and covers New England and the Chesapeake region from 1607 to 1660; volume 2, published in 2013, covers the middle colonies and the Carolinas from 1660 to 1730; and a third volume, taking the story to 1750, was published in 2016. Library catalog searches using the subject headings "law—United States—history" and "history—United States—Colonial Period, 1600–1775" either singly or together can lead to additional resources.

Legal Environment of the Colonies

The early law and legal system varied from colony to colony and differed greatly from the system that would develop after independence. The early differences, however, were those of degree and detail. Colonial residents saw themselves as English with their concurrent rights, subject to the crown and to Parliament. Exactly defining this relationship with Parliament contributed to the American Revolution, but before independence colonists accepted the right of the king or his representatives and of Parliament to make law with regard to the colonies.

The English government interacted with the colonies in a number of direct ways. The ultimate "right" to be a colony, or one of several forms, came from the executive power of the English government, either the crown or Parliament. Moreover, as Massachusetts demonstrates, the crown could change a colony from a corporate basis to a royal basis. The crown appointed governors of the royal colonies and, through the Privy Council, held ultimate power over most colonies by retaining the right to void colonial legislation and by acting as an ultimate court of appeals. Finally, the secretary of state for the Southern Department oversaw regular administration of the colonies until 1768, when the colonial or "American" secretary was appointed. Under the secretary of state, most of the day-to-day administrative work was entrusted to the Lords of Trade and Plantations, now called the Board of Trade.

Each of the thirteen colonies destined to become the United States operated under a charter, which set out the basic organization and governing rules. The three types of colony, each with a slightly different ultimate source of law, included proprietorship, corporate, and royal. The proprietorship colonies— Pennsylvania and Maryland—were owned by the Penn family and Lord Baltimore, respectively, under a personal grant from the king. Several colonies were organized under corporate grants—for example, a corporate body held the charters of Connecticut and Rhode Island up to independence—and the remainder were held as royal colonies, with the charter from the crown and with the crown holding a significant amount of residual rights. The underlying basis of each colony mattered in some issues and with regard to certain procedures but in other ways had little role in the daily lives of the colonists. Not every colony was organized the same way over the nearly two centuries of its colonyship. Massachusetts, for example, changed from being a corporate colony to being part of the Dominion of New England; after its charter was revoked in 1684, it resembled a royal colony during the lead-up to and through the Glorious Revolution. However, all colonies operated under a charter, had a colonial legislature, and had some sort of executive, whether a royal governor, proprietor, or corporate representative. Each had some sort of court system to adjudicate disputes that could appeal to the royal governor and, if the losing party could afford it, to the Privy Council. All colonies except Connecticut and

Rhode Island had to submit their laws to the Privy Council for approval.

The administration of the colonies created several kinds of documents, for example, correspondence between the individual colonies and the Lords of Trade, the secretary of state, and the Privy Council; the acts of the Privy Council that related to the colonies or disputes based in the colonies; and acts and sessional papers of the colonies that would have been sent to London for approval.

The *Calendar of State Papers, Colonial Series: American and West Indies* is the best resource for locating material up to 1738. It contains the text or abstract of the most important papers relating to the colonies. These volumes, printed in the nineteenth century, are available through British History Online, a subscription database; at larger libraries; or online through Google Books, the Internet Archive, and elsewhere. The full text of abstracted materials and other information related to the colonies can be found in the United Kingdom's National Archives, mainly in record groups CO1 (up to 1688) and CO5 (after 1688). Entry books or materials received, original correspondence, and the like may be found in other record groups. The National Archives has a very nice short guide to the title (http://www.nationalarchives.gov.uk/help-with-your-research/research-guides/america-west-indies-calendar-state-papers-colonial-1573–1739/). From 1738 through 1783, two British organs had the main responsibility for the colonies: the secretary of state for the Southern Department had the responsibility until 1768, and the American Secretary for the remainder of the period. Any difficulty in research due to the multiplicity of sources for material from the period after 1738 is made easier by C. M. Andrews's *Guide to the Materials for American History to 1783 in the Public Record Office of Great Britain* (1912), available online through Google Books and at many libraries. This guide provides clear descriptions of the materials at the National Archives; however, the National Archives has changed the referencing system since the early twentieth century, so researchers must translate the references in Andrews to the current referencing system.

Researchers interested solely in the era of the American Revolution should consult *Documents of the American Revolution, 1770–1783* (Colonial Office series), a twenty-one-volume set edited by K. G. Davies. This set is available in many academic libraries and can be searched, but not read, online through HathiTrust and Google Books.

While the rights and laws of England were the primary source of the laws of the colonies, local laws also governed. There was not a great deal of English publishing of American law, nor were there many publications that covered more than one colony. One significant exception was John Nicholson's *An Abridgement of the Laws in Force and Use in Her Majesty's Plantations: (viz.) of Virginia, Jamaica, Barbadoes, Maryland, New-England, New-York, Carolina, &c. Digested under Proper Heads in the Method of Mr. Wingate, and Mr. Washington's Abridgments,* published in 1704 in London. This resource is available at Eighteenth Century Collections Online and through the Law Library Microform Consortium's database, giving today's researcher a look at local laws of the time.

The charter of each colony set forth the limits of local authority and, possibly, the structure of local governance. But as seen in the case of Massachusetts, the charter could be revoked and replaced. Local legislatures could make law within the colonies, and they had mechanisms to settle disputes and a well-defined judiciary. These institutions developed in many ways over the course of the colonial era.

Because the underlying law was that of England, it is worth asking how the colonists knew the laws of England. To answer this, we first look at the number of lawyers in the colonies and the training they received. At the time, common law was not a university-based course of study. In England one apprenticed at the Inns of Court; in the colonies one apprenticed with an attorney. The first American law school did not appear until shortly after independence: William and Mary traces its law school to the appointment of George Wythe, with whom Thomas Jefferson apprenticed, as a professor of law in 1780. However, Tapping Reeve's expanded law school moved from his apprenticeship of lawyers to a lecture-based course of study at Litchfield, Connecticut, in 1784, and this has often been held as the first American law school. Overall, the number of trained lawyers in the colonies, while not known with great precision, was quite small, but it appears that at least the more important lawyers had access to English legal materials.

One of the great difficulties colonial lawyers faced was a lack of primary law books. No published reports of American courts were issued until 1789; no major legal treatises were published in the colonies until Blackstone's *Commentaries* was reprinted in Philadelphia in 1771–1772; and almost no technical legal doctrine existed until the controversy over the ratification of the federal Constitution. The law books of colonial America—north and south—were largely English imports. The dependence of the American colonial bench and bar on English publishing is dramatically evident from Herbert Johnson's study of the libraries of American lawyers, *Imported Eighteenth-Century Law Treatises in American Libraries, 1700–1799* (1978) and from a similar study of fourteen colonial Virginia lawyers' libraries by William Hamilton Bryson, *Census of Law Books in Colonial Virginia* (1978). The owners of most of these libraries (the two studies overlap somewhat) were wealthy and socially elite. There is, however, confirmation of the widespread distribution of law books in some general studies of reading in early America.

Johnson's study gives us a good idea of the wide range of the imported treatises, but he does not include court reports and statutes in his analysis. He does, however, include an appendix to his book with the complete inventories of five lawyers' libraries. Each contains a good collection of English reporters, and four of the five inventories also include at least one set of English statutes. Likewise, almost all of the Virginia libraries analyzed by Bryson contained a substantial number of court reports. In his Introduction, Johnson states:

> It is important to recognize that case reports formed the backbone of American law libraries ... [T]he law reports from the Westminster common law courts, as well as the reports of the English High Court of Chancery, were staple reading materials for American lawyers. ... Also included in American law libraries were statutory compilations. English statutes are most prominent in the colonial period, and they are usually supplemented by the appropriate colonial or state statutes. (*Imported Eighteenth-Century Law Treatises,* pp. xi–xii)

Finding tools, such as abridgments of cases and statutes and law dictionaries, were also present in virtually every library studied by Johnson and Bryson. The abridgments by Matthew Bacon and Charles Viner were the most popular, while Giles Jacob's *New Law Dictionary* was by far the most common dictionary. Each library also had several practice manuals and formbooks. The frequency with which works of legal history and philosophy appear—often by continental authors and sometimes in Latin or French—reflects the sophistication of these lawyers. Similarly, many of the libraries contained works on international law, civil law, and Roman law.

The findings of Johnson and Bryson are reinforced by the catalogs, broadsides, and newspaper advertisements of colonial booksellers. Further confirmation that law books were in considerable demand and English imports sold well can be drawn from descriptions of some of the founders' libraries at the now dormant group Libraries of Early America at LibraryThing. com (https://www.librarything.com/groups/PLEA). Note that although the group is dormant, the data is currently still available. This is a great example of one of the potential problems with crowd-sourced initiatives.

Publication of American law books came slowly from the earliest American printing presses. Not surprisingly, these first books were not carefully written legal treatises. There was, after all, very little American law to synthesize and analyze in the first years of settlement. They were instead publications of the colonial governments, often statutory, and "how-to" manuals and formbooks primarily designed for justices of the peace, law officers, and town officials.

In the chapter titled "Arts and Letters" in *Colonial America to 1763* (chapter 13), Thomas L. Purvis tracks the development of printing in the American colonies. He recounts that Cambridge, Massachusetts, was the home of American printing from 1639 to 1675. Additional presses were set up in Boston in 1675; Jamestown, Virginia, in 1682; Maryland in 1685; Philadelphia in 1685; and New York in 1693. By 1755 only an estimated twenty-one presses were in operation. Thirty-four presses operated in fifteen towns of ten of the American colonies by 1763. Specialized law publishing did not develop in America until Stephen Gould, who had started a printing business and bookshop in New York City in 1790, began in 1803 to concentrate on legal publications.

Colonial Charters and Legislation

As we have seen, each colony's charter or grant from the crown formed its basic law. In addition to these quasi-constitutional documents, many colonies were empowered to pass legislation that was binding in their territory. Most colonies had to send all such laws to the Privy Council for approval. In most instances, colonial legislation was published fairly quickly and in fairly close geographical proximity to the colony. The laws were published in chronological sets during the seventeenth and eighteenth centuries and were fairly widely available. These laws have been included online at *Early American Imprints* and HeinOnline. They can be easily found with a search for the title laws, using the name of the colony as the author. The full text of these laws can also be searched. Colonial charters can be found in Benjamin Perley Poore's *The Federal and State Constitutions, Colonial Charters, and Other Organic Laws of the United States* (1878) and F. N. Thorpe's *The Federal and State Constitutions, Colonial Charters, and Other Organic Laws of the United States, Territories and Colonies Now or Heretofore Forming the United States of America* (1909).

A major problem with chronologically printed material, whether cases or legislation, is that finding the law that relates to a particular topic in such material is fairly difficult. The process of publishing and tracking chronologically arranged legislation differs little from the eighteenth to the early nineteenth centuries; a more complete discussion of the process appears in chapter 5. The move toward the codification of the law did not gain steam in the United States until the nineteenth century; however, during the eighteenth century, legislatures occasionally organized and published laws in a topical arrangement. Often, they passed the rearrangement as a law, commonly with the added consequence of repealing the prior versions of the law. The repeal of prior laws would not cause much difficulty unless mistakes were made in creating the new arrangement or the new arrangement was not widely available. *Early American Imprints* also includes these rearrangements of the law, and they can be found with the same searches that uncover the chronological sets.

Statutory compilations were published for Massachusetts in 1648, 1660, and 1672, with supplements for the years in between. Major compilations were prepared and printed in America for most of the other colonies—Connecticut in 1673; New Hampshire, 1699; Maryland, 1700; Pennsylvania, 1714; Rhode Island, 1719; Virginia, 1733; Delaware, 1741; New York, 1752; and New Jersey, 1758. Compilations were also published in London for some of the colonies. In addition, session laws for individual legislative sessions were published in most of the colonies on a regular basis. In fact, government publications were quite extensive in many of the colonies and were largely legal in nature. The earliest state statutory compilations included the following:

- Connecticut: Book of General Laws (Cambridge, 1673)
- Delaware: Laws of Government (Philadelphia, 1741)
- Georgia: Digest of Laws (Philadelphia, 1801)
- Maryland: Abridgment of Laws (London, 1704; covers at least six other colonies as well) and Acts of Assembly (London, 1723)

- Massachusetts: Abstract of the Laws (London, 1641; never adopted) and Book of General Laws and Liberties (1648)
- New Jersey: Acts of the Province (Philadelphia, 1732)
- New Hampshire: Acts and Laws (Boston, 1716)
- New York: Laws and Acts (New York, 1694)
- North Carolina: Abridgement of Laws (London, 1704); see Maryland and Collection of Public Acts in Force (Newbern, 1751)
- Pennsylvania: Laws of the Province of Pennsylvania (Philadelphia, 1714)
- Rhode Island: Acts and Resolves (Newport, 1705)
- South Carolina: Laws of the Province (Charles-Town, 1736)
- Virginia: Laws of Virginia (London, 1662)

Eventually, all of the colonies had session laws and some sort of compilation of statutes. The compilations and session laws are available to researchers online through *Early American Imprints*. The *Acts of the Privy Council of England* can serve as a good backup for legislation that might be missing for any state except Connecticut and Rhode Island. When looking for the law of a particular jurisdiction, a search for the title "laws" and the name of the colony as the author will return the laws of the colony.

Royal Governors' Proclamations and Colonial Records

In the early twentieth century, Clarence Brigham collected the royal proclamations relating to the American colonies into a twelve-volume set, *British Royal Proclamations Relating to*

America, 1603–1783. The set includes only proclamations made by the king, with a few proclaimed by lord justices in the king's absence. Frequently reprinted, *Royal Proclamations* is organized chronologically with a brief index and is available at many libraries. It has also been digitized and is available online through the Internet Archive's collection of books.

Royal proclamations issued during the English Civil War can be found in the *Calendar of the Proceedings of the Committee for Compounding, etc., 1643–1660: Preserved in the State Paper Department of Her Majesty's Public Record Office.* Those issued at other times that were not royal but were approved by the Privy Council can be found in the *Privy Council Register.* During the nineteenth century, many states published collections of their colonial records, which may remain in the states' archives. For example, the *Public Records of the Colony of Connecticut* covering 1636–1776 was published in the last half of the nineteenth century. A good method for locating these is to conduct a subject search in WorldCat or another catalog using the subject "[state name]—history—Colonial period, ca. 1600–1775—sources." Be aware that searches for New York must specify state or city, "New York (state)—history," and so on. These collections, often available online through HathiTrust, Google Books, or the Internet Archive, are good sources for governors' proclamations.

Other Legal Materials Published in the Colonies

Among the earliest nonstatutory legal publications printed in the colonies was a collection of documents relating to English liberties prepared by or for William Penn and designed to assure new Pennsylvania settlers of their rights under English law. This potentially provocative compendium, *The Excellent*

Privilege of Liberty and Property Being the Birth-right of the Free-born Subjects of England, was printed in Philadelphia in 1687.

The influence of English law and legal publishing can be seen in other compilations of English documents enumerating rights, which the colonists later used against the crown and colonial administrations in their political struggles. Henry Care's *English Liberties, or the Free-Born Subjects Inheritance* was printed in London around 1680 for Benjamin Harris, who was forced to flee to America in 1686 in part for his publication of this book. Five thousand copies of it were confiscated by crown officers in England and destroyed, ironically, in view of its title and contents. *English Liberties* was reprinted in Boston in 1721 and in Providence in 1774, and many colonial lawyers had copies of the several earlier London editions.

One of the most interesting genres of colonial legal publishing is the practice manual. Many were compiled and published in the colonies and drew heavily from English justice of the peace manuals. Colonial justices and other officials, as well as educated citizenry, needed guidance in legal procedures and in managing the associated forms and documents. Widely used in England, practice manuals were even more important in the colonies where access to the few lawyers was often limited. An American manual typically included some narrative text summarizing the relevant law; excerpts from Blackstone, Coke, and other leading English writers; statutory excerpts and other important legal documents; a history of the office being served; and legal forms with instructions for their use. The content of the American manuals was strikingly similar to that of the English models. The early American versions drew heavily on and directly from Michael Dalton's *Country Justice* and William Nelson's *Office and Authority of the Justice of the Peace,* while later examples were based on Richard Burn's *Justice of the Peace.*

Perhaps the most popular American manual was *Conductor Generalis,* first published in New York in 1711 and then followed by seven later editions in New York, New Jersey, and Pennsylvania, before independence. Four more editions were issued after independence. Similar works, with different sources and configurations, appeared in Virginia in 1736, South Carolina in 1761, Massachusetts in 1773, and North Carolina in 1774. Interestingly, those in the southern colonies had more local content and were designed more for the particular colony of publication. These guides have been fully analyzed by John Conley in "Doing It by the Book: Justice of the Peace Manuals and English Law in Eighteenth Century America."

Colonial Court Decisions

Researchers must take care to distinguish between what attorneys consider court decisions and court records. Court decisions are most often the reports of courts considering matters of law. Court records include the materials filed and created during the process of a matter before a particular court.

Colonial court decisions are more easily treated. There was virtually no case reporting in the prerevolutionary colonies. A few judges' notebooks and other collections of the cases from particular courts for particular sessions were published during the time or have been published since. A catalog search using date restrictions and the subject term "law reports, digests, etc." and the name of the colony should produce them. Other case-finding tools described in chapters 5, 6, and 7 include some colonial cases.

Some of the few colonial reports include the following:

Ames, Susie M. *County Court Records of Accomack-Northampton, Virginia 1640–1645.* Charlottesville: University Press of Virginia, 1973.

Bond, Carroll T., Richard B. Morris, American Historical Association, Great Britain, Privy Council, Judicial Committee, Maryland, and Court of Appeals. *Proceedings of the Maryland Court of Appeals: 1695–1729.* Washington, DC: American Historical Association, 1933.

Connecticut, and Particular Court. *Records of the Particular Court of Connecticut, 1639–1663.* Hartford: Connecticut Historical Society, 1928.

Connecticut, Particular Court, and Annie Eliot Trumbull. *Records of the Particular Court of the Colony of Connecticut. Administration of Sir Edmond Andros, Royal Governor, 1687–1688.* Hartford, CT: Privately printed, 1935.

———. *Records of the Particular Court of the Colony of Connecticut. Administration of Sir Edmond Andros, Royal Governor, 1687–1688.* Hartford, CT: Privately printed, 1935.

Connecticut, Superior Court, William Samuel Johnson, John T. Farrell, and American Historical Association. *The Superior Court Diary of William Samuel Johnson, 1772–1773: With Appropriate Records and File Papers of the Superior Court of the Colony of Connecticut for the Terms, December 1772, through March 1773.* Washington, DC: American Historical Association, 1942.

Delaware (Colony) County Court (Kent County), and Léon Valinger. *Court Records of Kent County, Delaware, 1680–1705.* Washington, DC: American Historical Association, 1959.

Hoffer, Peter Charles. *Criminal Proceedings in Colonial Virginia: [Records of] Fines, Examination of Criminals, Trials of Slaves, Etc., from March 1710 [1711] to [1754], [Richmond County, Virginia].* Athens: University of Georgia Press, 1984.

Horle, Craig W., Colonial Society of Pennsylvania, and Welcome Society of Pennsylvania. *Records of the Courts of Sussex County, Delaware, 1677–1710.* Philadelphia: University of Pennsylvania Press, 1991.

Maryland (Colony) County Court (Prince George Co.), Philip Crowl, and Joseph Henry Smith. *Court Records of Prince Georges County, Maryland 1696–1699.* Washington, DC: American Historical Association, 1964.

Massachusetts, County Court (Essex County), George Francis Dow, Massachusetts, and Inferior Court (Essex County). *Records and Files of the*

Quarterly Courts of Essex County, Massachusetts. Salem, MA: Essex
Institute, 1911.

Massachusetts Superior Court of Judicature, Josiah Quincy, Samuel M.
Quincy, and Horace Gray. *Reports of Cases Argued and Adjudged in
the Superior Court of Judicature of the Province of Massachusetts Bay,
between 1761 and 1772.* Boston: Little, Brown, 1865.

Morris, Richard B., New York (State), Mayor's Court (New York), and
American Historical Association. *Select Cases of the Mayor's Court of
New York City: 1674–1784.* Washington, DC: American Historical As-
sociation, 1935.

Noble, John, John Francis Cronin, Massachusetts, and Court of Assistants.
*Records of the Court of Assistants of the Colony of the Massachusetts
Bay, 1630–1692.* Boston: County of Suffolk, 1901.

Parker, Mattie Erma Edwards, William S. Price, Robert J. Cain, North Caro-
lina, and Division of Archives and History. *North Carolina Higher-
Court Records.* Raleigh, NC: Department of Cultural Resources,
Division of Archives and History, 1968.

Pynchon, William, and Joseph Henry Smith. *Colonial Justice in Western
Massachusetts (1639–1702) the Pynchon Court Record; an Original
Judges' Diary of the Administration of Justice in the Springfield Courts
in the Massachusetts Bay Colony.* Cambridge: Harvard University Press,
1961.

Rhode Island, Vice-Admiralty Court, and Dorothy S. Towle. *Records of the
Vice-Admiralty Court of Rhode Island, 1716–1752.* Washington, DC:
American Historical Association, 1936.

South Carolina Court of Chancery, Anne King Gregorie, James Nelson Fri-
erson, and American Historical Association. *Records of the Court of
Chancery of South Carolina, 1671–1779.* Washington, DC: American
Historical Association, 1950.

Virginia (Colony) County Court (Northampton County), and Susie May
Ames. *County Court Records of Accomack-North-Hampton, Virginia,
1632–1640.* Washington, DC: American Historical Association, 1954.

Researchers should keep in mind that an eighteenth-
century lawyer would have had fewer local cases available for
reference. But as an active member of the bar in a small society,
a colonial lawyer would know about precedential cases and the
preferences of judges.

Colonial Court Records

While court decisions contain the reasoning of a court in coming to a conclusion, records of the courts will typically include the dockets, minutes, and file papers. The docket is a listing with brief descriptions of all documents filed and notice of all sessions held concerning a case. The minutes or records are generally brief descriptions of the matter, including the result. The file papers include materials filed at the court by the parties to the case. Generally, cases are organized chronologically by when they were filed. Most collections at courthouses or archives will have an index by party name. The dockets and minutes are often available in state archives, and a few have been reprinted.

The information available in the records varies widely by court and date. Case files present additional challenges. In the colonial era, because of cost, few papers would be generated regarding the underlying issue in a case. Also, fewer and shorter papers would likely be filed during the course of litigation. A researcher should not be surprised to see that the older a case file is, the smaller it is likely to be. Several other issues related to case files continue to this day. First, many courts return the materials to the litigants at the end of a case. Second, many courts destroy case files after a certain date. Finally, case files can be destroyed accidentally. As with everything, the farther back in time one goes, the more likely that materials may be missing or destroyed; but in general, a researcher can expect to have access to dockets and record books for many courts, and for some, case files may also be available. All of these materials will be held at state archives. More information about working with archives appears in chapter 8.

How might the law have been enforced in colonial America? Generally, a problem would be brought to a local governmental representative, often a sheriff or more likely a justice of the peace. These judicial officers were not trained in the law, but at least in the eighteenth century, they had access to justice of the peace manuals. Once a trained lawyer became involved, in the guise of either an advocate or a judge, they would likely have access to the colony's legislation and a good collection of English legal abridgments, case reporters, and other publications. Because the bar was small, local attorneys were likely to know a local judge's important interpretations of law. However, the underlying source of law, the laws of England, appears to have been fairly widely available in one form or another. It is when lawyers began to look for American law that the difficulties arose.

Research Example

Let us continue our research about witchcraft and the law from the previous chapter. We located English statutes that would have been in force in 1692, we found cases that may shed further light on the law, and we identified some publications that allow us to understand the tenor of the time. Here, we locate the Massachusetts laws about witchcraft. First, we determine whether Massachusetts statutes on witchcraft exist, then we look for available cases. Finally, we can search for books or news articles that might give us further flavor.

There are a few ways to look for statutory law. One method takes advantage of the "uniform authors" and "uniform titles" that catalogers assign to classes of books with inconsistent titles or authors. For example, no matter what a publisher calls a book containing session laws, the cataloger will assign it the uniform title of "laws, (etc.)." A book of laws is "written" by the legislature, so the name of the colony or state will be assigned as the uniform author. Consequently, a search at *Early American Imprints* for items published between 1600 and 1700 with the author "Massachusetts" and the title "laws" that also requires the truncated term "witch*" to appear in the text returns five documents. The first is the 1648 collection of the laws and liberties of Massachusetts. In the 1648 laws, the Second Capital law says that any man or woman who is a witch, who "consulteth with a familiar spirit," shall be put to death. The legal basis cites the Bible. The same law is repeated in the 1660 and 1672 versions of the general laws of the colony. From 1672 to 1692, the legislature did not address witchcraft. Therefore, before 1692, witchcraft was a capital crime in Massachusetts.

We can check several resources to find relevant cases from Massachusetts. Most of these, including the major collections of reported cases, will be treated with other case-finding tools in chapters 6 and 7. The list that our search above returned provides some case reports that cover our period. Of course, an attorney in Salem was unlikely to have access to them. Another way to identify case reports is to search WorldCat. A search for the subject "law reports, digests" and "Massachusetts" with a date restrictor eliminating cases published after 1700 is too limiting, since most reports from the colonial period were published long after. The same search with no date limitation returns more than five hundred items. We can look through the list and save the few that cover the seventeenth century. By displaying the chosen items in chronological order, we can quickly see the older items. Among the potentially interesting items is *Records and Files of the Quarterly Courts of Essex County, Massachusetts,* which includes Salem sessions.

After locating the statutes and searching for contemporary cases, we may want to look for contemporary news stories, pamphlets, or other publications from the colonies that discuss witchcraft. A search of *Early American Imprints* for all items that contain the term "witchcraft" and were published before 1701 returns twenty-four items. Of these, seven precede the Salem trials. The items printed before Salem include the laws of Massachusetts from 1660; a 1677 pamphlet written during King Philip's War by Increase Mather about the perfidy of the Native Americans; a 1684 essay by Increase Mather describing various times when God affected life in New England, including several cases of witchcraft; the 1685 laws of New Plymouth colony; an essay related to witchcraft and possessions by Cotton Mather from 1689; a 1689 essay by John Palmer in which witchcraft is mentioned, but not discussed; and two publications by George Keith, one from 1689 and the other from 1690, in which he argues strongly against the Mathers' accusations of witchcraft against various colonists during the preceding years.

The next five items contain four contemporary sermons and other printed pamphlets, three of them by Cotton Mather. The five also contain the laws passed by the session of the Massachusetts colonial legislature that began in June 1692 that contains "An Act Against Conjuration, Witchcraft, and Dealing with Evil and Wicked Spirits." The ten remaining items published in the seventeenth century begin the debate and recriminations. These include three more items by Increase and Cotton Mather as well as two by Thomas Maule arguing against the Mathers, one of which was titled *New-England pesecutors* [sic] *mauled with their own weapons.*

Readex's database *America's Historical Newspapers, 1690–2000* may contain some interesting material. However, the earliest mention of the term "witchcraft" found in a recent search was a 1721 item in the *American Mercury,* a

Philadelphia paper, with a London dateline reporting the results of trials under the Inquisition in Madrid. The first item that might be of interest to us is the second item, a dialog between a clergyman and layman published in the January 15–22, 1722, edition of the *New England Courant* in which the layman takes the clergyman to task, asking "who have been instruments of mischief and trouble both in church and state, from the witchcraft ... [W]ho is it that take the liberty to vilify a whole town in words too black to be repeated?"

By examining the pamphlet literature in *Early American Imprints* and the news in *America's Historical Newspapers,* we can see the Mathers' inciting the fear of witchcraft, we can see the government's reaction during the period of the trials, and we can watch the response to the horrors of the trials. We can see that thirty years after the trials, they were held against the clergy.

Further Reading

Cohen, Daniel A. "An Overview: The Succession of Genres, 1674–1860." In *Pillars of Salt, Monuments of Grace: New England Crime Literature and the Origins of American Popular Culture, 1674–1860,* 3–38. New York: Oxford University Press, 1993.

"The Common Law Right to Inspect and Copy Judicial Records: In Camera or on Camera." *Georgia Law Review* 16 (1981): 659–93.

Conley, John A. "Doing It by the Book: Justice of the Peace Manuals and English Law in Eighteenth Century America." *Journal of Legal History* 6 (1985): 257–98.

Farrand, Max. *The Laws and Liberties of Massachusetts: Reprinted from the Copy of the 1648 Edition in the Henry E. Huntington Library.* Cambridge: Harvard University Press, 1929.

Flaherty, David H. "The Use of Early American Court Records in Historical Research." *Law Library Journal* 69 (1976): 342–46.

Gersack, Dorothy. "Colonial, State, and Federal Court Records: A Survey."
       American Archivist 36, no. 1 (1973): 33–42.

James, Eldon R. *A List of Legal Treatises Printed in the British Colonies and the
       American States Before 1801.* Union, NJ: Lawbook Exchange, 2002.

Nelson, William Edward. *The Common Law in Colonial America.* New York:
       Oxford University Press, 2008.

Salmon, Marylynn. "Notes and Documents: The Court Records of Philadel-
       phia, Bucks, and Berks Counties in the Seventeenth and Eighteenth
       Centuries." *Pennsylvania Magazine of History and Biography* 107,
       no. 2 (1983): 249–91.

White, G. Edward. *Law in American History.* Oxford: Oxford University Press,
       2012.

Important Sources Mentioned in This Chapter

Andrews, Charles McLean. *Guide to the Materials for American History, to 1783
       in the Public Record Office of Great Britain.* Washington, DC: Carnegie
       Institution, 1912.

Brigham, Clarence S. *British Royal Proclamations Relating to America, 1603–
       1783.* New York: Franklin, 1965.

Bryson, William Hamilton. *Census of Law Books in Colonial Virginia.* Charlot-
       tesville: University Press of Virginia, 1978.

Chiorazzi, Michael G., and Marguerite Most. *Prestatehood Legal Materials: A
       Fifty-State Research Guide, Including New York City and the District of
       Columbia.* New York: Haworth Information Press, 2005.

*Conductor Generalis; Or, A Guide for Justices of the Peace, and Coroners, Con-
       stables, Jury-Men, Over-Seers of the Poor, Surveyors of High-Ways,
       Governors of Fairs, Gaolers, &c.: A Treatise Briefly Shewing the Extent
       and Latitude of the Several Offices, with the Power of the Officers
       Therein: To Which Is Added Copies of Warrants, Mittimusses, Recogni-
       zances, and Other Necessary Instruments.* New York, 1711. Davies, K. G.
       Documents of the American Revolution, 1770–1783. Colonial Office
       Series. Shannon: Irish University Press, 1972–.

Jacob, Giles. *A New Law-Dictionary: Containing the Interpretation and Defini-
       tion of Words and Terms Used in the Law* . . . Printed by E. and R. Nutt
       and R. Gosling in the Savoy, 1729.

Johnson, Herbert Alan. *Imported Eighteenth-Century Law Treatises in Amer-
       ican Libraries, 1700–1799.* Knoxville: University of Tennessee Press,
       1978.

Public Record Office (Great Britain), William Noel Sainsbury, J. W. Fortescue, Cecil Headlam, and Arthur Percival Newton. *Calendar of State Papers, Colonial Series* . . . London, 1860.

Public Records of the Colony of Connecticut [1636–1776] . . . *Transcribed and Published (in Accordance with a Resolution of the General Assembly) under the Supervision of the Secretary of State, with Occasional Notes, and an Appendix.* Hartford: Brown & Parsons, 1850.

4

Constitutional Law, 1780s

Although the Constitution of the United States is extremely important to U.S. law and legal history, researchers should keep in mind that it is not the only constitution in play, nor was it the first. This chapter examines sources for information about the U.S. and state constitutions; constitutional conventions, especially the Constitutional Convention of 1787; the ratification of the U.S. Constitution; and the ratification of the Bill of Rights and other amendments. It also looks at proposed amendments to the Constitution and will consider tools to help researchers understand what the Constitution meant to Americans of different eras.

First State Constitutions

Even before the Declaration of Independence was promulgated on July 4, 1776, states had begun to work on their own constitutions. State constitutional histories vary. Some states have had several constitutions, and some have had one. It is difficult to amend some state constitutions and easy to amend others.

However, common histories, tools, and themes run through the research into state constitutions. The first thing to notice about the earliest constitutions of the original thirteen states is that almost all date from the Revolution.

While many states have changed their constitutions since the eighteenth century, initial constitutions are often in demand by researchers, who can find them through several sources. For example, the website of the Center for Constitutional Studies at the National Humanities Institute (http://www.nhinet.org/ccs/docs.htm) provides access to the earliest constitutions of ten of the original thirteen states. Connecticut continued to operate under a version of the Charter of 1662, with the references to monarchy removed, available at the center's site, and Rhode Island under its 1663 charter, available at the Rhode Island Charter Museum (http://sos.ri.gov/divisions/Civics-And-Education/charter-museum). Georgia had three antebellum constitutions, of 1777, 1789, and 1798, all of which are available at the Digital Library of Georgia (http://georgiainfo.galileo.usg.edu/topics/government/articles/constitutions) at the University of Georgia Libraries.

These websites provide easy access to the first constitutions, but a researcher often needs more than the bare text. All of the first constitutions and more can be found in William Swindler's *Sources and Documents of United States Constitutions,* an eleven-volume set that includes constitutions and other documents for each state in chronological order, along with background notes, editorial comments linking provisions of preceding and following constitutions, selected bibliographies, and indexes.

Researchers who need more information about state constitutional conventions should examine *State Constitutional Conventions, Commissions, and Amendments (1776–1988),* a microfiche set available at many larger libraries originally from the Congressional Information Service. Access to the information is through printed bibliographies, such as C. E. Browne's *State Constitutional Conventions, from Independence to the Completion of the Present Union, 1776–1959: A Bibliography* (1973) as well as the Congressional Information Service's *State Constitutional Conventions, Commissions and Amendments, 1959–1978: An Annotated Bibliography* and *State Constitutional Conventions, Commissions & Amendments, 1979–1988: An Annotated Bibliography* (1989).

This microfiche set has recently been joined by a module of the *Making of American Law* series of databases, *Making of American Law: Primary Sources I and II,* which includes fully searchable copies of documents produced up to 1970 relating to, among other things, state constitutional conventions. It allows full-text and other searching, including author, title, subject, and back-of-the-book indexes. The database also allows researchers to limit their searches to constitutional convention material from among the variety of materials included in the database.

Two federal government documents published near the turn of the twentieth century pull together the organic laws of the states and territories: Benjamin Perley Poore's *The Federal and State Constitutions, Colonial Charters, and Other Organic Laws of the United States* (1878) and F. N. Thorpe's *The Federal and State Constitutions, Colonial Charters, and Other Organic Laws of the United States, Territories and Colonies Now or Heretofore Forming the United States of America* (1909).

The Constitutions of the States: A State by State Guide and Bibliography to Current Scholarly Research (1988) by Bernard D. Reams and Stuart D. Yoak is an important resource for finding recent scholarship on state constitutions. Researchers should also search library catalogs to locate monographs as well as the indexes and other tools that lead to periodicals from the historical and legal academies.

Guides to the Federal Constitution

Several excellent basic guides to the U.S. Constitution include David A. Schultz's *The Encyclopedia of the United States Constitution* (2009), David Spinoza Tanenhaus's *Encyclopedia of the Supreme Court of the United States* (2008), and Leonard W. Levy, Kenneth L. Karst, and Adam Winkler's *Encyclopedia of the American Constitution* (2nd ed., 2000). Kermit L. Hall's one-volume *Oxford Companion to the Supreme Court of the United States* (2nd ed., 2005) deserves a place on the bookshelves of anyone conducting research into the court or the Constitution. A recent multivolume treatise on U.S. constitutional law, Ronald D. Rotunda and John E. Nowak's *Treatise on Constitutional Law: Substance and Procedure* (5th ed., 2012), is geared to lawyers and law students and might not be "historical" enough for some researchers. However, treatises designed for lawyers or law students from the nineteenth or twentieth century may be just the resource for discovering how the U.S. Supreme Court interpreted the Constitution in different periods. The Oliver Wendell Holmes Devise *History of the Supreme Court of the United States* series is one of the best recent studies of the court and the Constitution. This series contains individual treatises by eminent legal historians, and each covers a period of the history of the court.

Several bibliographies contain materials on constitutional law; fairly recent ones of note include Kermit L. Hall's *A Comprehensive Bibliography of American Constitutional and*

Legal History, 1896–1979; its supplement, covering 1980–1987; and Bernard D. Reams and Stuart D. Yoak's *Constitution of the United States: A Guide and Bibliography to Current Scholarly Research* (1987). Others can be found by conducting a search in a library catalog, requesting the terms "constitution" and "bibliography." Researchers must take care to require that "bibliography" appear in the title of the work or in the subject assigned; otherwise, the search will also return books that merely contain a bibliography.

Two older but still often useful guides to the development of the federal Constitution are the U.S. Bureau of Rolls and Library's *Documentary History of the Constitution of the United States of America, 1786–1870* (5 vols., 1894–1905), and the Library of Congress Legislative Reference Service's *Documents Illustrative of the Formation of the Union of the American States* (1927).

There are many reasons for conducting research into the creation of the Constitution and the authors' interpretation. A legal researcher might be trying to discern the original intent of the framers regarding particular sections to make a legal argument; a legal scholar might be interested in the drafting history of the Constitution; a political historian might be interested in the process of ratification. No matter the purpose, a few tools can make the research process easier and more fulfilling.

Before getting too deeply into methods of constitutional research, recall that in research terms, there are several different constitutions. The first is the basic Constitution negotiated at the constitutional convention and adopted in 1789. Closely tied to this document, but with a slightly different history and therefore requiring slightly different research strategies, is the Bill of Rights, the first ten amendments to the Constitution. In addition, there are the other amendments.

Sources of the Constitution and Interpretive Materials

One of the first things to know when confronting a constitutional research issue is where to obtain a copy of the Constitution. Many copies are available: it has been reprinted repeatedly as a pamphlet; it has been included in many monographs; it even appears in most state codes. To a researcher, the source matters not so much because of textual differences, but because of the research tools provided with the Constitution. Which is the perfect fit?

The first source to consider is the *Code of Laws of the United States of America,* or the U.S. Code, the federal government's version of the statutory laws of the United States. It contains both the current federal laws of general import arranged topically and the Constitution. The U.S. Code was first published in 1926, is published every six years, and is supplemented annually. In law, it is the preferred citation source for federal statutes, though interestingly, not for the Constitution, for which no source is specified in the traditional legal citation manuals. The U.S. Code provides little more than the text of the Constitution.

A somewhat more helpful source is the *Constitution of the United States: Analysis and Interpretation.* This publication from the Congressional Research Service has been issued since 1952, with new editions and supplements published regularly. *Analysis and Interpretation* contains the text of the Constitution along with essays that describe how parts of the Constitution have been interpreted by the U.S. Supreme Court over the years. It includes a table of contents and a topical index and is available as a government document in some depository libraries and at HeinOnline. It can also be downloaded in PDF format for free at the Federal Digital System website (http://www.gpo.gov/fdsys).

While *Analysis and Interpretation* is a recent annotated version of the Constitution, it is not the only one. Over the past two hundred years, there have been several. Some available at HeinOnline include Andrew Jackson Baker's *Annotated Constitution of the United States* (1891) and Robert Desty's *Constitution of the United States, Annotated* (1879). Others can be located using searches of WorldCat or HeinOnline, such as "United States Constitution" with date restrictors, or a subject search for "constitutional law United States," or "Constitution" and "annotat*." Researchers may also find fruitful searching a smaller set of materials, such as the database *Making of Modern Law: Legal Treatises.*

These sources provide access to the text of the Constitution and references to the important U.S. Supreme Court cases that have interpreted it. Other tools can direct a researcher to books, articles, or cases that can help with a constitutional research problem. The most comprehensive are the two annotated versions of the U.S. Code. Both Lexis and Westlaw provide online and print access to the Constitution within their versions of the U.S. Code. Along with the full text, broken down by clause, these versions provide references to law review articles, practice guides, legal encyclopedias, and other research resources that treat the relevant constitutional clause, as well as cases from all levels of courts that interpret it.

The annotated versions of the Constitution provide short descriptions of how a case and the relevant aspect of the Constitution relate and a citation to the case. Because many cases are listed under almost every part of the Constitution, case annotations are organized into an outline designed around the topics that each clause raises.

There are no good analogs for constitutional encyclopedias or *Analysis and Interpretation*–style publications for state constitutions, but annotated versions of the state constitutions do exist. Either Lexis or Westlaw, or frequently both, publish print and online annotated versions of every state's current constitution. These appear in each state's code in print and in the state's code database, as well as in a database devoted to the constitution.

Some state constitutions are amended with great frequency, and many states have had more than one constitution. This makes it sometimes difficult but always imperative to verify that the resource references the correct form of the constitution in question. The date of publication of the case or article can help with this but is not always a reliable indicator. Beyond historical treatments of a constitutional policy, cases are frequently litigated under law that has later been changed, as long as the change does not moot or otherwise necessitate dismissal of the case. Therefore, it is possible that a case will have been decided with a slightly different version of a constitution in effect than that being litigated. Since there have been so few amendments to the federal Constitution, this should be a lesser concern to researchers working with it.

When the research is about the meaning of the Constitution or its interpretation, the main issue that arises relates to canons of statutory or constitutional interpretation: What material can and should be used to interpret the Constitution, and what weight will it be given? Within this issue reside many others, including the use of drafting and adoption history, the definition of terms, which cases to use, whether and how much to use nonlaw material, and what sort of material to use.

The next step in constitutional research is to understand the Constitution, so we turn to how to find canons of interpretation, drafting and adoption history, and some case-finding tools. Determining the definition of terms at various times, finding and using nonlaw material, and other issues are discussed in chapters 10 and 11.

Developing an understanding of the canons of interpretation, other methods of interpretation, and the controversies surrounding them requires study. One method for locating treatises that can serve as entrees into the discussion is to search a law library or other major library catalog using the subject "law—United States—interpretation and construction." A search for legal periodicals treating statutory or constitutional interpretation would also yield useful information. The *Index to Legal Periodicals* returns more than three thousand articles each for searches for the subject phrase "statutory interpretation" or "constitutional interpretation." With such results, a researcher must differentiate the best articles and books from the others. Several methods for determining the most useful materials are discussed during the treatment of secondary sources in chapter 6.

One way to approach interpretation is to use material related to the creation of the Constitution and writings by the founders lobbying for its adoption. Some sources are clearly related to the writing and adoption of the Constitution. Philip B. Kurland and Ralph Lerner's *The Founder's Constitution* (1986), available in print and online, brings together a variety of these materials and organizes them by constitutional clause.

The first part of *The Founder's Constitution* covers the major themes of the Constitution, starting with the preamble and continuing through the text and the Bill of Rights. For example, Article 1, Section 10, Clause 1, "No State shall enter into any Treaty, Alliance, or Confederation . . ." is annotated by, among other items, reference to *Deering v. Parker*, 4 Dall. App.

xxiii (P.C. 1760), James Madison, Notes for Speech Opposing Paper Money, 1 Nov. 1786; Records of the Federal Convention, Luther Martin, Genuine Information, 1788; James Madison, Federalist, no. 44, 299–302, 25 Jan. 1788; Charles Pinckney, South Carolina Ratifying Convention, 20 May 1788; Edmund Randolph, Virginia Ratifying Convention, 6 June 1788; Thomas Jefferson to W. H. Torrance, 11 June 1815; James Madison to Charles J. Ingersoll, Feb. 1831; and Joseph Story, Commentaries on the Constitution 3:§§1351, 1353–57, 1365–66, 1370–94, 1833. Researchers can browse *The Founder's Constitution* or employ one of the indexes (short titles, authors and documents, cases, constitutional provision) in either the print or online version. In addition, the online version can be searched.

Materials Related to the Constitutional Convention

Sources of information about the Constitutional Convention of 1787 include materials about the Continental Congress, which, when appropriate, will be included in the discussion of materials related to the convention.

At the close of the convention, secretary William Jackson presented to the convention president, George Washington, the materials that he had gathered. Washington, in turn, passed them on to the Department of State in 1796. There they remained until 1818 when Congress ordered the publication of material from the convention in the *Journal, Acts and Proceedings of the Convention, Assembled at Philadelphia, Monday, May 14, and Dissolved Monday, September 17, 1787, which Formed the Constitution of the United States.* Included within this publication are the *Formal Journal of the Proceedings of the Convention,* the *Journal of the Proceedings of the Committee of the Whole House,* the *Voting Record of the Convention: The Ayes, Noes, and*

Divided Votes, and loose sheets containing additional voting records. Jackson also provided two endorsed copies of the "Virginia Plan" (or "Randolph Plan"); an annotated (by Washington) copy of the August 6, 1787, draft Constitution reported to the convention by the Committee of Detail; a draft of the letter from the convention to Congress that was to accompany the Constitution; a signed duplicate letter from citizens of Rhode Island "Concerning Representation at the Philadelphia Convention"; a letter from James McHenry to George Washington; a letter to the president of the convention by William Rawle enclosing a "Resolve by the Directors of the Library Company of Philadelphia"; and a letter from Jonah Phillips to the president and members of the convention. These documents are all contained in *Documentary History of the Constitution of the United States of America, 1786–1870* (vol. 1, 1894, pp. 262–283).

Secretary of State John Quincy Adams saw that the material was organized and published in 1819 as the *Journal, Acts and Proceedings of the Convention.* In 1830 the convention material was reedited and republished by Jonathan Elliot as *The Debates, Resolutions, and Other Proceedings, in Convention, on the Adoption of the Federal Constitution.* In 1894, the State Department began the publication of the *Documentary History of the Constitution of the United States,* the first volume of which contains the transcript of the convention journals.

Over time some additional documents from the convention appeared and have become a part of its legacy. Among them are the papers of David Brearley that were provided to the secretary of state by his executor in 1818, the Credentials of the Delegates, and the "Gerry Motion." These, and the materials provided by Jackson, have been published by the U.S. National Archives as a microform publication, "The Records of the Constitutional Convention of 1787." In addition, other contemporaneous materials created by delegates have become a part of the records of the convention. Among the most regarded are James Madison's notes. Also important are Robert Yates's *Secret Proceedings and Debates of the Convention Assembled at Philadelphia* (Websters and Skinners, 1821) and notes and papers by Rufus King, James McHenry, William Pierce, William Patterson, Alexander Hamilton, Charles Pinckney, and George Mason as well as materials from the Committee of Detail.

In the early twentieth century, Max Farrand collected the previously published materials and all others that he could locate, organized them into one chronology, and published *Records of the Federal Convention of 1787.* The first three volumes were published in 1911. A new edition, published in 1937, included a fourth volume containing additions and corrections. In 1987, James H. Hutson supplemented the *Records* with a fifth volume. The first three volumes are available in print at many libraries and online through a variety of places, including Hein-Online and the Library of Congress's Century of Lawmaking website (a part of the American Memory project), which contains a number of useful resources for early constitutional research. The first two volumes cover the proceedings chronologically, and the last two include supplementary material. Access to the data is improved by the chronological arrangement. A topical index to the first three volumes appears at the end of volume 3. The fifth also contains an index.

Researchers interested in a narrative account of the proceedings of the convention may be disappointed by the journals. These are like early legislative journals, that is, not a description of all of the discussions and events, but a record of the decisions. An excellent discussion and description of the records of the convention is provided by a recent article by Mary Sarah Bilder,

"How Bad Were the Official Records of the Federal Convention?," available through the Social Science Research Network, a website that contains a number of prepublication versions of scholarly papers and other scholarly essays and working papers. Madison's notes, published separately many times, stand as the single most complete contemporary narrative description of the convention and are included in Farrand's *Records*. Madison's handwritten notes are housed at the Library of Congress and are available online in Series 5 of the *Papers of James Madison* in the American Memory collection.

Letters of Delegates to Congress, 1774–1789, another resource that provides insight into the development of the Constitution, was published in 1976 and incorporates an earlier collection by Edward Burnett, *Letters of Members of the Continental Congress*. *Letters of Delegates* is available at many libraries in print and online for free at the Library of Congress's Century of Lawmaking website. The set is organized chronologically with a table of contents listing the parties to the correspondence; there is also an index, and the set may be searched online.

It should be noted that the *Journals of the Continental Congress* describes the business of the congress. It contains the texts of the resolutions and records of attendance and votes, but it does not include discussions, speeches, and other information. Between 1904 and 1937, the Library of Congress gathered the material together and published *The Journals of the Continental Congress, 1774–1789*. The *Journals* are available in print at many libraries and online, for free, at the Library of Congress's Century of Lawmaking website. It can be browsed by date, and there is a short topical table of contents and a short topical index. Another useful website is the Library of Congress's Documents from the Continental Congress and the Constitutional Convention, 1774–1789. In addition to the more traditional materials, this site provides access to two collections of broadsides related to the Continental Congress and the constitutional convention.

Materials Related to the Adoption of the Constitution

While comparatively little material is available from the actual constitutional convention, a great deal of information from the process of the Constitution's ratification exists. The ratification played out in front of the nation. The most famous items, the *Federalist Papers,* were initially published in the press. Two types of materials can enlighten researchers: articles and pamphlets arguing for or against the proposed Constitution and debates at the state legislatures.

For new researchers approaching the ratification of the federal Constitution, a great place it start is Paul Leicester Ford's *Bibliography and Reference List of the History and Literature Relating to the Adoption of the Constitution of the United States, 1787–8.* Originally published in 1888, it has recently been reprinted and is available online through HathiTrust and Google Books.

The major articles published in the press arguing for the adoption of the Constitution are more commonly known as the *Federalist Papers* and have been published many times and are widely available. The articles arguing against adoption have less frequently been published, but a search of WorldCat for "anti-federalist papers" will return many examples, including T. Harry Williams and Milton Longhorn's *The Anti-Federalist: Excerpts from Papers of Leading Opponents of the Federal Constitution,* which was published under the auspices of the Works Progress Administration and the University of Wisconsin in the

1930s. The full text of this version is available online through HathiTrust. Another recent collection is Bernard Bailyn's *The Debate on the Constitution: Federalist and Antifederalist Speeches, Articles, and Letters During the Struggle over Ratification* (1993).

The most complete collection of information about ratification appears in a set still being produced by the Wisconsin State Historical Society, *The Documentary History of the Ratification of the Constitution.* Begun in 1976 and originally edited by Merrill Jensen, the set now contains twenty-eight volumes, with more scheduled. Completed volumes include *Constitutional Documents and Records, 1776–1787, Commentaries on the Constitution,* and ratification debates in Pennsylvania, Delaware, New Jersey, Georgia, Connecticut, Massachusetts, Virginia, New York, Rhode Island, North Carolina, Maryland, South Carolina, New Hampshire, and Vermont; still to come are volumes on ratification in North Carolina and on the ratification of the Bill of Rights in the states. This is an invaluable set and is held by most libraries associated with institutions of higher learning and many larger public libraries. An online version is also available as a subscription database that provides a wide variety of search capabilities as well as the indexes available in the print version, a chronology, and other means of access to the data.

The Debates in the Several State Conventions on the Adoption of the Federal Constitution was compiled by Jonathan Elliot and published in 1827, though the second edition published in 1836 is preferred. In addition to the documents pertinent to a discussion of ratification, the Declaration of Independence, the Articles of Confederation, and the journals of the constitutional convention (though a less complete version than that published as the *Journals of the Federal Convention of 1787*), and the text of the proposed Constitution, this volume contains the text of the debates in the state legislatures. Elliot provides a topical index and a speaker's name index; the work is available at many libraries and online through HathiTrust, Google Books, the Internet Archive, and the Century of Lawmaking website.

The articles and pamphlets that make up the *Federalist* and *Anti-Federalist Papers* can also be found in their original contexts. Many first appeared in newspapers of the day (newspaper research is discussed in chapter 11). Some of the papers were published as pamphlets, and many of those can be found using *Early American Imprints*. Finally, a researcher who wishes to find broadsides relating to the ratification should begin with the *Continental Congress Broadside Collection* and the *Constitutional Convention Broadside Collection* consisting of 256 and 21 titles, respectively, placed online by the Library of Congress through its American Memory project.

On July 26, 1788, New York became the eleventh state to ratify the Constitution, and on March 4, 1789, the Constitution came into effect. On September 25, 1789, Congress proposed the Bill of Rights. The adoption and ratification of ten of the first twelve proposed amendments followed a different course than the Constitution did on its road to ratification. The most useful sources for tracking the ratification of the Bill of Rights are Neil H. Cogan's *Complete Bill of Rights* and Bernard Schwartz's *The Bill of Rights, A Documentary History*. In addition, *The Founder's Constitution* has also gathered contemporaneous documents relating to the amendments.

Materials Related to Constitutional Amendments

Since 1789, there have been many further attempts to amend the Constitution. After the Bill of Rights, seventeen amendments, including Prohibition and its repeal, were successfully added to the Constitution, though there have been more than ten thousand proposed amendments. For the history and ratification of amendments after the first ten, the first place to look is the *Encyclopedia of Constitutional Amendments* by John Vile. A new series, titled *The Complete Reconstruction Amendments,* by Neil H. Cogan, will gather materials related to the reconstruction amendments. The first will be published in early 2018 and will cover the Fourteenth Amendment. Later collections will cover the Thirteenth and Fifteenth Amendments. This series, published by Oxford University Press, will do for the reconstruction amendments what Cogan's *Complete Bill of Rights,* mentioned above, did for the first ten amendments.

Other than these sets that cover a unified series of amendments, most research into the other amendments requires a researcher to look for materials on specific amendments, for example, Thomas Ripy's *Ratification of the Sixteenth Amendment* (1985), Everett Brown's *The Ratification of the Twenty-First Amendment* (1935), and Sarah Slavin's *The Equal Rights Amendment: The Politics and Process of Ratification of the Twenty-Seventh Amendment to the U.S. Constitution* (1982). Common subject headings used for these types of resources include "United States—Constitution—16th Amendment" or "Constitutional Amendments—United States—Ratification."

Information about proposed but unsuccessful amendments is harder to come by. Vile has collected congressional documents listing all proposed amendments and has updated the list. However, *Proposed Amendments to the U.S. Constitution* provides little more than the bare minimum information about each amendment—merely date, title, and possibly document number. Further information can be obtained only by conducting legislative research as described in chapter 6.

Research Example

As an opportunity to examine the constitutional resources more fully, we will look for discussion during the Constitutional Convention of 1787 and during ratification of whether the common law should be specifically adopted and what effect the Constitution might have on the common law. We first turn to the index of Farrand's *Records of the Federal Convention of 1787;* in the print version, the index is in volume 4. Under "common law" are the entries, in alphabetical order, "and Constitution," "and definition of felony," "and federal code," "jurisdiction of federal courts," and "jury trial." Note that if we go to Farrand at the Library of Congress website, volume 4 is not available, and the index is much less complete. There, the index entry offers "common law, II, 431, 637." That entry leads to the discussion of the common law and the jurisdiction of the federal courts, noted above, and part of the discussion on the common law and the Constitution, also noted above. The Library of Congress site does allow full-text searching.

When we ask that the terms "common" and "law" and "constitution" all appear in one document at the Library of Congress site, we get two results. One is to the index, which we have already seen. The other is to text related to the common law and the Constitution, which the print index—but not the online index—referenced. Using both means of searching in the online version, index and full-text searching, we got the same results as the better index in the print version of supplementary volume 4 of Farrand.

For the subject "common law and Constitution," the print index and online searches direct us to volume 2, page 637, and volume 3, page 130. The first presents some notes by George Mason containing his objections to the Constitution that were written on the blank pages of his copy of the September 12 draft and that he circulated to several people (Farrand explains that the notes are from Kate Mason Rowland's *Life of George Mason,* vol. 2, pp. 387–90 [1892]). Mason's objections were that "[t]here is no Declaration of Rights, and the laws of the general government being paramount to the laws and constitution of the several States, the Declaration of Rights in the separate States are no security. Nor are the people secured even in the enjoyment of the benefit of the common law which stands here upon no other foundation than its having been adopted by the respective acts forming the constitutions of the several States."

Volume 3, page 130, presents a letter from James Madison to George Washington dated October 18, 1787. In the letter Madison directly responds to Mason's objections, writing, "What can he mean by saying that the Common law is not secured by the new Constitution, though it has been adopted by the State Constitutions. The Common law is nothing more than the unwritten law, and is left by all the Constitutions equally liable to legislative alterations." Madison then goes on to explain why the convention was right to avoid an express adoption of the common law for the nation.

To determine whether issues related to the place of the common law in relation to the Constitution played a role in the adoption of the Constitution, we can check three resources. The first is Jonathan Elliot's *The Debates in the Several State Conventions on the Adoption of the Federal Constitution: As Recommended by the General Convention at Philadelphia in 1787* (1836). In examining the index for each volume, we find no entries under "common law" in volumes 1, 2, 4, and 5. In volume 3, there are two entries: "Bill of Rights more necessary in this Government than in any other, 445. Common law of England;

Punishments, &c., ... 446." On page 445, we find a speech by Patrick Henry discussing the need for a Bill of Rights.

To determine whether the issue was discussed in a particular state, for example, Massachusetts, we can look at the *Documentary History of the Ratification of the Constitution*. The online version allows full-text searching, but it also contains an index for each section of the series. Turning to the index that covers the Massachusetts volumes, we find five entries: "bill of rights originates from," "Congress can alter," "Constitution does not rest upon," "serves as a bill of rights for those states without one," and "will not work under Constitution." Turning to the last of these we come to a letter to the Massachusetts Convention from "Agrippa" published in the *Massachusetts Gazette* on January 15, 1788. This is the second part of a three-part series by "Agrippa" published on January 11, 15, and 18. In this section, "Agrippa" argues that a Bill of Rights is necessary because the common law can be changed by the states and there is no guarantee of the principles that "we hold sacred" recognized by the common law in the Constitution. The reader is further informed of a speech on this issue by James Wilson on October 6 at a public meeting in Philadelphia and the fact that the speech was printed in Massachusetts October 24–November 15, 1787.

Finally, we can turn to the *Federalist Papers*. Many editions are indexed, and one print version refers nine times to "common law": *Federalist* nos. 37, 42, 43, 81, 83, and 84.

From these items, we can see that the protections of the common law were considered during the writing of the Constitution and that the discussion fed into the larger discussion of the need for a Bill of Rights. This simple research question can lead to a more complete understanding of the thinking that led to the Bill of Rights.

Further Reading

Bilder, Mary Sarah. "How Bad Were the Official Records of the Federal Convention?" *George Washington Law Review* 80 (2011): 1620–82.

Gummere, Richard M. "The Classical Ancestry of the United States Constitution." *American Quarterly* 14, no. 1 (1962): 3–18.

Hutson, James H. "Creation of the Constitution: The Integrity of the Documentary Record." *Texas Law Review* 65 (1986): 1–39.

Maier, Pauline. *Ratification: The People Debate the Constitution, 1787–1788.* New York: Simon & Schuster, 2010.

Richardson, William A. "Chief Justice of the United States or Chief Justice of the Supreme Court of the United States." In *The New England Historical and Genealogical Register,* 49, no. 195 (1895): 275–79.

Wood, Gordon S. *The Creation of the American Republic, 1776–1787.* Chapel Hill: University of North Carolina Press, 1969.

Important Sources Mentioned in This Chapter

Browne, Cynthia E. *State Constitutional Conventions, from Independence to the Completion of the Present Union, 1776–1959: A Bibliography.* Westport, CT: Greenwood, 1972.

Cogan, Neil H. *The Complete Bill of Rights: The Drafts, Debates, Sources, and Origins.* New York: Oxford University Press, 1997.

Congressional Information Service. *State Constitutional Conventions, Commissions and Amendments.* Bethesda, MD: Congressional Information Service, 1973.

———. *State Constitutional Conventions, Commissions and Amendments, 1959–1978: An Annotated Bibliography.* Washington, DC: Congressional Information Service, 1981.

———. *State Constitutional Conventions, Commissions & Amendments, 1979–1988: An Annotated Bibliography.* Bethesda, MD: Congressional Information Service, 1989.

Elliot, Jonathan, ed. *The Debates in the Several State Conventions on the Adoption of the Federal Constitution.* Washington, DC: Printed by and for the Editor, 1836 and 1845.

Farrand, Max, ed. *The Records of the Federal Convention of 1787.* New Haven, CT: Yale University Press, 1911.

Ford, Paul Leicester. *Bibliography and Reference List of the History and Literature Relating to the Adoption of the Constitution of the United States, 1787–8.* Brooklyn, NY: 1888.

Hall, Kermit L. *A Comprehensive Bibliography of American Constitutional and Legal History, 1896–1979*. Millwood, NY: Kraus, 1984.

Jensen, Merrill, John P. Kaminski, and Gaspare J. Saladino. *The Documentary History of the Ratification of the Constitution*. Madison: Wisconsin Historical Society Press, 1976.

Kurland, Philip B., and Ralph Lerner. *The Founders' Constitution*. Chicago: University of Chicago Press, 1987.

Schwartz, Bernard. *The Bill of Rights: A Documentary History*. New York: Chelsea House, 1971.

Smith, Paul Hubert, and Ronald M. Gephart. *Letters of Delegates to Congress, 1774–1789*. Washington, DC: Library of Congress, 1986–.

Swindler, William Finley. *Sources and Documents of United States Constitutions*. Dobbs Ferry, NY: Oceana, 1973.

United States and Bureau of Rolls and Library. *Documentary History of the Constitution of the United States of America, 1786–1870*. Washington, DC: Department of State, 1901.United States, U.S. Supreme Court, Library of Congress, Legislative Reference Service, Library of Congress, and Congressional Research Service. *Constitution of the United States of America: Analysis and Interpretation: Annotations of Cases Decided by the Supreme Court of the United States . . .* Washington, DC: GPO, 1953–.

Vile, John R. *Encyclopedia of Constitutional Amendments, Proposed Amendments, and Amending Issues, 1789–2015*. Santa Barbara, CA: ABC-CLIO, 2015.

———. *Proposed Amendments to the U.S. Constitution, 1787–2001*. Clark, NY: Lawbook Exchange, 2003.

Databases

Gale. *The Making of Modern Law*. http://www.gale.com/primary-sources/the-making-of-modern-law.

Kurland, Philip B., and Ralph Lerner. *The Founders' Constitution*. http://press-pubs.uchicago.edu/founders//

Library of Congress. *A Century of Lawmaking for a New Nation: U.S. Congressional Documents and Debates*. https://memory.loc.gov/ammem/amlaw/.

———. *Documents from the Continental Congress and the Constitutional Convention, 1774 to 1789*. http://bit.ly/2t3sRud.

5
The Early Republic, 1790s–1870s

By the 1790s, at least fourteen governments were making law in the United States, but questions remained. How much of the pre-Revolution colonial and English law would be recognized or relied upon? If the United States was to remain committed to the common law, then a collection of precedents had to be found. How was the law, including legislation and court opinions from federal and state governments, to be published and distributed? In addition to these important legal and more prosaic issues, the nation was also deciding issues about the relative powers of the various branches of government and the relations between the states and the federal government.

Reception Statutes

Before the Revolution, the law under which the colonies had operated consisted of colonial statutes, English statutes, and common law. But as independence became the goal of the rebellion, the question arose about the place colonial and English law would play. Americans were familiar with the common law system and, although there had been a political breakdown, the cause was not a breakdown of the common law; the legal system had generally worked well during the eighteenth century. After independence, the United States chose to retain the common law system. However, one of the most important ingredients in a common law system is a body of law from which to work.

To "create" a body of law, most states passed "reception statutes," which generally allowed English law as of a certain date to be considered a part of the state's laws. Some statutes held that the law that had operated in the colony as well as acts of the colonial legislature and courts would remain in effect until changed by the legislature or courts, unless they were, as the Massachusetts Constitution held, "repugnant to the rights and liberties contained in this constitution."

Virginia's Reception Statute from 1776 states:

> And be it further ordained, That the common law of England, all statutes or acts of Parliament made in aid of the common law prior to the fourth year of the reign of King James the first [1607, when Jamestown was founded], and which are of a general nature, not local to that kingdom, together with the several acts of the General Assembly of this colony now in force, so far as the same may consist with several ordinances, declarations, and resolutions of the General Convention, shall be the rule of decision, and shall be considered as in full force, until the same shall be altered by the legislative power of this colony. ("An ordinance to enable the present magistrates and officers to continue the administration of justice," Ordinances Passed at a

General Convention of Delegates and Representatives, from the Several Counties of Virginia, Held at the Capitol, in the City of Williamsburg on Monday the 6th of May, anno Dom: 1776. Williamsburg, VA: Alexander Purdie, 1776)

Massachusetts treated reception in its constitution, which still holds that "all the laws which have heretofore been adopted, used, and approved in the Province, Colony, or State of Massachusetts Bay, and usually practiced on in the courts of law, shall still remain and be in full force, until altered or repealed by the legislature" (ch. vi, art. vi).

Even with the reception statutes, however, not a lot of law was yet made in many of the states or in the United States as a whole. Therefore, for several decades, U.S. court decisions continued to rely on English law. Through much of the nineteenth century, English legal treatises sold well in the United States, and many went through several American editions. For example, at least twenty-two full editions and fifteen abridgments of Blackstone's *Commentaries* were published in the United States before 1897. For a complete picture of the law in the early nation, reference to both American and English sources is necessary.

In considering nineteenth-century sources, a researcher should keep in mind that legal publishing was not very advanced, even in the largest of the new states. Before the Revolution, several colonies had contracted with local printers to print their statutes. In those colonies, the publication of statutes continued relatively seamlessly. In others and as states were added to the nation, printers would be found. However, a larger problem remained. In a common law system, legislation is important, but case law is critical.

Organization of the Government

Before delving into the law of a state or the federal government of a particular time, researchers must develop an understanding of the governmental structure and especially of the court system at the time period they are considering. Researchers should also be aware of the publication systems that were in use.

The structures of the federal and state court systems have changed over time. A state legal research guide can offer the history of a state's government and courts structure. New York is a good jurisdiction to use as an example. Today, at its simplest, New York has a three-layered court system, with the Court of Appeals as the highest court. The intermediate appellate court is the Appellate Division of the Supreme Court; there are four appellate divisions, each with jurisdiction over a different geographical part of the state. Finally, there is a fairly complicated trial court system with several courts of limited jurisdiction and with the Supreme Court acting as the court of general jurisdiction.

The history of New York's court system is fairly complex, yet it demonstrates many of the common issues that a researcher may encounter when looking into the early years of the original thirteen states. New York's court system went through several changes in the seventeenth century, but the Act of 1691 set up the system, parts of which lasted until the nineteenth century. Under this act, a Supreme Court of Judicature was created. This court had original jurisdiction for civil and criminal cases. It consisted of a chief justice and four puisne (equivalent to today's associate) judges. The court sat in New York City, and it also held circuit sessions in the various counties. Additionally, the court held special sessions when it was in circuit to hear more serious matters; these were the Courts of Oyer and Terminer. Once a year, one of the judges would sit with three specially commissioned justices of the peace in each county to act as a Court of Common Pleas to hear matters triable at common law. Appeals from the Supreme Court of Judicature went to the governor and his council, sitting as a Court of Errors, and then to the king and the Privy Council.

The Court of Chancery was also created by the Act of 1691, but its history is a bit more checkered. It was allowed to lapse in 1699 and was revived by the governor in 1701, but it remained a fairly unimportant court until the nineteenth century.

The New York Constitution of 1777 mandated a change in the court structure to replace the governor as the place of appeals. The appellate structure was set by the legislature in 1784 when the Court for the Correction of Errors, made up of the president of the senate, the senators, the chancellor of the Chancery Court, and the judges of the existing Supreme Court, was established.

In 1821 the Supreme Court of Judicature became the intermediate appellate court with appeals to the Court for the Correction of Errors. In addition, in the 1820s, eight judicial circuits were created and staffed with judges.

By the early nineteenth century, the Court of Chancery developed into an extremely important court, most especially under the leadership of Chancellor James Kent. However, by the 1840s, dissatisfaction with the length of time that appeals in chancery could take and with the fact that senators dominated the Court for the Correction of Errors was so great that the court system was revamped again in the Constitution of 1846. The structure put in place in the 1840s closely resembles that of today. The Constitution of 1846 eliminated the Court of Chancery and gave its jurisdiction to the Supreme Court.

The Court for the Correction of Errors was eliminated and replaced by the Court of Appeals. The Supreme Court, which had acted as the Court of Appeals, was given initial responsibility for cases in both law and equity. The new structure also created eight, later reduced to four, general terms of the Supreme Court to act as the intermediate appellate court. This became the Appellate Division of the Supreme Court that exists today. There have been some changes to the system since the 1840s, but the current system still looks much as it did in 1850.

Researchers must be aware that the history of the judiciary in many states is as, or even more, complicated as that of New York, and they must be careful to understand what the judiciary looked like in the state and time being researched. They must also understand the appellate process of the time.

Examining changes in the federal court system over time is also instructive. Article III, Section 1 of the Constitution created the U.S. Supreme Court and "such inferior Courts as the Congress shall from time to time ordain and establish." By the Judiciary Act of 1789, Congress divided the nation into thirteen judicial districts and established a district court in each to act as the trial court for admiralty and maritime cases as well as for some minor criminal cases. Congress also established circuit courts that were to act as appellate courts for appeals from the district court and as trial courts for most federal criminal cases, civil suits initiated by the United States, and civil suits between citizens of different states. The circuit courts convened in the districts and were designated by the names of the districts. Rather than create circuit judgeships, the act stipulated that the circuit court panel would consist of the local district court judge and two members of the Supreme Court. In 1793, Congress reduced the number of Supreme Court justices necessary for a panel to one.

In 1801, Congress established six federal judicial circuits each with its own circuit court and circuit judges. Supreme Court justices were no longer required to sit on circuit panels. In 1802, however, a new Congress revisited the federal courts. The Judiciary Act of 1802 retained the six numbered circuits but abolished the circuit judgeships. Panels reverted to a district judge and a Supreme Court justice, though district court judges could sit as a circuit court for all matters except appeals from their district courts.

Through the nineteenth century, Congress expanded the number of circuits and rearranged the states in the circuits to retain population parity. As the number of circuits increased, so did the Supreme Court, so there was generally one justice per circuit. In 1869 Congress created a circuit judgeship for each circuit. At that time, a panel could consist of two or three people, the circuit judge, the justice designated for that circuit, or the district court judge. In 1891, the circuit courts of appeal were created, thereby stripping the circuit court of its appellate jurisdiction. The circuit judges were assigned to both their circuit courts and circuit courts of appeal. The Judicial Code of 1911 eliminated the circuit courts (though not the circuit court of appeals).

The trend in the twentieth century was for the Circuit Court of Appeals—renamed the Court of Appeals for the designated circuit, the First Circuit, for example, in 1948—to expand its jurisdiction while the right of appeal to the Supreme Court was limited. The Court of Appeals for the District of Columbia was established in 1893 and the Tenth Circuit in 1929. Finally, in 1980, the Eleventh Circuit was created by splitting the Fifth Circuit. The U.S. Court of Customs and Patent Appeals and the U.S. Court of Claims were merged in 1982 into the U.S. Court of Appeals for the Federal Circuit.

The states in each circuit changed over time; Table 5.1 lists each circuit and shows, for each time period, the states that made up the circuit.

Table 5.1. States within each circuit over time

Circuit	Years	States
Eastern	1789–1790	Connecticut, Massachusetts, New Hampshire, New York
	1790–1791	Connecticut, Massachusetts, New Hampshire, New York, Rhode Island
	1791–1801	Connecticut, Massachusetts, New Hampshire, New York, Rhode Island, Vermont
Middle	1789–1801	Delaware, Maryland, New Jersey, Pennsylvania, Virginia
Southern	1789–1790	Georgia, South Carolina
	1790–1801	Georgia, North Carolina, South Carolina
First	1801–1802	Maine, New Hampshire, Massachusetts, Rhode Island
	1802–1820	Massachusetts, New Hampshire, Rhode Island
	1820–1915	Maine, Massachusetts, New Hampshire, Rhode Island
	1915–present	Maine, Massachusetts, New Hampshire, Puerto Rice, Rhode Island
Second	1801–present	Connecticut, New York, Vermont
Third	1801–1802	Delaware, New Jersey, Pennsylvania
	1802–1866	New Jersey, Pennsylvania
	1866–1948	Delaware, New Jersey, Pennsylvania

(Continued)

Table 5.1. Continued

Circuit	Years	States
	1948–present	Delaware, New Jersey, Pennsylvania, Virgin Islands
Fourth	1801–1802	Maryland, Virginia
	1802–1842	Delaware, Maryland
	1842–1862	Delaware, Maryland, Virginia
	1862–1864	Delaware, Maryland, North Carolina, Virginia
	1864–1866	Delaware, Maryland, North Carolina, Virginia, West Virginia
	1866–present	Maryland, North Carolina, South Carolina, Virginia, West Virginia
Fifth	1801–1802	Georgia, North Carolina, South Carolina
	1802–1842	North Carolina, Virginia
	1842–1862	Alabama, Louisiana
	1862–1866	Alabama, Florida, Georgia, Mississippi, South Carolina
	1866–1948	Alabama, Florida, Georgia, Louisiana, Mississippi, Texas
	1948–1980	Alabama, Canal Zone, Florida, Georgia, Louisiana, Mississippi, Texas
	1980–1982	Canal Zone, Louisiana, Mississippi, Texas
	1982–present	Louisiana, Mississippi, Texas
Sixth	1801–1802	Kentucky, Ohio, Tennessee
	1802–1842	Georgia, South Carolina
	1842–1862	Georgia, North Carolina, South Carolina
	1862–1866	Arkansas, Kentucky, Louisiana, Tennessee, Texas
	1866–present	Kentucky, Michigan, Ohio, Tennessee

Seventh	1807–1837	Kentucky, Ohio, Tennessee
	1837–1862	Illinois, Indiana, Michigan, Ohio
	1862–1863	Indiana, Ohio
	1863–1866	Michigan, Ohio
	1866–present	Illinois, Indiana, Wisconsin
Eighth	1837–1862	Kentucky, Missouri, Tennessee
	1862–1863	Illinois, Michigan, Wisconsin
	1863–1866	Illinois, Indiana, Wisconsin
	1866–1867	Arkansas, Iowa, Kansas, Minnesota, Missouri
	1867–1876	Arkansas, Iowa, Kansas, Minnesota, Missouri, Nebraska
	1876–1889	Arkansas, Colorado, Iowa, Kansas, Minnesota, Missouri, Nebraska
	1889–1890	Arkansas, Colorado, Iowa, Kansas, Minnesota, Missouri, Nebraska, North Dakota, South Dakota
	1890–1896	Arkansas, Colorado, Iowa, Kansas, Minnesota, Missouri, Nebraska, North Dakota, South Dakota, Wyoming
	1896–1907	Arkansas, Colorado, Iowa, Kansas, Minnesota, Missouri, Nebraska, North Dakota, South Dakota, Utah, Wyoming
	1907–1912	Arkansas, Colorado, Iowa, Kansas, Minnesota, Missouri, Nebraska, North Dakota, Oklahoma, South Dakota, Utah, Wyoming
	1912–1929	Arkansas, Colorado, Iowa, Kansas, Minnesota, Missouri, Nebraska, New Mexico, North Dakota, Oklahoma, South Dakota, Utah, Wyoming
	1929–present	Arkansas, Iowa, Minnesota, Missouri, Nebraska, North Dakota, South Dakota

(Continued)

Table 5.1. Continued

Circuit	Years	States
Ninth	1837–1842	Alabama, Arkansas, Louisiana, Mississippi
	1842–1862	Arkansas, Mississippi
	1862–1866	Iowa, Kansas, Minnesota, Missouri
	1866–1889	California, Nevada, Oregon
	1889–1890	California, Montana, Nevada, Oregon, Washington
	1890–1900	California, Idaho, Montana, Nevada, Oregon, Washington
	1900–1912	Alaska, California, Hawaii, Idaho, Montana, Nevada, Oregon, Washington
	1912–1951	Alaska, Arizona, California, Hawaii, Idaho, Montana, Nevada, Oregon, Washington
	1951–1977	Alaska, Arizona, California, Guam, Hawaii, Idaho, Montana, Nevada, Oregon, Washington (note that in 1959 Alaska and Hawaii became states)
	1977–present	Alaska, Arizona, California, Guam, Hawaii, Idaho, Montana, Nevada, Northern Mariana Islands, Oregon, Washington
Tenth	1863–1865	California, Oregon
	1865–1866	California, Nevada, Oregon
	1866–1929	Abolished
	1929–present	Colorado, Kansas, New Mexico, Oklahoma, Utah, Wyoming
Eleventh	1980–present	Alabama, Florida, Georgia
California Circuit	1855–1863	California

Case Reporting

In England case reports had been published for several centuries, but toward the end of the eighteenth century, there were still no case reporters in America. That doesn't mean that there are no "reports" of preindependence American cases. As mentioned in chapter 3, some judge's notebooks and other material describing judicial proceedings were kept, and some were published. However, most eighteenth-century lawyers would not have had access to these. A list of the reports that were printed before the nineteenth century can be found in Wilfred J. Ritz's *American Judicial Proceedings First Printed Before 1801.* Other resources that can direct a researcher to early materials include *Early American Imprints,* for materials up to 1819, and the *Bibliography of Early American Law.* Of course, simply because the reports were printed, does not mean they were widely available.

As the court systems developed, a system for case reporting also took shape but remained a nongovernmental activity until into the nineteenth century. During the 1790s and after, reporting in each state progressed a little differently; however, by the early nineteenth century, the most important decisions of the most important courts in each state and in the federal system were being noted and, in some sense, published using the private reporter model.

During the nineteenth century there was a slow move toward the kind of case reporting that we see today. Initially, private reporters took down the arguments of counsel and the opinions delivered orally by the court and then arranged printing and distribution. Over time, judges began to offer written opinions and to choose which cases got "reported." As a part of this process, reporters shifted from freelance work to a government job: the Reporter of Decisions. While the story of reporting is different in each state, there were no American case reports in 1788; by the early to mid-nineteenth century all states reported the opinions of most of the cases decided by the highest courts of the states and many federal cases. By later in the century the private system evolved into a government function.

Historians will find that it was not uncommon for a historically significant lower court case to go unreported. Once judges gained control of reporting, they chose cases that would become the building blocks of the law and ignored cases that merely repeated well-settled law. Historians will often want to read a case to get insight into the people involved, whereas lawyers care only about the law involved. Today, reported and many unreported cases are available to most attorneys online via Lexis or Westlaw. In the past, the main distinction between reported and unreported opinions was availability. Today, the main distinctions are in the citations and the rules about how the opinions may be used at a particular court.

The first American case reporter was by Ephram Kirby of Connecticut, who published *Reports of Cases Adjudged in the Superior Court of the State of Connecticut from the Year 1785 to May, 1788, with Some Determinations in the Supreme Court of Errors in 1789.* It covered cases from the Superior Court and some from the Supreme Court of Errors decided between 1785 and 1788. Kirby's reports were followed by Jesse Root's and Thomas Day's reports before *Connecticut Reports* began in 1814. In 1790, Alexander J. Dallas published the first volume of his reports, which would eventually mark the beginning of the *United States Reports*. By volume 2, *United States Reports* was recording the decisions of the

U.S. Supreme Court and included Dallas's notes of the opinions delivered by the Court. The first volume is a little different: as a way to develop a common law for the United States, it contained mainly Pennsylvania cases from before the Revolution and no U.S. Supreme Court cases. Dallas was followed in reporting the U.S. Supreme Court by several private reporters, some working under an understanding with the Court, until the mid-nineteenth century when the justices began to write and distribute their opinions and the office of Reporter of Decisions became a governmental position. An interesting description of the system and how and why it changed can be seen through the lens of the Supreme Court case of *Wheaton v. Peters* (33 U.S. [8 Pet.] 591 [1834]) as described in Craig Joyce's "Wheaton v. Peters: The Untold Story of the Early Reporters" (1985 Yearbook of the Supreme Court Historical Society 35 [1986]: 35–92).

As the Court moved to a more regularized reporting system, the earlier nominative reports were added to the beginning of the new publication, the *United States Reports*. Thus, volume 1 of Dallas's reports became volume 1 of the *United States Reports*. Volume 1 of *Cranch's Reports* (William Cranch was the author of Supreme Court opinions immediately following Dallas) became volume 5 of the *United States Reports;* volume 1 of Henry Wheaton (the reporter following Cranch) became volume 14 of the *United States Reports*. A table in *The Bluebook: A Uniform System of Citation* lays out the nominative reporters and the volumes they cover.

Researchers should understand that until the reports became a clerical product, not every case in a covered court is necessarily included in the reports. For example, if the author/reporter was absent and could not get notes, the case would not appear. Researchers should also be aware that the case reports were not a verbatim transcript of the proceedings or of the orally delivered opinion of the court. The early reports generally contained, for the cases covered, a summary of the arguments of both attorneys and a summary of the court's opinion. By the turn of the nineteenth century, reporters covered the highest court in most of the states. While it might be assumed that the quality of the reports varied depending on the skills of the reporter, there are few instances in which several reports of the same case are reported for comparison.

State courts experienced a similar history, with various nominative reporters publishing the opinions from the highest courts in the states. As the system became regularized and the responsibility moved to the court, many of these earlier reporters gathered together to create a single run of the opinions of the state's highest court and, perhaps, of other courts. These official state reports continued to be published into the twentieth and twenty-first centuries. HeinOnline offers a *State Report Checklist* by Keith Weise and Karen Fiederowicz that lists all of the reporters published for a state's cases, which will set researchers up to search for specific reporters.

By sometime in the nineteenth century, a regular system was in place for publishing the opinions of the most important courts of each state and the U.S. Supreme Court. It wasn't until West started publishing the *Federal Reporter* that there was a regular series for the lower federal courts. In the states, the system generally became a governmental activity as with the U.S. Supreme Court. The reporting of the other federal courts remained a private matter, although by the late nineteenth century, the number of reporters had declined and reporting was much more systematic. See chapter 6 for a discussion of this later nineteenth-century development.

Access to Nineteenth-Century State Case
Law Today

Several publishers have attempted to collect and provide access to the case reports from the early nineteenth century. Bloomberg Law, Lexis, and Westlaw include the cases covered in the major state reporters, including the nominative reporters that retrospectively became a part of the state reports. However, the farther back one goes, the less complete the holdings. The coverage for the courts from some states can differ by publisher and are sometimes less than comprehensive. For example, the South Carolina Constitution, adopted in 1776, created a high court for law and a high court for equity. Opinions from these courts were reported in a number of nominative reports from 1783 and 1784, respectively, until 1868. At that time, the courts were combined and a reporter, *South Carolina Reports*, containing the opinions from the South Carolina Supreme Court, started publication. Westlaw includes the following cases from South Carolina: Supreme Court, 1868 to the present; Courts of Common Pleas and General Sessions of the Peace, 1783–1795; Constitutional Court of Appeals, 1791–1824; and Court of Appeals, 1983 to the present. Lexis includes South Carolina Court of Appeals cases from 1983, South Carolina Supreme Court cases from 1867, and South Carolina unpublished cases from 2007. Bloomberg includes Supreme Court of South Carolina opinions from 1868 to the present and South Carolina Court of Appeals opinions from 1983 to present. Each database lacks some part of a court's work. Westlaw does not cover the Court of Equity from 1784, and Lexis and Bloomberg cover none of the antebellum courts.

Table 5.2 shows states with the date of the earliest widely available published high court opinions and the earliest date of

Table 5.2. Date of earliest cases included in selected online databases for each state where any database does not include from the earliest

State (date of earliest commonly available high court decisions)	Bloomberg	Lexis	Westlaw
Alabama (1820)	1840	1820	1820
Connecticut (1785)	1814	1785	1785
Delaware (1792)	1790	1814	1792
Iowa (1837)	1839	1855	1839
Louisiana (1809)	1809	1809	1813
Maryland (1770)	1851	1770	1787
Michigan (1805)	1847	1843	1805
Nebraska (1860)	1860	1871	1871
New Mexico (1852)	1883	1852	1852
New York (1791)	1796	1794	1799
North Dakota (1867)	1890	1867	1867
Ohio (1809)	1852	1821	1821
Pennsylvania (1754)	1845	1791	1791
South Dakota (1867)	1890	1867	1867
Tennessee (1791)	1791	1791	1811
Texas (1840)	1846	1840	1840
Utah (1861)	1872	1861	1861
Vermont (1789)	1826	1826	1789
Virginia (1779)	1790	1730	1729
Washington (1854)	1889	1854	1854

case coverage when at least one of Bloomberg, Lexis, or Westlaw databases does not include the earliest cases.

An example will illustrate why a researcher should look for cases that may not be in the major databases. In 1824, the U.S. Supreme Court decided *Gibbons v. Ogden* (22 U.S. 1 [1824]), which held that Congress was granted the right to regulate interstate commerce by the Commerce Clause of the Constitution. Someone interested in the case might want to see any opinions from lower courts as the case made its way to the Supreme Court or the related cases heard in New Jersey at the same time. The first opinion in the case that became the Supreme Court case was written by Chancellor James Kent at the New York Court of Equity and was reported at 4 *Johns. Ch.* 150 (1819). That case was appealed to the New York Court for the Correction of Errors. The decision of the Court for the Correction of Errors was reported at 17 *Johns. Ch.* 488 (1820). This was the case that was appealed to the U.S. Supreme Court.

When researchers look for cases related to *Gibbons v. Ogden* in the three major databases, they will get slightly different results. From the Supreme Court case, it is easy to find the two New York cases. The case history at Lexis, the direct history at Bloomberg Law, and the direct history at Westlaw list the two prior New York opinions. Bloomberg Law and Westlaw provide the full texts of both New York opinions as well. Lexis provides the full text of the opinion of the Court for the Correction of Errors, but not of the Chancery Court's opinion. While the issue was litigated in New York, similar litigation among the same parties was taking place in New Jersey. While not a parent or child of the Supreme Court case, the New Jersey cases are related and may well be of interest to a researcher. Neither Lexis nor Westlaw makes these cases apparent. Bloomberg Law includes them as related cases in the history. If researchers using Lexis wanted to obtain Chancellor Kent's opinion, they might look at Westlaw or Bloomberg, or they might turn to one of the sources that contain many reporters not covered by Bloomberg Law, Lexis, or Westlaw.

Researchers can use three good tools to determine what reports might have existed. The easiest and most likely to hand in a law environment is the *Bluebook*. It contains a list for each state that includes its main courts and indicates the main reporters that cover each court, as well as the years of coverage. The *Bluebook* is, however, the least complete of the tools. The second option is to examine *Hein's State Report Checklist*, which brings together several bibliographic tools that list the various reports for each state and their years of coverage. Researchers can then look for the cases in the online databases or a library catalog. If a reporter has been identified, researchers will conduct an author and/or title search. The library catalog is the third major tool for identifying state reporters. Searching in the catalog for the subject "law reports, digests, etc." and a subdivision by the geographical jurisdiction, or using the geographical jurisdiction as a second search term, should return the opinions of the highest courts in each jurisdiction.

Some of the reporters not included in the later state reporter series, and therefore more difficult to find, have been digitized and made available online by the Law Library Microform Consortium (LLMC; see more at www.llmc.com). Researchers can also use HathiTrust, the Internet Archive, and Google Books for locating reporters online.

Access to Nineteenth-Century Federal Case Law Today

As we have seen, the modern concept of case reporting developed over the course of the nineteenth century. Coverage of the U.S. Supreme Court started with Alexander Dallas, an unofficial reporter who transcribed oral decisions and sold them. This continued until Henry Wheaton received the exclusive right to publish and sell the opinions from 1817 to 1827. Following Wheaton, Richard Peters began the process that changed the report style from transcriptions with scholarly additions, which could be very slow to appear, to the quickly published texts of the justices' opinions, further accelerated when Peters reprinted some of Wheaton's work. In the resulting Supreme Court case, *Wheaton v. Peters*, the Court held that there is no copyright in Supreme Court opinions. The same volume of the *Reports* contained an order from the Court directing the justices to file their opinions in written form (33 U.S. [8 Pet.] vii [1834]). Thus, by the 1830s Supreme Court reporting looked substantially like it does today.

All of the reported Supreme Court cases are available through online resources. They can be found at the for-fee databases Bloomberg Law, HeinOnline, Lexis, and Westlaw as well as many other databases. They are also available for free through Google Scholar, and a variety of places, including the Legal Information Institute at Cornell Law School and FindLaw, offer incomplete collections for free.

Comprehensive reporting of lower federal court opinions did not begin until West started publishing its *Federal Reporter* in 1880. Reporting from the lower federal courts was far less complete than even the sometimes haphazard Supreme Court reporting. Reporter coverage of the federal courts before 1880 was unorganized and spotty. However, West compiled all existing reports of federal cases from courts other than the Supreme Court to 1880 and published them in *Federal Cases*. While many cases were never reported, any that were are very likely included in *Federal Cases*. This set, unlike any other reporter, is organized alphabetically.

During the early nineteenth century, the circuit court was the main federal court. Because the jurisdiction of the district court was more limited than it is today, the circuit court acted as a trial court and an appellate court. The district court was the trial court for smaller federal civil cases and for admiralty cases. The circuit court served as the trial court for most federal criminal cases, civil cases between citizens of different states, and civil cases initiated by the United States. The circuit court could hear appeals from most district court cases.

Table 5.3 lists all of the reporters that include cases from the federal courts, excluding the Supreme Court, to 1880.

Table 5.3. Reporters covering federal courts other than the Supreme Court to 1880

Court	Reporter	Years
First Circuit	Gallison	1812–1815
	Mason	1816–1830
	Sumner	1829–1839
	Story	1839–1845
	Woodbury and Minot	1845–1847
	Curtis	1851–1856
	Ware	1822–1866
	Lowell	1865–1877
	Clifford	1858–1878
	Holmes	1870–1875
	Haskell	1866–1881
Second Circuit	Paine	1810–1840
	Blatchford	1845–1887
	Blatchford's Prize Cases	1861–1865
Third Circuit	Wallace	1801
	Peters	1803–1818
	Washington	1803–1827
	Fisher's Prize Cases	1812–1818
	Baldwin	1827–1833
	Wallace, Jr.	1842–1862
Fourth Circuit	Brockenbrough	1802–1836

	Taney	1836–1861
	Chase	1865–1869
	Hughes	1792–1883
Fifth Circuit	Woods	1870–1879
Sixth Circuit	McLean	1829–1855
	Bissell	1851–1883
	Bond	1856–1871
	Flippin	1859–1880
Seventh Circuit	McLean	1829–1855
	Bissell	1851–1883
	Woolworth	1863–1869
Eighth Circuit	Hempstead	1839–1855
	Woolworth	1863–1869
	Dillon	1870–1879
	M'Crary	1877–1888
Ninth Circuit	McAllister	1855–1859
	Deady	1861–1869
	Sawyer	1870–1891
District of Columbia	Cranch	1801–1840
	Hayward and Hazelton	1840–1849
All circuits	Wharton's State Trials	1789–1801
	Brunner's Collected Cases	1789–1860
	Abbott's U.S. Reports	1856–1871
	National Bankruptcy Register	1867–1879
Patent reports and decisions	Robb	1789–1850
	Fisher's Patent Reports	1821–1851
	Cranch's Patent Decisions	1841–1847
	MacArthur's Patent Cases	1841–1859
	Fisher's Patent Cases	1848–1878
	Banning and Arden	1874–1880
District Court Reports		
District of Maine	Ware	1822–1866
	Haskell	1866–1881

(Continued)

Table 5.3. Continued

Court	Reporter	Years
District of Massachusetts	Bee's Admiralty	1792–1809
	Fisher's Prize Cases	1812–1818
	Ware	1822–1866
	Sprague	1841–1864
	Lowell	1865–1877
District of Vermont	Benedict	1865–1879
District of Connecticut	Benedict	1865–1869
Southern District of New York	Van Ness (Prize Cases)	1814
	Blatchford and Howland	1827–1837
	Olcott (Admiralty)	1843–1847
	Abbott's Admiralty	1847–1850
	Blatchford's Prize Cases	1861–1865
	Benedict	1865–1879
Northern District of New York	Benedict	1865–1879
Eastern District of New York	Benedict	1865–1879
Eastern District of Pennsylvania	Peter's Admiralty	1789–1807
	Fisher's Prize Cases	1812–1813
	Gilpin	1828–1836
	Crabbe	1836–1846
Western District of Pennsylvania	Newberry's Admiralty	1820–1849
District of Maryland	Peter's Admiralty	1789–1807
District of South Carolina	Bee's Admiralty	1792–1809
District of Arkansas	Hempstead	1820–1849
Southern District of Ohio	Bond	1856–1871
Southern districts	Hughes	1792–1883
	Newberry's Admiralty	1842–1857

Western districts	Newberry's Admiralty	1842–1857
	Bissell	1851–1883
	Brown's Admiralty	1859–1875
	Flippin	1859–1880
Pacific state districts	Hoffman (land cases)	1853–1858
	Deady	1861–1869
	Sawyer	1879–1893
All districts	Abbott's United States Reports	1865–1971
	National Bankruptcy Register	1867–1879

Please note that there are far fewer reports than may first appear. The reports are listed under each jurisdiction from which cases were pulled. Consequently, many are listed several times. In addition, many of the reports cover a number of courts for many years in only a few volumes. For example, Robert William Hughes, *Reports of Cases Decided in the Circuit Courts of the United States for the Fourth Circuit* (Washington, DC: W. H. and O. H. Morrison, 1877–1883), covers all southern district courts and the Fourth Circuit for ninety years in only five volumes.

Case Finding in the Early Nineteenth Century

Case reports tend to be organized chronologically and, until West's reports, often cover only one court. This publishing scheme makes a great deal of sense as a means of collecting and printing the material, but it makes case finding very difficult. Searching for cases that deal with a particular legal issue becomes even more difficult because appellate cases are rarely about only one legal issue. When an appeal is made, all possible issues on which the case can be overturned are pled and argued together. The court will address all of the arguments that merit comment in its opinion. A researcher, then, is left with bits of law sprinkled throughout a set of books organized chronologically. The obvious problem is how to find the law that relates to a particular topic. Today we have access to most of the early cases in the databases of Bloomberg Law, Lexis, and Westlaw.

As we saw in chapter 2, the English solved this issue first by abridgments, then by proto-treatises, and then by comprehensive *Institutes* and digests; finally, the nineteenth and early twentieth century saw the rise of the modern legal treatise. In the United States, the first efforts to enable case finding were the inclusion of short topical indexes for each volume of reports. A lawyer could find cases in the few early volumes relatively easily, but as the quantity of law increased, it became clear that volume indexes would not remain a reasonable solution.

The early nineteenth century featured the development of research tools that enabled U.S. lawyers to find cases by topics. As we will see in chapter 6, West created digests of cases and retrospectively digested early cases. Those tools made early-nineteenth-century case law available to later researchers. The tools developed then are still available and can be useful today.

During the nineteenth century, U.S. legal treatises were written and steadily improved in quality and importance. However, for much of that time the importation and use of English treatises was common, and American editions of English treatises became increasingly popular.

In the 1820s, one of the most important early American law books was published; *Commentaries on American Law* by

Chancellor James Kent of New York has the same sort of breadth and depth that one would expect in an *Institute* in other nations. Kent's *Commentaries* covered international, federal, and state law generally and included the major legal issues: the law of war, the rights of the person, rights in personal property, and rights in real property. The *Commentaries* was extremely influential; however, for most practicing lawyers, it did not resolve the day-to-day issues of practice in an increasingly industrialized nation.

Kent's *Commentaries* has been reprinted and digitized by several groups and is widely available for free on the Internet, as are most of the important English and U.S. legal treatises from this period, which are available with controlled vocabulary catalog-style and full-text searching through Gale's *Making of Modern Law: Legal Treatises*. Another database that contains similar material is West's *Rise of American Law*. Since this database includes only treatises published by West, its nineteenth-century coverage is much slighter than that of *Making of Modern Law*; but it continues well into the twentieth century, far beyond *Making of Modern Law*.

Other bibliographies that can help a researcher identify early legal treatises include the *Bibliography of Early American Law; Early American Imprints;* J. G. Marvin's *Legal Bibliography, or a Thesaurus of American, English, Irish and Scotch Law Books: Together with Some Continental Treatises*, which has been digitized by Google; and *American Law Publishing, 1860–1900*.

An American version of another important research tool developed in England during the mid-eighteenth century—the legal digest—appeared in the early nineteenth century and included John Anthon's *A Digested Index to the Reported Decisions* (1813–1814) and Nicholas Baylies's *A Digested Index to the Modern Reports* (1814). Today, legal researchers often think of digests as case digests only, but in the early nineteenth century, there was a broader common understanding of the term "digest" to include statutes as well as cases. Digests of the law contain brief descriptions, topically arranged, of cases or statutes and citation references to the law. When researchers identify the section of a digest that covers their topic, they are directed to all of the relevant law covered by the digest. A digest generally breaks down the case or statute into pieces, each covering a legal issue; it then takes the pieces of law published in chronological order in case reporters or session laws and reorganizes them topically. Legislative digests are no longer necessary because of the adoption of topically arranged codes by all U.S. states and by Congress.

The first modern digest, John Comyns's *Digest of the Laws of England,* was published in 1762. The first and most important early American digest is Nathan Dane's *A General Abridgement and Digest of American Law,* a nine-volume set published between 1823 and 1829. Many other digests published in the nineteenth century covering specific topics or specific courts were popular. Comyns's, Dane's, and others are available to researchers today and can be found online at the Legal Classics and Spinelli's Reference libraries at HeinOnline. One useful title is Frederick C. Brightly's *Digest of the Decisions of the Federal Courts, from the Organization of the Government to the Present Time, 1789–1873* (1868–1873).

None of the early digests was comprehensive, nor did they have the level of detail that a modern researcher would recognize. The first step toward a more comprehensive digest was taken by Theron Metcalf, J. C. Perkins, and George Ticknor Curtis when *Digest of Decisions of the Courts of Common Law and Admiralty in the United States, 1754–1846* was published by Hilliard in Boston between 1840 and 1846. The second and subsequent editions were published by Little Brown between 1848 and 1888. Between 1848 and 1870 is was published in noncumulative annual volumes. At that point, it was reimagined by Benjamin Vaughan Abbott to compile cases from the beginning to 1867 in one cumulative set. This was published in 1876 as the *Digest of the Reports of the United States Courts and the Acts of Congress.* It was supplemented through 1888 by annual noncumulative volumes called the New Series.

In 1887, West started the *American Digest.* In the 1890s, West purchased the copyrights of the *United States Digest* and the *Digest of the Reports of the United States Courts* from Little Brown and Abbott. The resulting publication was initially considered another series of the *United States Digest,* but by 1894 the series along with the supplementation and additional cases were collected into the *Century Edition,* the first part of West's American Digest System. The *Century Edition* covers the years 1658–1896 and, as we will see in the next chapter, laid the foundation for West's national system.

Another nineteenth-century innovation was the selective reporter covering several jurisdictions. One of the most important, *The American Decisions: Containing All the Cases of General Value and Authority Decided in the Courts of the Several States, from the Earliest Issue of the State Reports to the Year 1869,* was published by Bancroft-Whitney between 1878 and 1888. This was an effort to find, collect, and print the most important cases from around the nation to enable attorneys from any state to find cases that related to a legal issue. This reporter was not comprehensive, but the cases were deemed to be the best. *American Decisions* was followed in the early twentieth century by *Ruling Case Law,* a set that pulled cases from many American and English reporters. One final selective reporter that remains an important legal research tool is *American Law Reports,* which includes a research essay, called an annotation, that discusses in depth the main legal issue raised in a case, in addition to the case report. The annotation also includes references to cases that stand for any of the propositions that appear in the annotation.

Researchers interested in the U.S. Supreme Court may also consider more recent histories of the Court and the important cases it has heard. One collection that deserves special mention is the series of histories of the U.S. Supreme Court, funded by the Oliver Wendell Holmes Devise, including Julius Goebel Jr.'s *Antecedents and Beginnings to 1801* (1971); George Lee Haskins and Herbert A. Johnson's *Foundations of Power: John Marshall, 1801–15* (1981); G. Edward White and Gerald Gunther's *The Marshall Court and Cultural Change, 1815–35* (1988); Carl Brent Swisher's *The Taney Period, 1836–64* (1974); Charles Fairman's *Reconstruction and Reunion, 1864–88* (1971– 1987) and *Five Justices and the Electoral Commission of 1877* (1988); Owen Fiss's *Troubled Beginnings of the Modern State, 1888–1910* (1993 and 2006); Alexander M. Bickel and Benno C. Schmidt Jr.'s *The Judiciary and Responsible Government, 1910–21* (1984); and William M. Wiecek's *The Birth of the Modern Constitution: The United States Supreme Court, 1941–1953* (2006). Each is well researched and footnoted.

Case Files

To conduct research for court materials other than an opinion of the court, a researcher must examine court journals and dockets. A court's journal will provide a very brief description of the reason for the suit or appeal and will note the outcome. The docket will list documents filed in the case as well as other events. The documents mentioned in a court's docket may be available through federal or state archives, but in many instances the documents will have been lost, discarded, or destroyed.

The minutes and dockets for the U.S. Supreme Court from 1829 to the early twentieth century were published by the National Archives in a microform set held by many libraries. Materials from before 1829 are in the National Archives, Record Group 291. Finding the journals and dockets from other courts, at least those from before the past few years, may be more difficult and usually requires contacting either state archives or a federal archive.

Researchers may find useful another kind of material related to cases—the brief. When a case is appealed, the litigants make most of the arguments through briefs. The parties file them on a variety of issues raised by the case, and, on occasion, friends of the court may file amicus briefs arguing for a legal position. These can open an important window into a case and the development of the law. United States Supreme Court briefs from the 1830s onward are fairly readily available. Supreme Court briefs from before the 1830s may be included in one of two microform sets published by the National Archives: *Appellate Case Files from the Supreme Court of the United States, 1792–1831* or *Case Papers of the Supreme Court of the United States, 1790– 1807*. Briefs from other courts may raise additional research issues. A microform set and the *Making of American Law: Supreme Court Briefs, 1832–1978* contain many, but not all, briefs filed with the Supreme Court. Several law libraries are depositories for Supreme Court briefs and are identified in *A Union List of Appellate Court Records and Briefs: Federal and State,* by Michael Whiteman and Peter Scott Campbell.

To determine what briefs related to a particular case might exist, a researcher will examine the docket entries associated with it. The dockets from the U.S. Supreme Court are available at many libraries on microform. The dockets and briefs from other courts are more difficult to find. Many have been filmed and are available at some libraries; the *Union List* can also help a researcher locate this material. Researchers familiar with modern court dockets will likely find early dockets somewhat disappointing. Even after a nineteenth-century docket has been examined, it can be difficult to determine what material might have been filed in a case. If the material has not been filmed, state or federal archives are the best places to search (see chapter 8 for archival research).

More recently, the federal government has made many dockets and their accompanying documents available through Public Access to Court Electronic Records (PACER) (http://www.pacer.gov). The coverage of PACER and the other tools mentioned here is not long; it extends little past the 1990s. PACER is a fee-based system, although several crowdsourcing tools are available that can make using PACER cheaper. PacerPro has a free tier that allows PACER searching, and it allows the free downloading of any PACER document that anyone in the PacerPro system has ever downloaded. Any document that a researcher downloads becomes part of the database. PacerPro makes its money on docket tracking tools. RECAP, from the Free Law Project (https://free.law/recap/), is a browser plugin that tells researchers and provides a link when its database contains a free document, and it adds any document that a researcher downloads to its database. Bloomberg, Westlaw, and Lexis have made federal and some state dockets available. They start with the PACER data and add some briefs to their databases that they acquire through their document retrieval businesses. Researchers with sufficient funding can hire these document retrieval businesses to acquire documents not included in the database.

In addition, Lexis and Westlaw have also added some other court documents and oral arguments to their databases.

An interesting resource for the U.S. Supreme Court is the Oyez project (http://www.oyez.org), a multimedia archive of the Court. For many cases it includes a summary, the opinions, and a recording of the oral argument.

Publication of Legislation

During the eighteenth and most of the nineteenth centuries, colonies/states published their legislative enactments as session laws: that is, laws passed by the legislature during a particular session arranged chronologically, then occasionally organized topically. For several states, the ongoing legislative publications seamlessly moved from the colonial government to the state government. As the nineteenth century progressed, the production of the session laws and the organization of the laws became more regularized. The organized version began to be approved by the legislature, and the organizational structure began to last longer between revisions. This process is the American version of codification. In the United States, codes are the topical arrangement, generally adopted by state, of the permanent acts of the legislature of general import.

The development of session law publication was rapid; however, the development of codification progressed differently in each state and at the federal level. Not only did each state adopt a code at a different time, but each state also organized its codes differently, and many states periodically recodified their statutory law. A state research guide should indicate the dates of recodification and the coverage of a state's session laws. In general, session laws are available from very early in the history of a state or colony and continue to the current day. The historical session laws are available at HeinOnline and some law libraries. More recent session laws are available online through Lexis and Westlaw and often a state legislature's website.

At the federal level, all early efforts to publish and organize the law were private. During the early years of the Republic, Congress authorized certain collections of federal statutes. The first published was the *Laws of the United States of America* (1796–1797), compiled by Zephaniah Swift, printed by R. Folwell (the Folwell edition), and authorized by Congress in 1795; it covers three Congresses in three volumes. It was continued with a new volume for every Congress through the tenth, ending in 1809. It was superseded by the *Laws of the United States of America* (1815), printed by John Bioren and W. John Duane (authorized in 1814), which covers the first to twenty-eighth Congresses in ten volumes (1789–1845). Other collections include *Public and General Statutes Passed by the Congress of the United States of America* (1827–1848), by Joseph Story and George Sharswood, which covers from 1789 through 1847. These and other collections are available at HeinOnline and some libraries, and certain volumes are available online through HathiTrust and Google Books.

Finally, during the 1840s the federal government began publishing session laws in the *Statutes at Large.* These contain public laws, private laws (laws that affect a single person or a small group of specified people), presidential proclamations, treaties with foreign countries (until 1950), and treaties with Native Americans. At the beginning, the *Statutes at Large* was designed to replace the earlier federal statutory publications, so the first eight volumes included the laws from the first Congress to the 1840s. Volumes 1 through 5 contain public laws; volume 6 contains private laws; volume 7, treaties with Native

Americans; and volume 8, treaties with foreign powers. From volume 9 forward, all types of material are included in each volume. Within a volume, material is organized by type, and within each type, by chronological order. Each volume also contains a subject index.

If a researcher has a citation to the *Statutes at Large,* finding the act of Congress is very straightforward: locate the *Statutes at Large,* turn to the volume included in the citation, and then turn to the page included in the citation. As a government document, the *Statutes at Large* is widely available in print. The volumes that cover up to 1875 are available at the Century of Lawmaking website of the Library of Congress; volumes covering from 1789 through 1950 are available at the Library of Congress at https://www.loc.gov/law/help/statutes-at-large/. The Library of Congress website contains a link to the GPO site that has volumes covering from 1951 forward. All volumes are also available online through HeinOnline, ProQuest Congressional, and LexisNexis.

The codification movement in the United States did interact with the movement in Europe. One of the leaders of codification, Jeremy Bentham, contacted James Madison with an offer to codify American law. In addition, Louisiana and New York moved along the codification path faster and farther than many other states. The codification movements in Louisiana during the 1820s and 1830s, led by Edward Livingston, and in New York during the 1850s, led by David Dudley Field, were influential locally and in Europe; but U.S. codes, while more structured and official than in other common law jurisdictions, are not the complete statements of the law that the European codes became. It is important to recognize this influence to understand the development of legal materials during the nineteenth century.

In Europe the organization of law, often led by scholars and other outsiders, was embraced by the government. Interestingly, several topically arranged collections of U.S. state laws were published in the late eighteenth century. For example, in 1784, the Connecticut legislature organized all of the law then in effect and passed the organized version as a single law. In doing so, it repealed all of the prior law that made up the collection. Thus, in 1784 Connecticut had a collection of legislation that looks like a step on the path to codification. Although several other states continued and expanded on these efforts, most publishing, even at the state level, remained a private enterprise.

One hundred years after Connecticut's 1784 collection of legislation, the federal government completed its first effort at codification. Before 1870, a researcher looking for federal legislation could find it in the *Statutes at Large* or in one of the privately published collections. The major privately published sets as well as the *Statutes at Large* are available at HeinOnline. In 1875, after a ten-year effort, Congress passed the *Revised Statutes of the United States* into law. Confusingly, this is often called the "Revised Statutes of 1873" because it contained all statutes of a general and permanent nature in effect on December 1, 1873, or the "Revised Statutes of 1874" because it was authorized by Congress on June 20, 1874.

One of the sections included in the *Revised Statutes*, section 5596, had two very important effects. First, it repealed all of the statutes passed before 1873, and second, it made the *Revised Statutes* "legal evidence of the laws and treaties." Shortly after the passage and publication of the *Revised Statutes*, complaints about errors contained in the *Statutes* and about the difficulty in using it led to a second edition of the *Revised Statutes* published in 1878. This edition repaired some of the errors in the first edition and included laws passed since 1873. However, the act passing the second edition of *Revised Statutes* in 1878 did not repeal any prior law and is considered to provide only "prima facie evidence of the law." Both editions of the *Revised Statutes* have been separately published, and they have been published within the *Statutes at Large*. They are both available at HeinOnline.

Congress authorized supplements to the *Revised Statutes* in 1881 and 1891, and from then, after every Congress. However, these supplements were not widely adopted by users, and they can be difficult to locate. Nonetheless, private publishers continued to publish collections of the statutes as well as finding aids, and the government continued to publish *Statutes at Large*.

Finding Legislation

A savvy researcher can immediately see a problem with a chronological publication pattern. When one looks at a law, it is not immediately apparent whether any sections have been amended or repealed. Often, many volumes have to be consulted together to determine the law on a particular topic. Several attempts to solve this problem included Connecticut's choice to restate the law in 1784 and repeal prior laws. In 1784 a researcher would need to consult only one volume, but as more laws passed, the number of individually indexed volumes increased. The collections of federal laws published in the late eighteenth and early nineteenth centuries offered a second solution—printing the laws in chronological order but including an index to the entire corpus. A researcher could consult one index but potentially have many laws to examine and put together to determine the state of the law. Another solution saw separately published index/digests of the federal statutes, prepared in the early nineteenth century. One of these is Asbury Dickens's *Synoptical Index to the Laws and Treaties of the United States of America, from March 4, 1789 to March 3, 1851* (1852). This and others are available at law libraries and HeinOnline.

Another important index to early federal statutes is the *Index-Analysis of the Federal Statutes Together with a Table of Repeals and Amendments* (1908–1911) by George Winfield Scott, et al. Volume 1 covers from 1878 to 1907, and volume 2, from 1789 to 1873. The first volume was revised several times so that it eventually covered from 1878 to 1925, when the United States Code was created. The volume that covers from 1789 to 1873 directs a researcher to the *Statutes at Large,* and the volume that covers from 1878 directs a researcher to the 1873 *Revised Statutes* and any later changes appearing either in the second edition of the *Revised Statutes* published in 1878 or a later volume of the *Statutes at Large.* Researchers have to put the law together from these, adding, revising, and deleting parts of the implicated session laws.

Indexes and digests of legislation as well as the alternative versions of the statutes are available at many libraries as well as the U.S. Code library at HeinOnline. One of the nicer features of Hein's collection is a table that allows the researcher to sort the publications by a variety of criteria, including dates of publication and dates of coverage.

Until the 1870s, federal statutory law was available only in a chronologically arranged form. Topical indexes and digests existed, but there was no place to find a topical arrangement of federal law. However, by 1870 several states had organized their laws topically. Louisiana, influenced by the *Code Napoleon,* had adopted codes in 1808, 1825, and 1870. Massachusetts had organized its laws into a topical arrangement as early as the

Revised Statutes of 1836. New Jersey had an unofficial, though highly regarded and cited, organized version of its statutes in *Elmer's Digest* in 1838. As early as 1801, New York's laws were organized topically in the *Laws of the State of New York* by James Kent and Jacob Radcliff, and by 1829 the *Revised Statutes* was in effect. These early state laws can be found at many law libraries, and many of the volumes are also available online through Google Books and HathiTrust.

The federal government was a little slower in moving toward a code. In 1875, the federal government published the *Revised Statutes of the United States*, which organized into a logical arrangement the general and permanent public laws in force as of December 1, 1873. The law that made the *Revised Statutes* the law also repealed prior laws. However, there were a number of errors in the *Revised Statutes*, so Congress ordered a second edition prepared, which was published in 1878. The *Revised Statutes, Second Edition* did not repeal the first edition. Both editions of the *Revised Statutes* were published within the *Statutes at Large*, as volume 18, part 1 (1878) and part 2 (1873). They are available where the *Statutes at Large* can be found. They have also been separately published many times. Lawyers practicing from the 1880s to the 1920s would have used the *Revised Statutes*, supplemented by the second edition and by any session laws passed from 1874. As we have seen, the *Index-Analysis of the Federal Statutes* would facilitate this process. Congress finally adopted a successful organization of its laws in the 1920s.

Private Laws

In addition to public laws, legislatures often passed private laws, which affect a limited group of people or a single person. Private laws frequently dealt with issues such as the immigration status of a single person or the rights of a particular person to a federal pension. While researchers today may not find private laws very interesting, in the nineteenth century, they were extremely important, and in many cases their import lives on. Before around the 1870s, corporations were created by the legislature passing a private law. By the end of the nineteenth century, the creation of corporations became a matter of filling out a form and filing it with the secretary of the state. However, research on the origins of a corporation created before then will go back to private laws.

Usually, private laws were published alongside public laws. When they do not appear together, however, a researcher can conduct a separate search for private laws from the session of interest or look for a collection of private laws for a particular jurisdiction and time period. These collections usually have a topical index as well as a table of contents and are available at many law libraries; some are also available online through Google Books and HathiTrust.

Research Example

We will work with several questions here in order to demonstrate several sources. We first look at legislation dealing with Congress's power to regulate commerce. We can begin by using a nineteenth-century topical collection of statutes, for example, Frederick C. Brightly's *Analytical Digest of the Laws of the United States.* This volume, published in 1857, covers laws passed between 1789 and 1857. It is organized by large topics, and it has a fairly detailed index. When we look in the index for "commerce, Congress's power to regulate," we are sent to page 4. Not surprisingly, page 4 contains Article I, Section 8, Clause 4 of the Constitution.

To make the research a little more interesting, let us try to find laws passed up to 1850 related to the gathering and dissemination of statistical information about foreign commerce. Using Brightly again, except this time selecting the main heading "commerce," we find that the entire first section is about statistics. The statistics portion of commerce is broken down into twenty-four parts, the last of which creates, within the office of the secretary of state, the position of superintendent of statistics.

Let us now try to find federal cases about Congress's power to regulate commerce. To make the search more interesting, we can also decide to work as a mid-nineteenth-century lawyer may have worked and consult Brightly's *Digest of the Decisions of the Federal Courts, from the Organization of the Government to the Present Time* (1868). In the index under "commerce, power to regulate," we are directed to page 151, which is within the discussion of cases related to the section covering constitutional law on the regulation of commerce. We could have found the same material by browsing to the main section of "Constitution," looking through the categories into which Brightly divided constitutional law, then turning to "regulation of commerce." There, Brightly presents forty-nine brief blurbs about cases decided before 1857 that dealt with Congress's power to regulate commerce. Each blurb provides a citation to the case as well as a brief idea of how the case treated the legal topic.

We next use the *Index-Analysis of the Federal Statutes* to find the federal laws relating to the reporting of U.S. Supreme Court opinions. When we turn to "Supreme Court, reports," we are directed to "reports of the Supreme Court of the United States" on page 859. There we learn that we might also like to examine "public documents" at page 808. If we

look at "distribution," we see that there are five laws, ranging
in date from 1817 to 1866, that in part deal with the topic. To
determine what the law is, we need to examine all five laws.
Funnily enough, directly below the entry for distribution is
an entry for "furnished to Department of Justice for distribution to Officers of Court." This law appears at volume 17 of
the *Statutes at Large* on page 578 and became law on March 3,
1873.

Further Reading

Aumann, Francis R. "American Law Reports: Yesterday and Today." *Ohio State University Law Journal* 4 (1938): 331–45.

Bloomfield, Maxwell. "William Sampson and the Codifiers: The Roots of American Legal Reform, 1820–1830." *American Journal of Legal History* 11 (1967): 234–52.

Boyd, Anne Morris, and Rae Elizabeth Rips. "Congressional Publications, Continued: Colonial Period and Early U.S. Congresses." In *United States Government Publications*, 76–81. New York: Wilson, 1950.

Cohen, Morris L. "Legal Forms: From Clay to Computers." *Yale Law Report* 31 (1985): 25–28.

Dwan, Ralph H., and Ernest R. Feidler. "The Federal Statutes—Their History and Use." *Minnesota Law Review* 22 (1937): 1008–29.

Friedman, Lawrence M. *A History of American Law.* New York: Simon and Schuster, 1973.

———. "Law Reform in Historical Perspective." *Saint Louis University Law Journal* 13 (1968): 351–72.Helmholz, R. H. "Use of the Civil Law in Post-Revolutionary American Jurisprudence." *Tulane Law Review* 66 (1991): 1649–84.

Hezel, George M. "Influence of Bentham's Philosophy of Law on the Early Nineteenth Century Codification Movement in the United States." *Buffalo Law Review* 22 (1972): 253–68.

Hoeflich, M. H. "Law Blanks and Form Books: A Chapter in the Early History of Document Production." *Green Bag, 2d* 11 (2008): 189–201.

———. "Legal Ephemera: A Window on Society and Law." *American Bookman: A Quarterly of Criticism and Theory of the Public Arts* (March 1997): 785–88.

Horwitz, Morton J. *The Transformation of American Law, 1780–1860.* Cambridge, MA: Harvard University Press, 1977.

Howe, Daniel Walker. *What Hath God Wrought: The Transformation of America, 1815–1848.* New York: Oxford University Press, 2007.

Joyce, Craig. "A Curious Chapter in the History of Judicature: Wheaton v. Peters and the Rest of the Story (of Copyright in the New Republic)." *Houston Law Review* 42 (2005): 325–91.

———. "Wheaton v. Peters: The Untold Story of the Early Reporters." *1985 Yearbook of the Supreme Court Historical Society* 35 (1986): 35–92.

McFarland, Carl. "David Dudley Field, Codification of Statutes, and Administrative Law." *Montana Law Review* 10 (1949): 1–12.

Nelson, Bonnie R., and Marilyn Lutzker. "Historical Research with Primary Sources: Nineteenth Century America." In *Criminal Justice Research in Libraries and on the Internet,* 185–96. Westport, CT: Greenwood, 1998.

Newmyer, R. Kent. "Spreading the Word: Codifier as Publicist." In *Supreme Court Justice Joseph Story: Statesman of the Old Republic,* 271–304. Chapel Hill: University of North Carolina Press, 1985.

Richardson, William A. "Chief Justice of the United States or Chief Justice of the Supreme Court of the United States." In *The New England Historical and Genealogical Register* 49, no. 195 (1895): 275–79.

Stein, Peter. "The Attraction of the Civil Law in Post-Revolutionary America." *Virginia Law Review* 52 (1966): 403–34.

Surrency, Erwin C. "Law Reports in the United States." *American Journal of Legal History* 25 (1981): 48–66.

Wagner, Wienczyslaw J. "Codification of Law in Europe and the Codification Movement in the Middle of the Nineteenth Century in the United States." *Saint Louis University Law Journal* 2 (1952): 335–59.

Wood, Gordon S. *Empire of Liberty: A History of the Early Republic, 1789–1815.* Oxford: Oxford University Press, 2009.

Important Sources Mentioned in This Chapter

Bioren, John, and William J. Duane. *Laws of the United States of America: from the 4th of March, 1789, to the 4th of March, 1815, including the Constitution of the United States, the old Act of Confederation, treaties, and many other valuable ordinances and documents; with copious notes and references. Arranged and published under the authority of an act of Congress, In Five Volumes.* Philadelphia, 1816.

Boutwell, George S. *Revised statutes of the United States, passed at the first session of the Forty-third Congress, 1873–'74; embracing the statutes of the United States, general and permanent in their nature, in force on the first day of December, One thousand eight hundred and seventy-three, as revised and consolidated by commissioners appointed under an act of Congress; and as reprinted, with amendments, under authority of an act of Congress approved the second day of March, in the year one thousand eight hundred and seventy-seven, with an appendix.* Washington, DC: GPO, 1878.

Dane, Nathan. *A General Abridgement and Digest of American Law with Occasional Notes and Comments.* Boston: Cummings, Hilliard, 1823.

Kent, James. *Commentaries on American Law.* New York: O. Halsted, 1826.

Marvin, J. G. *Legal Bibliography, or a Thesaurus of American, English, Irish, and Scotch Law Books: Together with Some Continental Treatises.* Philadelphia: T & J. W. Johnson Dennis, 1953.

McKinney, William Mark. *Ruling Case Law.* Northport, NY: E. Thompson, 1929.

Proffatt, John, and A. C. Freeman. *The American Decisions: Containing All the Cases of General Value and Authority Decided in the Courts of the Several States, from the Earliest Issue of the State Reports [1760] to the Year 1869 . . .* San Francisco: A. L. Bancroft, 1878.

Ritz, Wilfred J. *American Judicial Proceedings First Printed Before 1801: An Analytical Bibliography.* Westport, CT: Greenwood, 1984.

Scott, George Winfield, Middleton G. Beaman, and Agnes (McNamara) Munson. *Index-Analysis of the Federal Statutes (General Permanent Law), 1789–1873 [1873–1907].* Washington, DC: GPO, 1908.

Story, Joseph, and George Sharswood. *Public and general statutes passed by the Congress of the United States of America from 1789 to [1847] inclusive, whether expired, repealed, or in force: arranged in chronological order, with marginal references, and a copious index: to which is added the Constitution of the United States, and an appendix.* Boston: Wells and Lilly, 1827.

United States. *Appellate Case Files of the Supreme Court of the United States, 1792–1831.* Washington, DC: National Archives and Records Service, 1962.

———. *Case Papers of the Supreme Court of U.S., 1790–1807.* Washington, DC, 1790.

———. *Index to the Appellate Case Files of the Supreme Court of the United States, 1792–1909.* Washington, DC: National Archives and Records Administration, 1963.

————. *The Laws of the United States of America: In three volumes. . . . Published by Authority.* Philadelphia, 1796.

————. *Revised Statutes of the United States, passed at the first session of the Forty-third Congress, 1873–'74: embracing the statutes of the United States, general and permanent in their nature, in force on the first day of December, One thousand eight hundred and seventy-three, as revised and consolidated by commissioners appointed under an act of Congress: with an appendix containing "An act to correct errors and supply omission."* Washington, DC: GPO, 1875.

————. *Statutes at Large, From the United States.* Washington, DC: GPO, 1845–.

————. *United States Reports. Cases adjudged in the Supreme Court.* Washington, DC: GPO, 1790–.

Whiteman, Michael, and Peter Scott Campbell. *A Union List of Appellate Court Records and Briefs: Federal and State.* Littleton, CO: F. B. Rothman, 1999.

Wiese, Keith, and American Association of Law Libraries. *Hein's State Report Checklist.* W. S. Hein, 2015.

Databases

Gale. *Making of Modern Law: U.S. Supreme Court Records and Briefs, 1832–1978.* http://www.gale.com/c/making-of-modern-law-us-supreme-court-records-and-briefs-1832-1978.

Law Library Microform Consortium. LLMC Digital. http://www.llmcdigital.org/.

Readex. *Early American Imprints, Series I: Evans, 1639–1800.* http://www.readex.com/content/early-american-imprints-series-i-evans-1639-1800.

————. *Early American Imprints. Series II: Shaw-Shoemaker, 1801–1819.* http://www.readex.com/content/early-american-imprints-series-ii-shaw-shoemaker-1801-1819

6

Research Gets Organized, 1880s–1930s

Toward the end of the nineteenth century several trends in legal bibliography, as well as the development and refinement of several legal research tools, created a better-organized world of legal research. The federal government made its first attempt at codification in 1873. At roughly the same time, West Publishing Company began producing a comprehensive collection of state and federal case reporters, which came to be known as the National Reporter System. West also applied the concept of case law digests to the National Reporter System, thus offering legal researchers a comprehensive collection of cases and tools that provided a consistent topical arrangement of case law. By listing every reported case that cited a given case and indicating how the subsequent treated the earlier, citators became a valuable research tool for attorneys. Until the late nineteenth century, attorneys created their own citators by marking up their personal reporter volumes. In the 1870s, Frank Shepard began selling lists of cases citing earlier reported cases, soon compiled into books that provided lawyers with both information about the status of a specific case and another means of finding cases relevant to a particular issue. The era reached its climax of successful federal law codification with the publication in 1925 of the United States Code, using the organization developed for the federal government by West.

Aside from the not inconsequential rise of administrative law and the associated research tools, legal research changed little in the fifty years after 1930. The development of computerized databases in the 1960s and 1970s began to change legal research, but into the twenty-first century most online research tools matched those developed at the turn of the twentieth century.

Selective Reporters and *American Law Reports*

In 1847, J. I. Clark Hare and H. B. Wallace started publishing *Select Decisions of American Courts*. In later editions, *Select Decisions* became *American Leading Cases*. Whatever the title, *Select Decisions* was the first American example of a selective case reporter. Selective reporters relied on editors to collect the best cases, mainly from state courts but in some instances from federal courts as well. Several competitors joined *American Leading Cases,* including the "Trinity Series" published in the early twentieth century by Bancroft-Whitney, made up of the 100-volume *American Decisions: Cases of General Value and Authority Decided in the Courts of Several States,* the 60-volume *American Reports: Containing All Decisions of General Interest Decided in the Courts of Last Resort of the Several States,* and the 140-volume *American State Reports, Containing the Cases of General Value and Authority Subsequent to Those Contained in the American Decisions and the American Reports Decided in the*

Courts of Last Resort of the Several States. Highly important from the mid-nineteenth century, selective reporters remained so after West began printing cases more comprehensively, as many lawyers in the twentieth century found the quality of the selective reporters more attractive for research purposes than West's comprehensive reporters. The later development of online searching and the normalization of easy access to everything marked the end of the reporting side of selective reporters.

But even today, selective reporters are used. In 1919, the Lawyers Cooperative Publishing Company started publishing *American Law Reports* (ALR), which is published today by Thomson Reuters, the company that also publishes the West reporters. For much of its life ALR provided lawyers with two valuable services: it continued as a selective reporter in the mold of *American Leading Cases,* and it provided lawyers with annotations. ALR annotations, essays that provide detailed discussion of the major issue raised in each selected case, are valuable even though ALR is no longer an important case reporter. ALR had a sister publication that, because of antitrust rules, is now owned by Lexis. *United States Reports, Lawyers' Edition* reports U.S. Supreme Court cases and provides researchers with occasional briefs and research annotations.

ALR is in its seventh series for state law issues and second for federal, and the methods for finding and updating annotations have changed over time. A brief examination of these changes can provide insight into the process of legal research during the twentieth century. The first three ALR series cover both state and federal law, and the only differences among the series are the years covered. With the fourth series, ALR spun off federal annotations into a series called ALR Fed that is itself in a second series, ALR Fed. 2d. ALR's fourth through seventh series cover only state law.

To find an annotation in the first series of ALR using print resources, researchers have two options: use a digest that ALR created for the first series, or use a one-volume index to the annotations. To find annotations in the later series, researchers can examine a different digest or use a multivolume *Index to Annotations*.

Finding out about changes to annotations with the print version is a two-step process. First, researchers must determine whether the annotation has been supplemented or superseded; to do this, they will consult the "Table of Annotations Supplemented or Superseded." The table will direct them to a later annotation to use instead of or in conjunction with the original annotation. Next, for the third series and after, including both federal series, researchers should check the "pocket part," a small paperback pamphlet that fits into the back cover of the main volume. Organized like the main volume, the pocket part contains changes to the main volume. Further updating can still be done by telephone. To find changes and new materials for annotations from the second series, researchers need to examine the *ALR Later Case Service,* several bound volumes that contain newer material for a range of volumes of *ALR, Second Series.* These volumes are replaced occasionally and updated through pocket parts. To update the first series of ALR, researchers must examine the *ALR Blue Book of Supplemental Decisions.* Each volume contains updates to the entire run of *ALR, First Series.* As the volumes do not cumulate, each must be checked to bring the ALR up to date.

ALR is available online through Lexis and Westlaw; the digest and index are available through Westlaw (neither of these is available through Lexis). However, the annotation titles are very descriptive, so searches limited to the title can be quite effective. Because annotations are updated online, researchers do not need to consult additional sources for updates. Within an annotation researchers will find a helpful section that lists related annotations for further study.

Comprehensive Case Reporting

During the nineteenth century, case reporting developed from a haphazard practice in which lawyers, and often scholars, took down counsels' arguments and judges' opinions to a system in which an employee of the court collected judges' opinions, increasingly written down, and published them in government-sanctioned reporters. Since these reporters tended to cover one court, publication occurred after the completion of a court's session, when enough material had been gathered. Selective reporters published the most important cases, often years after those cases had been decided. Reporting of cases from the lower federal courts relied on circuit-based reporters and the national selective reporters.

West Publishing saw the market for near contemporaneous publishing of cases. By combining the opinions of several courts and several states, John West realized he could gather enough opinions to publish a reporter volume quickly, getting the cases into lawyers' hands in weeks rather than months or years. West's innovation not only sped up the distribution of cases but also substantially increased the market for any one reporter. *The Syllabi,* the pamphlet that grew into the *North-Western Reporter,* the first of West Publishing's case reporters, began in 1876. Within little more than a decade West was publishing seven regional reporters (Atlantic, North Eastern, North Western, Pacific, South Eastern, Southern, South Western) that covered all states, as well as one that covered the U.S. Supreme Court and another that covered other federal courts. In addition,

West collected the available federal cases from before 1880 and published them in another reporter, *Federal Cases* (see chapter 5). Almost every case that could set precedent in the United States was published quickly in a West reporter. In the late twentieth century, West made all of its published cases, the cases published by other publishers that predated West's publishing business, and all of the digest data available online through Westlaw.

West Digests

Comprehensive case reporting was not the only innovation that helped West to leap to the top of the legal publishing world. The company also expanded the digest as a case-finding tool, making it comprehensive and nationally consistent. For centuries, authors had distilled and digested the law into small statements and cited the most important cases that stood for a legal statement. West's digests were a little different: West digested every reported case, and West's organizational scheme was implemented throughout the country.

West's editors read each case, extract every point of law, and then describe the application of the law in a single sentence. Next they classify the sentence into their topical scheme. The topic description and sentence are together called a "headnote," which is included at the top of each case in the West reporter. Headnotes serve a bit like a table of contents to the case. The headnotes are then collected and arranged in West's topical order and published in many digests.

West publishes digests for almost every state, for four of the seven regions used in the National Reporter System, for the federal courts, for the U.S. Supreme Court, and for the entire country. There are no digests for the northeastern, southern, or southwestern regions; the Dakotas appear in one digest; and there is no digest for Delaware, Nevada, or Utah, although their cases are covered in the regional and complete (decennial) digests. While West did not reprint older state cases, it did digest them, so each digest includes references to cases from the beginning of case reporting in the jurisdiction forward. Also, West printed the *Century Digest*, which contains headnotes from state cases that predate West's publishing.

The national consistency of West digests made them very useful. A lawyer could look up any relevant case from any jurisdiction, identify the proper classification reference—called the Topic and Key Number—and then take the number to the digest covering the jurisdiction and find all reported cases about the same issue.

West has divided U.S. law into hundreds of Topics, and each Topic has many Key Numbers arranged topically under it. When using a digest, researchers must understand the Topic and Key Number classification scheme and find the section that treats their issue.

The next step is to use the proper print digest or database to find the cases from the right court or era. Researchers can use several methods to identify the proper Topic/Key Number. The easiest is to find a case through another source, such as a treatise, and then find the case in the West reporter or online through Westlaw. The relevant section of the case will have been assigned a Topic/Key Number. In the absence of a case, three additional methods can be used to find a Topic/Key Number. First, all print digests have an index, called the "Descriptive Word Index," that allows researchers to use index terms to find a Topic/Key Number. A second method takes advantage of the fact that West's classification scheme is arranged topically. Researchers can browse through the outline, in a digest, online through Westlaw, or in the separately published *West's Analysis of American Law: Guide to the American Digest System* to find the right Topic/Key Number. The Descriptive Word Index is not available online; however, researchers can browse the Digest Outline and search for terms in the outline at Westlaw. The third method for finding a Topic/Key Number is a variation of the first: using Westlaw or another online case database, researchers can conduct Boolean or relevance searches for a relevant case and look it up at Westlaw or in a West reporter.

Shepardizing

In a common law system, lawyers rely on past cases to determine the law, so it is very important to know whether and how courts have treated cases since they were decided. A lawyer who relies on a case that has been reversed by an appeals court or overruled by a later case will likely lose the case and almost certainly encounter a great deal of trouble. Until the middle of the nineteenth century, a lawyer's solution to this problem entailed reading the available new cases and, when he or she encountered a citation to a case that had been found in another reporter, making a notation next to the cited case to indicate its later treatment. On occasion, researchers today can see these notations in reporters housed in libraries and scanned into Google Books or other book-scanning projects.

In the nineteenth century, some businesses in larger cities had employees who traveled from law office to law office, inserting these references into their copies of the reporters. Frank Shepard held this job in Chicago during the 1870s. In the mid-1870s he started a company that offered to mail law offices lists of citing references, with shorthand notations indicating how the later case treated the earlier case. The recipient would then insert Shepard's adhesive list into the reporter volumes. Soon Shepard moved from sending adhesive lists to sending books made up of the lists. Lawyers found Shepard's system so efficient and worthwhile that it changed little until it was digitized and added to Lexis in the 1980s.

"Shepardizing" cases offers lawyers two important benefits: the assurance that a case found is still "good law" and the identification of cases that are relevant to a legal issue. A case will cite an earlier case when the court is making a statement of law and the case cited has something to say about that issue of law. The later court may be relying on the case cited, using it to bolster the statement or disparaging the case that it cites. No matter how the court treats the earlier case, merely by citing it, the court is asserting that it says something relevant.

In *Effective Legal Research* (4th ed., 1979), Miles O. Price, Harry Bitner, and Shirley R. Bysiewicz write, "Authority alone is that which is capable of binding a court on a given issue.... Its discovery, therefore, underlies and motivates all legal research" (p. 2). But not all authority will do; it must be relevant authority. Legal researchers use several shorthand methods to discover relevant authority among the law. With case finding, researchers may rely on editors to assign the same classification to the legal statement within a case that they will choose. Another class of methods relies on the presence or relationship of certain words that researchers select within the case. Using Shepard's Citations for research relies on the fact that when a court cites a case, it is claiming that there is legal relevance between the cases.

Until Shepard's Citations was digitized, the process of Shepardizing a case was onerous and tedious. Researchers would start by identifying the set of Shepard's Citations that covered the jurisdiction of the case in hand's origin. However, for much of the late nineteenth and twentieth centuries, cases might be printed in several reporters. For much of its history, Shepard's Citations provided researchers with different information depending on which citation they used for access. Therefore, the second step in Shepardizing a case was to determine which citation to Shepardize and then determine which volumes of the set selected would provide all cases that cited the case in hand. Since cases are constantly being decided, a set of Shepard's Citations would generally contain some volumes that covered a reporter or more for a long period of time. There then may be one or more hardbound supplementary volumes that would bring coverage from the close of the main bound volume(s) forward to some date. Then, one to three or more paperback pamphlets would likely bring coverage from the end of any supplementary volumes forward in time. The modern researcher should note that none of these bound or paper volumes overlapped; each must be checked. Further, Shepard's Citations did not list each citing case only once. It included a notation for every page on which the cited case was mentioned. Researchers would generally start at one end of the chronology; the authors generally started at the most recent pamphlets and worked backward, though either direction works. Researchers would find the case in each volume of Shepard's first by reporter, then by volume, and then by page. After checking every volume of Shepard's, researchers would have encountered every later case that cited their case.

The tediousness of Shepard's Citations did not end with the collection of volumes, or with the fact that researchers would get different information if they Shepardized the same case by a different citation, or even with the fact that the Shepard's volumes in a library did not cumulate, making checking every volume a necessary part of the exercise. The lists of citations were also very difficult to read. Shepard's contains an immense amount of data. To fit all the data into a reasonable number of pages, Shepard's abbreviated and compacted the data a lot. Each page of a Shepard's volume contained six columns consisting of a number, an abbreviation, and another number with no spaces between. Occasionally, a letter might appear to the left of the first number. This combination of numbers and letters was the citation to the case that cited the one being Shepardized. Shepard's provides nothing more than the volume of the citing case, a compacted reporter abbreviation, and the page of the case on which the cited case was mentioned. The letter to the left of the citation indicated either that the citing case had an effect on the history of the cited case or that it treated the case in some identifiable way.

In the 1990s, Shepard's Citations was digitized and joined by a digital competitor from West, KeyCite. The products are analogous. Shepard's is now available as a tool at Lexis, and KeyCite as a tool at Westlaw. They both list the cases that cite the case that was entered; they both indicate later treatment; and they both allow for faceted limiting of a list of citing references by limits such as jurisdiction, length of discussion, point of law discussed, and date. They even allow a researcher to search within the text of the citing cases. An examination of the documentation provided by each service can provide more information about the differences between the services and more information about how to use each of them.

United States Code

Chapter 5 addressed the nineteenth-century efforts in Congress to organize federal legislation. Through the mid-1920s, the *Revised Statutes* remained the law, and researchers might use it in conjunction with the *Revised Statutes, Second Edition* and the following *Statutes at Large* to find federal legislative law. Alternatively, they might use one of the privately published law-finding tools, such as the *Index-Analysis of the Federal Statutes* by George Winfield Scott or one of the topically arranged collections of federal legislation that were privately published in the early twentieth century. *Federal Statutes Annotated* was compiled by William M. McKinney and published by Thompson Publishing from the early twentieth century. It went through two editions and was annually supplemented. West published John A. Mallory's *United States Compiled Statutes, Annotated* in 1916. It was regularly, though not annually, supplemented. Today, another good resource is the *Index to the Federal Statutes, 1874–1931*, published by the GPO in 1933.

By the mid-1920s Congress realized that the system for finding federal legislative enactments by subject needed to be addressed. Mindful of the problems it had encountered the last time it had attempted to codify the law, Congress approached the problem a little differently. First, it hired a contractor to develop the organizational structure of the code (the choice is not surprising: West Publishing Company), and it determined to take the process of enacting the code into law and repealing the predecessor law very carefully. It also soon developed a revision schedule and created an in-house committee and professional staff to oversee the codification, revision, and passage into "positive law" of the code.

Since the creation of the United States Code, about half of the titles have been considered and passed into positive law. Unless a researcher is tracking the history of a Code section, positive law means little. To lawyers who do not need to track the history of a section, the only potential issue may arise if there is a difference between the text of the Code and the text of the session law: for titles that have been passed into positive law, the U.S. Code rules; otherwise, the session law is the law.

The U.S. Code contains all public laws of a general and permanent nature organized into titles, chapters, and sections. It is revised and republished every six years. Every year between those six years, a cumulative supplement is published that includes all changes since the last of the six-year revisions. Many libraries will have the entire run of the Code as well as all of the supplements. HeinOnline also has all editions of the Code and the supplements. Beneath each section of the Code is a parenthetical that lists the original session law that created the section as well as every session law that amended it. This information is critical to researchers who want to track how a law has evolved over time.

Consider the law on the transportation of liquor into a state that prohibits its sale, codified today at Title 18, Section 1262, or 18 U.S.C. 1262. Below the text of the law there is a parenthetical that is included for all sections in all versions of the Code that lists all of the amendments back to the first appearance of the law. Below Section 1262 in the most recent edition of the Code, the parenthetical is: "June 25, 1948, ch. 645, 62 Stat. 761; May 24, 1949, ch. 139, §32, 63 Stat. 94; Pub. L. 101–647, title XXXV, §3540, Nov. 29, 1990, 104 Stat. 4925; Pub. L. 103–322, title XXXIII, §330016(1)(H), Sept. 13, 1994, 108 Stat. 2147." According to this, the law was passed in 1948 and was amended in 1949, 1990, and 1994. But in 1948, Congress took up and passed the entire Title 18 into law. That action reset the oldest law listed in all of the parentheticals to that 1948 law. Therefore, when looking at Section 1262 in any Code after 1948, the oldest citation listed in the parenthetical is to *that* law, not the first time that the law which later became Section 1262 was passed.

To find the history of the law before 1948, the researcher's first step is to look at the "Historical Notes" section that appears immediately below the parenthetical in all editions of the Code. The note in the current edition provides: "Based on sections 222, 223 of title 27, U.S.C., 1940 ed., Intoxicating Liquors (June 25, 1936, ch. 815, §§2, 3, 49 Stat. 1928)." Here the researcher can see that this law existed as far back as the 1930s. It is also clear that the law moved in 1948 from Title 27, Sections 222 and 223, to Title 18, Section 1262. The 1940 and the 1946 editions of the Code provide the following information below 27 U.S.C. 222 (Definitions): "(June 25, 1936, ch. 815, §2, 49 Stat. 1928)." And below 27 U.S.C. 223 (Transporting into State where sale prohibited; penalty; State definition of intoxicating liquor adopted): "(June 25, 1936, ch. 815, §3, 49 Stat. 1928)." This confirms that the law which today appears in Section 1262 originated in the 1936 law.

Any law on this topic that existed before 1936 is unrelated to the current law. To find any such law, researchers will need to use the topical law-finding tools and methods discussed above. As is clear from this example, the parenthetical from an edition of the Code older than the passage of a title into positive law will bring the researcher back to the initial passage of the law, the 1926 initial passage of the U.S. Code, or, in some cases, to the *Revised Statutes* of 1873. The *Revised Statutes* and earliest editions of the Code provide good histories for each section. If researchers are stuck between 1873 and 1926, the early-twentieth-century indexes or annotated Codes can help take them back to the *Revised Statutes*. Of course, a person researching a section of Title 18 that made its first appearance after 1948 will not encounter the positive law issue: the historical parenthetical will contain the complete record of the section's history.

All of the versions of the Code provide the law, the parenthetical, and the history notes, but attorneys want more. They are interested in finding the cases that interpret the legislation and the law review articles and treatises that explain the legislation. They also want to find forms and other tools that can help them practice in the area of law that the legislation affects. All of this information is made available in one of the two annotated versions of the Code: the *United States Code Annotated* (USCA), published by West (now Thomson Reuters), and the *United States Code Service* (USCS), for years published by Lawyers Cooperative Publishing but now published by Lexis. The annotated versions of the Code are updated annually by pocket parts and more frequently by supplements. The USCA is available online through Westlaw, and the USCS is available through Lexis. To find the law as of a particular date, researchers need only use the last edition of the Code before the date that interests them and then, since the annual supplements cumulate, the supplement for that year.

There are several methods that a researcher can use to find Code sections. Often, a secondary source such as a legal treatise or law review article will cite the Code. If the researcher has already located a relevant case, that case will often cite the Code. There are four additional methods that a researcher can use. First, all versions of the U.S. Code include a detailed subject index. Second, all of the versions also contain several useful tables; the most important lists every session law and indicates where in the Code its parts were codified. The third method uses the fact that statutes often pick up a popular name—for example, the "Sherman Antitrust Act," the "Robinson-Patman Act," or the "Securities and Exchange Act"—during or after passage that can be used as an entree for research. Two tools are available to help researchers find the law when all they have is the popular name. From 1925, the various versions of the U.S. Code have tables of acts by popular name, and these are available in both their print and online versions. Shepard's Citations also produces a tool called *Shepard's Acts and Cases by Popular Name*, available only in print. Finally, since the Code is topically arranged, a researcher can browse the Code.

The era that saw the development of the U.S. Code, Shepard's Citations, and West's digests and reporters was, in many ways, the heyday of legal publishing. The era also generated a terrific literature in legal research. Hornbooks such as *How to Find the Law, Legal Research in a Nutshell,* and *Fundamentals of Legal Research* all give in-depth bibliographic introductions to the materials mentioned above.

Developments in the States

It should come as a relief that the development of legal publishing and the appearance of legal research tools in the states mirrored the development at the federal level. In some areas, for example, codification, states were far ahead of the federal government; in others, mainly because of smaller markets, they lagged. However, West reporters and digests, Shepard's citators, and annotated codes existed for almost every state from roughly the same time as for the federal system. Many of the same editors, compilers, and publishers worked in both venues. States lagged in legislative histories, treatises, law reviews, legal encyclopedias, and restatements. Other than restatements, each of these exists at the state level, but less will be available than at the federal or national level.

Legislative History

A legislative history gathers the materials that a legislature generated when considering proposed legislation. Generally, a history is conducted for bills that became law. It might be conducted in an attempt to determine the legislature's intent when passing some legislation. Often, however, historians, political scientists, and others are interested in tracking the process of legislation as it works its way through a legislature for other reasons. Federal legislative history is far more robust than state legislative history; what follows is a description of the federal system and federal documentation. State systems will be similar but often with far less information available to researchers. Congressional publishing practices and congressional publications are also important because, for most of the nineteenth century, Congress was the most prolific and important government publisher in the United States. Many important documents from federal departments outside of Congress are most readily available in the form published by Congress.

A quick review of the legislative process will help explain the kinds of documents a researcher will encounter when conducting a legislative history. When a bill is filed in either the Senate or House of Representatives, it is referred to a committee. The committee may hold hearings, and it may request various studies to help the members better understand the issues. After the committee has considered the bill and made any changes it feels are necessary, it may recommend that the bill should become law, though most legislation does not make it out of committee. If the committee recommends the passage of a bill, it will generally include an accompanying report. From the committee, the bill goes to the floor of the chamber, where it may again be debated. As at the committee, the bill can be amended on the floor. Eventually, the bill may come to a vote and may pass the chamber.

If during the same legislative session, the identical bill also passes in the other chamber of Congress, it goes to the president for signature or veto. If it is signed, then it is law. If it is vetoed, it is returned to Congress and must pass both chambers by a supermajority to override the veto.

When two similar, but not identical, bills are passed by the two chambers, the leadership of the House and Senate will bring together a conference committee. This conference committee will agree to a compromise bill, which will then be sent back to the two chambers for an up-and-down vote. When an identical bill passes both chambers, either through the conference process or otherwise, the bill will go to the president for signature or veto. When a president signs or vetoes a bill, he will often make a statement expressing why the bill was necessary or why he is vetoing the bill.

As a bill wends its way through Congress, documents are created that may provide some insight into the debates surrounding the passage of the law. The major documents that typically make up a legislative history are committee reports (conference reports are considered especially valuable), floor statements, hearings, and committee prints or other documents. All of these may interest a historian. To lawyers interested in making an argument based on the legislative history, the most important documents are committee reports.

The various congressional documents are often printed and distributed to libraries designated as government document repositories. In addition, since 1815, the federal government has published the *United States Congressional Serial Set,* which includes the reports and other documents from Congress. The *Serial Set* does not include the text of hearings or floor debate.

American State Papers predates the *Serial Set.* It includes materials surrounding the major functions of the federal government from 1789 to 1832. *American State Papers* also included congressional reports and other congressional documents.

Together, the *Serial Set* and *American State Papers* contain many of the reports that form the backbone of a legislative history.

Although *American State Papers* is an extremely useful resource, it misses some materials from Congress. A bibliography by A. W. Greely, *Public Documents of the First Fourteen Congresses, 1789–1817*, is a Senate document and therefore is included in the *Serial Set*; it is more complete than *American State Papers*.

Neither *American State Papers* nor the *Serial Set* includes texts of floor debates and congressional hearings. Floor debates have been regularly published since 1789, but for much of the first century, the debates were summarized rather than being verbatim records. The floor debates have been published successively in the *Annals of Congress*, the *Register of Debates*, the *Congressional Globe*, and the *Congressional Record*. The *Annals of Congress* cover from 1789 to 1824, though the *Annals* were compiled between 1834 and 1856 and not published contemporaneously. The *Annals* were compiled using the best records available, primarily newspaper accounts. The speeches in the *Annals* are not a verbatim record but are paraphrased. The *Register of Debates* covers 1824 to 1837. Again, it is not a verbatim account of the proceedings but a summary of the "leading debates and incidents"; it was published by commercial publisher Gales and Seaton contemporaneously with the proceedings. The *Congressional Globe*, also published contemporaneously, covers from 1833 to 1873. Initially, the *Globe* contained a "condensed report" of the proceedings, but beginning in 1851, the contents approach being verbatim. Finally, the *Congressional Record* began publication in 1873 and continues today. It is far more comprehensive than its predecessors and contains a corrected verbatim report of the proceedings of Congress.

Congressional hearings are traditionally the most difficult congressional documents to obtain. While often printed by the GPO and available in some depository libraries, until recently they were not generally included in other sets of congressional materials or databases. Today, they are often available online through the ProQuest Congressional and ProQuest Legislative Insight databases.

Another type of document, committee prints and documents, do not often provide much insight into congressional deliberations, but they nonetheless can be a researcher's best friend. Prints and documents are materials that a committee may consider or may have created to facilitate its work, so they are often documents that also facilitate a researcher's work. The aforementioned *Constitution of the United States of America: Analysis and Interpretation* is an example of a Senate committee document. Often, Congress will have legislative histories created and will publish them as committee prints. Researchers should consider examining documents and prints when they find them.

The final congressional items that researchers may find useful are the texts of bills. Historically, bill texts have occasionally been included in legislative journals or in the records of floor debates. Often, the records of floor debates are the best source for amendments made on the floor. ProQuest recently produced a microform set of bills and resolutions from 1933 and even more recently, it released an online version for bills and resolutions from 1789 forward. The Library of Congress has a full set, and several other libraries have significant runs of bills. The Library of Congress collects legislative information from the Office of the Clerk of the House of Representatives, the Office of the Secretary of the Senate, the Government Publishing Office, the Congressional Budget Office, and the Congressional

Research Service and uses it to create Congress.gov, "the official website for U.S. federal legislative information (https://www. congress.gov/about). It contains information from 1973 to present.

It is often glibly said that the first rule of compiling legislative histories is: don't. Compiling a legislative history can be difficult and time-consuming, and there are many existing legislative histories covering many of the most important laws. Researchers can consult one of several guides to discover whether a legislative history has been compiled. The first to consider is *Sources of Compiled Legislative Histories* by Nancy Johnson, available in print at many libraries and HeinOnline. This lists federal acts by date and popular name. It also includes the bibliographic information for the legislative history as well as some indication about what the legislative history includes. The easiest tool to use is ProQuest's Legislative Insight, which provides full-text searchable access to many legislative histories. Not every law is included in Legislative Insight, but it is often the best resource for those that are. ProQuest Congressional includes the legislative histories that the Congressional Information Service (CIS) has compiled for every law since the mid-1980s. In addition, the search functions allow researchers to compile their own legislative histories in ProQuest Congressional.

Another useful tool is a library catalog or WorldCat, searched for the phrase "legislative histories" and either the public law number, bill number, name of the act, or subject of the act. A third source, the *United States Congressional Serial Set*, will be discussed below. The final source is the collection of indexes created by the CIS, now owned by ProQuest. Since the mid-1980s, CIS has compiled a legislative history for all laws passed by Congress and has published them online at ProQuest

Congressional and on microform. Beginning in the 1970s, CIS created detailed indexes to congressional and executive documents as well as a full-text microform collection of congressional documents. Most, but not yet all, of the indexes and documents have been moved online and are now included at ProQuest Congressional; however, researchers should be aware of the wide variety of the excellent CIS indexes and the accompanying microform set. Some of the important index titles include *CIS US Congressional Committee Prints Index from the Earliest Publications Through 1969; CIS Index to Executive Branch Documents, 1910–1932, not Published in the U.S. Serial Set;* and *CIS Executive Orders and Proclamations, March 4, 1921–December 31, 1983.* Most law libraries have the indexes in print, and much of the material is available in the ProQuest databases. A search of a library catalog for "Congressional Information Service" as an author will lead a researcher to the indexes. Much more information about locating material published by the federal government, other than Congress, is included in chapter 7.

A resource that can help a researcher conduct a partial legislative history for laws passed since the late 1940s is the *United States Code, Congressional and Administrative News* (USCCAN), West's federal session law publication. In addition to public and private laws and proclamations and executive orders, USCCAN contains a legislative history section for each law passed. This section reprints part or all of the most important reports related to a law and a list of the days that a bill was considered on the floor of the House of Representatives and the Senate.

The *Serial Set* is available in print at university and some major public libraries. The print index to the *Serial Set,* published by CIS, is available at many libraries. The Library of

Congress's American Memory: A Century of Lawmaking website contains some of the reports and documents from the *Serial Set* organized by Congress. The site offers limited searching
of the descriptions of some of the documents.

Two online versions of the *Serial Set* allow full-text searching and provide page images of the documents. The Readex
version allows browsing by subject, type of document, name
(personal, geographic, and act), committee, and Congress. It
also allows searching for full text, searching for bill number,
and searching within the browsing categories as well as the
ability to limit results to documents that contain tables, maps,
or illustrations. The ProQuest version also allows full-text
searching, with the ability to limit searches to particular fields,
by type of document, and by whether the document contains
illustrations or statistical tables. A separate search in the Pro-
Quest version, which can be combined with the search of the
rest of the *Serial Set*, allows searching for *Serial Set* maps.

While the great bulk of publicly available congressional
materials can be found in the *Serial Set*, hearings are separately published and can be identified either with the CIS *U.S.
Congressional Committee Hearings Index* and the indexes to
Unpublished U.S. Senate Committee Hearings and *Unpublished
U.S. House of Representatives Committee Hearings* or by using
ProQuest Congressional. Since hearings tend to be very long,
the complete testimony from some hearings never gets published. In research terms, there are three classes of hearings:
those officially published, those unofficially published, and
those never published. A researcher should also be aware of
what part of a hearing was actually published. Many times, the
witness statements provided to the committee will be published
but not the transcripts of what was said. Officially and unofficially published hearings can be found using the CIS indexes

and by using ProQuest Congressional. Some materials related to hearings that have never been published may be available from the committee or at the National Archives or the Library of Congress.

Some private enterprises attend committee hearings and transcribe the testimony. This material often can be purchased from major database providers or the transcription company as a part of a congressional information package. However, any stenographic materials created by a private enterprise are the property of the enterprise and not the government.

When using the *Congressional Record,* researchers should be aware of one major complication: there are two versions of it, and the page numbers differ. When initially published, the *Congressional Record* is in its "daily" version. Pages reflecting the debates in the House of Representatives bear an "H" prefix; those in the Senate bear an "S" prefix; and the "extension of remarks" section, materials requested to be published "in the record," bears an "E" prefix. Eventually, corrections are made and the *Congressional Record* is published in its "final" version. Here, the pages bear sequential numbers through the session. Researchers must take care to note which version they are using. No easy translation tables exist to take researchers from the "daily" page number to the "final" page number or vice versa. The easiest way to find the correct page is to note the debate date and approximate time and browse through the debates.

The serials that report Congress's debates are available in a variety of sources: in print and microform with annual indexes, and online. The online versions vary in their efficacy. The Library of Congress provides free access to an indexed and searchable version from 1789 through 1875. The serials are also available at HeinOnline and ProQuest Congressional, where the full text can be searched.

Often, researchers will want to locate discussion related to particular bills. Indexes and full-text searching can help them locate these discussions, but another method can be effective. By using the journals of the House and Senate, researchers can find the dates on which any bill was discussed on the floor of either chamber. They can then turn to that day's report and scan for the discussion.

Another type of congressional publication is the work product of the Congressional Research Service (CRS), which prepares and/or updates reports for members of Congress on whatever issue is requested. ProQuest Congressional has made available many of these reports, dating to the early twentieth century.

One important issue that often arises is whether a researcher has all of the session laws and all of the codes from a jurisdiction. It helps to know when and how frequently a legislature meets, but special sessions can wreak havoc for a researcher. As we saw with cases, state legal research guides are especially useful here. In addition, Hein publishes a checklist of legislative materials published for each state, which will help a researcher know what materials will make a complete set.

In tracking the work of a legislature, one of the most important resources is the legislative journal, usually published for each legislative body. There, a researcher can find a description of a legislature's business. The journal will record all bills submitted, all bills sent to a committee, all votes, other business, and when these things took place. The journals are one of the best places to track everything that happens at a legislature. But they do not report the words spoken on the floor of the legislative body, nor do they usually contain the full text of the legislation.

Finding the text of early bills is problematic. Although there are collections of federal bills that go well back into the eighteenth century, the farther back in time, the less complete they are. It is not until the early 1930s that a complete collection of federal bills is available. To investigate within the bills, a researcher should start with an appropriate tool. For a law that has been passed, several legislative history tools, described above, will indicate the bills related to the law. For laws that did not pass, a researcher will use the journals of the House or Senate in conjunction with other secondary sources to determine the dates and numbers of bills related to a particular subject. With the dates or sessions of Congress in which a bill was submitted and the bill number in hand, a researcher can then locate the bill in one of the collections of bills.

State legislative histories vary widely. All states have legislative journals that allow researchers to find basic information about the process of a bill through the legislature. But the type and quantity of material available vary by state. A state legal research guide is often the best starting point, but almost always researchers will have to use the state law library and often the state archives. Researchers should be forewarned that even after diligently digging for material related to a state law, they may unearth nothing.

Treatises

The mid-twentieth century was the heyday of the modern treatise. Legal treatises have gathered around most major areas of law. The main treatises are many volumes in length, were written by eminent legal scholars, and are kept up to date today by legal practitioners, by other scholars, and sometimes by the publisher's staff. These treatises pull together most of what a person interested in a particular area of law would need. They provide a statement of the law, an explanation, citations to cases and statutes, practice tips, forms, and any other information lawyers may need. Treatises can be located in most law libraries by using the library catalogs. Perhaps the best way to determine the most important treatises in a particular area is to use the following criteria.

First, the Association of American Law Schools has published *Law Books Recommended for Libraries,* initially printed in the 1950s and updated again in the 1970s. This volume is available at many libraries and HeinOnline. The American Bar Association published James A. McDermott's *Recommended Law Books* with a second edition in 1986. This slim volume lists the best treatises in each area of law. Although somewhat out of date, it is still useful because many treatises have valuable brand recognition; a particular title will remain as *the* treatise through many decades and many authors. Another way to determine the best, or most important, treatises is to see which bear the names of the most eminent scholars and which have been published over the decades and have gone through many editions. An earlier edition of a treatise is a valuable means of determining the state of the law at the time.

Looseleafs are a unique kind of legal publication. They get their name from their print format: most were published in binders, with new pages replacing older pages. Looseleafs were therefore kept up to date with regular supplementation, sometimes as often as weekly. A looseleaf pulls together everything necessary for someone to practice in a particular area of law. They often serve as the place to find administrative decisions and also contain statutes, cases, rules and regulations, commentary, finding aids, and citators. In addition, looseleafs often contain practice tips and discussions of the law. They don't exist for every area of law; they typically exist around the areas that involve a large amount of money.

They can be found through catalog searches in a recent series, *Legal Looseleafs in Print*, published by Infosources since 1981 that lists virtually all looseleafs; many are also included in *Legal Information Buyer's Guide & Reference Manual*, by Kendall F. Svengalis, published since 1996.

Most currently published looseleafs are available online with some historical content. Most looseleafs continue for decades, and since noncurrent material is discarded, they can be a difficult place for a researcher to get an understanding of the law in the past. They are still valuable for old administrative decisions and cases, but the commentary is likely to be current. One looseleaf stands out as an important exception. The *Standard Federal Tax Reporter* is reissued every year. While pages are added and removed throughout a year, the set represents the state of the law at the close of the year.

Law Reviews and Periodical Indexes

A great many innovations in legal research tools and methods occurred around the turn of the twentieth century, including the development of a new species of legal literature: the dedicated academic law review. In general, many serious serial publications developed during the nineteenth century. Before the advent of law reviews, serious articles about legal topics often appeared in periodicals of interest to the general educated reader. Journals such as the *North American Review* contained articles by judges and lawyers that, while they may have been of interest to the typical reader, were of special interest to the attorney-reader. In 1852, the *American Law Register* from the University of Pennsylvania Department of Law began publication. The era of student-edited law reviews, now the dominant paradigm, perhaps started with *Albany Law School*

Journal in 1875. This journal, of which only one issue survives, lasted one year but was followed by the *Columbia Jurist* (1885–1887), the *Harvard Law Review* (1887–), and the *Yale Law Journal* (1891–).

When conducting research in law reviews, a researcher's main difficulty is finding articles about a particular topic. During the nineteenth century and for much of the twentieth, most law reviews were general in nature and published articles on almost any legal topic. Later in the twentieth century, specialized law reviews appeared. For most of the twentieth century, relevant law review articles could be identified through a periodical index. Periodical index searching presents different issues for researchers than does full-text searching. Index searching is much more like catalog searching; there are fewer words in a record and there is generally a controlled vocabulary. Also, like catalogs, where more recent records have tables of contents that can be searched, more recent index entries may have abstracts and sometimes even the full text that can be searched. With index searching, researchers will want to construct broader searches with fewer proximity constraints, and they will want to include controlled vocabulary terms. One common problem with some indexes is that the controlled vocabulary can be too broad; for instance, the controlled vocabulary term "constitutional" doesn't help all that much in a legal periodical index.

The most important index was and is the *Index to Legal Periodicals* by H. W. Wilson Co. (now the *Index to Legal Periodicals and Books*). The *Index to Legal Periodicals* has been published since 1908 and indexes articles by author, title, and topic. As with most topically arranged sources, it occasionally cumulates several volumes into a larger volume. More recent material is in smaller, sometimes paper issues or volumes that cover shorter periods of time. To get a complete listing of articles on a topic over time, a researcher must consult all volumes. The *Index to Legal Periodicals* is available online through Lexis and Westlaw. EBSCO has released Legal Source, a database that includes all of the data from the *Index to Legal Periodicals* as well as the law-related data from EBSCO's full-text databases. Today, Legal Source is the preferred index for all but the oldest articles.

In 1980, the *Index to Legal Periodicals* was joined by the *Current Law Index*. Available online in a slightly expanded version called LegalTrac, the *Current Law Index* covers many of the same journals as the *Index to Legal Periodicals*, but it adds more practitioner-oriented periodicals and some bar journals and legal newspapers. It also indexes articles by author, title, and topic. One difference in the indexing is that the *Current Law Index* uses Library of Congress subject headings for its first-level indexing while the *Index to Legal Periodicals* uses its own index terms. The *Current Law Index* is also available through both Lexis and Westlaw.

Starting in 1887, *An Index to Legal Periodical Literature* was published. It continued to 1937. This index, compiled by Leonard A. Jones and Frank E. Chipman and thus commonly known as Jones-Chipman, covers material, albeit a little idiosyncratically, from the eighteenth century to 1937. Jones-Chipman is available online as a part of the Nineteenth Century Masterfile database. This is probably the best index for articles about the law published up to 1908.

The other main method for finding law review articles is through full-text searching. Lexis and Westlaw have the full text of many law reviews since the 1990s and for the most important journals from the 1970s. HeinOnline includes the full text of many law reviews from the beginning of law journals. However, Hein may not have the most recent issues.

The digital library JSTOR has a smaller collection of the most important law reviews, and its coverage goes back to the earliest journals.

Researchers wishing to conduct a full-text search on Lexis or Westlaw are limited by the dates of coverage. On JSTOR they are limited by the number of titles and on HeinOnline by some of the issues with Hein's searching and the possibility that the most recent issues will not be included in the search.

Another difficulty with full-text searching for law review articles is that it can be very difficult to restate a legal idea in a search that will return relevant articles. Some legal issues are always described in common parlance using the same terms, but others are described in many different ways. Constructing comprehensive searches for the latter topics can be challenging. Since researchers can search the indexes by author, title, and a controlled vocabulary subject, it is often easier to locate articles *about* a particular topic rather than articles that mention a particular topic or words. The downside to index searching is that overly broad subjects are often assigned to articles, causing a search to return an unmanageably large collection of articles. For example, the search for "constitutional law—United States" as a subject in Legal Source returns more than sixty-eight hundred articles published since 1902.

Legal Encyclopedias

Another development from around the turn of the twentieth century was the legal encyclopedia, filled with articles designed mainly for attorneys. National legal encyclopedias attempt to describe all U.S. law, while state-based legal encyclopedias attempt to describe the law of a particular state. As with other encyclopedias, legal encyclopedias are broken down by alphabetically arranged topics. Under each topic the discussion is broken down in an arrangement of sections that makes sense for the topic. Legal encyclopedias are available in print and online, where researchers can search by full text or browse by topic and section. Indexes to the encyclopedias generally and to each topic are available in print and online through Westlaw. A researcher interested in the law raised in a particular case or by a particular statute can also turn to tables of cases and statutes in legal encyclopedias.

Legal encyclopedias offer a snapshot of an area of law at the time that a volume was published and are updated in print through pocket parts. Changes will accumulate, but the year-by-year changes are lost as pocket parts are discarded annually. On occasion a replacement volume is published that incorporates the changes reflected in the pocket parts, thereby offering a new snapshot.

There are two national legal encyclopedias: *American Jurisprudence, 2nd* (Am Jur) and *Corpus Juris Secundum* (CJS). Until fairly recently, Am Jur was published by Lawyers Cooperative Publishing and CJS by West. Thomson Reuters now publishes both. Many states have legal encyclopedias, but not all. Most of the state encyclopedias are titled by the state name followed by "Jurisprudence." States that do not have encyclopedias will often have a series of treatises geared to practitioners in a "practice" series. They will have a series title with the state's name followed by "Practice."

A researcher should know about a few older encyclopedias as well. First, both Am Jur and CJS had first editions. Am Jur was published between 1936 and 1952, while *Corpus Juris* was published by the American Law Book Company between 1914 and 1937. *The American and English Encyclopedia of Law* was published between 1887 and 1896, and its second edition was published between 1896 and 1905. *Ruling Case Law* was published between 1914 and 1921.

Restatements and Uniform Laws

In the 1920s, legal scholars and practitioners founded the American Law Institute to develop a series of restatements of the law. These restated the common law as it was practiced in various states. The restatements were not and are not the law but were designed to act almost as a national code of common law. The gathered academics and practitioners carefully worked through and debated several drafts written by experts in a field. Eventually, a restatement was adopted. The basic statement of the law was accompanied by comments and examples written by the drafters. Eventually, cases that adopted and interpreted the restatement were added to the publication.

There have been three series of restatements. The first, adopted and published between 1923 and 1944, covered the law of agency, conflict of laws, contracts, judgments, property, restitution, security, torts, and trusts. Beginning in the 1950s, a second series of restatements were published that updated the first and included more commentary and the rationale for the decisions made by the drafters. Currently, the third restatement series, begun in 1987, is being published. Thus far, the third series has further updated all or parts of several restatements and has added or is adding new restatements. The third series currently consists of restatements of agency, foreign relations, law governing lawyers, property (mortgages, servitudes, wills, and other donative transfers), restitution and unjust enrichment, suretyship and guaranty, torts (product liability, apportionment of liability, and physical and emotional harm), trusts, and unfair competition. The American Law Institute is also working on restatements of employment law and the U.S. law of international commercial arbitration.

The restatements are available in print and online through Lexis and Westlaw. In both versions, researchers can find the restatement of a law, notes regarding its origins and meaning, illustrations, and lists of jurisdictions that have adopted the restatement formulation. One of the changes made in restatements over the years is that today, they tend to state what the scholars believe the law should be rather than to restate what the law is. Nevertheless, the restatements provide a window to twentieth-century law and its development.

The archives of the American Law Institute are housed at the University of Pennsylvania's Biddle Law Library. The various drafts and other versions of the restatements are available at many law libraries and HeinOnline.

In the late nineteenth and early twentieth centuries many lawyers and legislators recognized that some of the variations in state law caused difficulties. In 1892, the lawyers eventually founded the National Conference of Commissioners on Uniform State Laws, renamed the Uniform Law Commission (ULC) in 2007. It has proposed a series of uniform laws that it encourages states to adopt. The ULC currently consists of 350 commissioners appointed by the states. The commissioners are lawyers and often legislators, judges, and legal scholars. The commissioners go through a long drafting process and eventually propose a uniform state law. It is then up to the states to decide whether to consider or adopt the law. If adopted, it can be altered. The uniform laws represent the commissioners' take on the ideal law to garner political support. To date, well over one hundred uniform laws have been proposed. The most successful, adopted in all fifty states, is the Uniform Commercial Code. Drafts of uniform laws are available at HeinOnline, and

Thomson Reuters publishes an annotated version of the uniform laws. The set, also available online through Westlaw, provides information about the states' adoption of the law as well as some of the cases interpreting the law. Once the law leaves the ULC, state legislative, state legislative history, and state case research will have to be undertaken.

Research Example

Let us look at the law related to espionage. In 1917 Congress passed the Espionage Act. Since the U.S. Code wasn't published until 1925, we first look at the law in the session laws and the codes before 1925 and then within the first editions of the Code. But before that, we should determine the depth to which we want to go in our research. Initially, some basic information will suffice, so we can start by consulting a legal encyclopedia or even Wikipedia.

In fact, the Wikipedia entry is quite good, providing the citation to the Espionage Act, including the Public Law and *Statutes at Large* citation. It also discusses amendments and proposed amendments to the act as well as the background to the act and some information about its enforcement. In addition Wikipedia provides a link to information about *Schenck v. United States* (249 U.S. 47 [1919]), the Supreme Court case interpreting the act that discussed Charles T. Schenck's speech in opposition to World War I, stating, "[t]he most stringent protection of free speech would not protect a man falsely shouting fire in a theater and causing a panic."

We can then turn to Am Jur, available online through Westlaw. If we search in the index for "espionage," we find the word within headings and as a heading. Looking it up first as a heading, we note that the discussions tend to be within the topic "sedition." We then decide to look at "defenses" and "definition." These are classified as "sedition section 31" and "sedition section 13." First turning to "definition," we get a West Topic and Key Number and references to several articles that touch on the definition of espionage. We then find a short section describing the definition of espionage. At least each sentence, and sometimes each clause, has a reference to a court opinion that stands for the proposition expressed.

When we turn to the section on "defenses," we get some of the same information—the same Topic and Key Number, for example—but also references to a treatise on federal procedure, a treatise on trial strategy when defending people accused of participating in a conspiracy, and form books that deal with defenses to espionage.

To find the law, we can work from the reference that Wikipedia provided and look for 40 Stat. 217. Using HeinOnline we find the law as it was passed. To follow the law forward, we want to discover where it was codified when the U.S. Code was created in 1925, so we look at the 1925 edition and examine the "Table of Cross References Under Which the Statutes Contained in This Code Are Classified." We find "espionage" and are referred to page 620, where we are further referred to Title 50 War. After turning to Title 50, we see that chapter 4 deals with espionage. In 1925, the topic "espionage" is housed in 50 U.S.C. Sections 31–42. We know that the sections have moved over time, and the easiest way to track that move might be to go to the most recent U.S. Code and look for "espionage" in the index. Today, espionage is generally within Title 18 and located at Sections 792 *et seq.* although some topics are placed in other locations in the Title and the Code.

By looking at a more recent version of the Code, we can find secondary sources and cases interpreting the espionage sections. In print, we can choose to ignore materials published after a particular date, and online we can choose not to see them.

Another direction we can take is to put *Schenck* through a citator. If we Keycite *Schenck,* we find 767 cases; we could limit the display according to a variety of characteristics. If we use Google Scholar's citator, we get 646 cases; if we use Bloomberg Law's, we get 736 cases. Shepard's Citation at Lexis gives us 805 citing decisions. The differences are likely because the systems have slightly different collections of unreported cases and state lower court opinions. The differences at the appellate level (excluding Google) are likely illusory.

Further Reading

Bogert, George Gleason. *How to Find the Law.* Chicago: Blackstone, 1916.

deLong, Suzanne. "What Is in the United States Serial Set?" *Journal of Government Information* 23, no. 2 (1996): 123–35.

Foster, George N. *Lawyers Legal Search: Rules and Problems of Search Illustrated by Diagrams or Geometric Charts.* Rochester, NY: Lawyers Cooperative, 1920.

Hendrickson, A. M., and Charles Lesley Ames. *The Practitioners' Manual of Legal Bibliography: Specially Compiled for Use in the Practitioners' Correspondence Course.* St. Paul: n.p., 1910.

Hicks, Frederick Charles. *Materials and Methods of Legal Research.* Rochester, NY: Lawyers Cooperative, 1923.

Horwitz, Morton J. *The Transformation of American Law, 1870–1960: The Crisis of Legal Orthodoxy.* New York: Oxford University Press, 1992.

Hurst, James Willard. *Law and the Conditions of Freedom in the Nineteenth-Century United States.* Madison: University of Wisconsin Press, 1956.

Jarvis, Robert M. "John B. West: Founder of the West Publishing Company." *American Journal of Legal History* 50 (2008): 1–22.

Kiser, Donald J. *Principles and Practice of Legal Research.* Brooklyn, NY: American Law Book, 1924.

Lile, William Minor, Henry S. Redfield, Eugene Wambaugh, A. F. Mason, James E. Wheeler, and Nathan Abbott. *Brief Making and the Use of Law Books.* St. Paul, MN: West, 1906.

Price, Miles O., and Harry Bitner. *Effective Legal Research: A Practical Manual of Law Books and Their Use.* New York: Prentice-Hall, 1953.

Townes, John Charles. *Law Books and How to Use Them.* Austin, TX: Austin Print, 1909.

West Publishing Company. *Manual; American Digest and National Reporter Systems: Effective Use of the Key-Number, the Tables of Cases and Descriptive-Word Index. How to Search for the Case in Point.* St. Paul: West, 1924.

Important Sources Mentioned in This Chapter

American Law Institute. *Restatement of the Law of Torts as Adopted and Promulgated by the American Law Institute at Washington, D.C., May 11, 1934.* St. Paul: American Law Institute Publishers, 1934.

Bancroft-Whitney Company. *American Jurisprudence: A Comprehensive Text Statement of American Case Law as Developed in the Cases and Annotations in the Annotated Reports System: Being a Rewriting of Ruling Case Law to Reflect the Modern Developments of the Law.* San Francisco: Bancroft-Whitney, 1936.

Congressional Information Service. *CIS Annual/Congressional Information Service: Abstracts of Congressional Publications and Legislative Histories of US Public Laws.* Bethesda, MD: CIS, 1985.

———. *CIS Index to U.S. Executive Branch Documents, 1789–1909: Guide to Documents Listed in Checklist of U.S. Public Documents, 1789–1909, not Printed in the U.S. Serial Set. Pt. 3 Supplementary Indexes.* Bethesda, MD: CIS, 1992.

Frank Shepard Company. *Shepard's Citations: A Detailed Presentation of the Scope and Uses of Citation Books, with Illustrative Examples of Their Use, and an Analysis of Their Relation to Other Methods of Legal Research.* New York: Frank Shepard Co., 1931.

Jones, Leonard A., and Frank Ellsworth Chipman. *An Index to Legal Periodical Literature.* Boston: Boston Book, 1888.

Lawyers Cooperative Publishing Company. *American Law Reports Annotated.* Rochester, NY: Lawyers Cooperative, 1919.

Mack, William, and Donald J. Kiser. *Corpus Juris: Being a Complete and Systematic Statement of the Whole Body of the Law, as Embodied in and Developed by All Reported Decisions.* New York: American Law Book, 1934.

United States. *United States Congressional Serial Set.* Washington, DC: GPO, 1817–. Note: Before the 97th Congress, the *Serial Set* had no official name; it was popularly known as the "Congressional Serial Set." The set has also been known as "Serial Number Set," "Congressional Edition," "Congressional Set," "Congressional Series," "Congressional Series of United States Public Documents," "Congressional Document Series," "Sheep set" or "Sheep-Bound Set" (owing to its distinctive sheepskin binding), and "Serial set."

United States, Lawyers Cooperative, and LexisNexis. *United States Code Service.* Rochester, NY: Lawyers Cooperative / Charlottesville, VA: LexisNexis, 1972–.

United States, West Publishing Company, Thomson/West, and Thomson/Reuters. *United States Code Annotated.* St. Paul, MN: West / New York: Thomson/Reuters. 1927–.

United States Congress. *American State Papers.* Washington, DC: Gales and Seaton, 1834.

West Publishing Company, Thomson/West, and Thomson/Reuters. *Corpus Juris Secundum.* St. Paul, MN: West / New York: Thomson/Reuters, 1936–.

———. *National Reporter System.* St. Paul, MN: West / New York: Thomson/Reuters, 1885–.

———. *West's Digest System.* St. Paul, MN: West / New York: Thomson/Reuters, 1885–.

Databases

EBSCO. *Index to Legal Periodicals and Books.* https://www.ebsco.com/products/research-databases/index-to-legal-periodicals-and-books.

———. *Index to Legal Periodicals Retrospective: 1908–1981.* https://www.ebsco.com/products/research-databases/index-to-legal-periodicals-retrospective.

———. *Legal Source.* https://www.ebsco.com/products/research-databases/legal-source.

Paratext. *Nineteenth Century Masterfile.* http://paratext.com/19th-century-masterfile/.

ProQuest. *ProQuest Congressional.* https://www.proquest.com/libraries/academic/databases/proquest-congressional.html.

———. *Proquest Legislative Insight.* https://www.proquest.com/products-services/legislativeinsight.html.

Readex. *United States Congressional Serial Set.* http://www.readex.com/content/us-congressional-serial-set–1817–1994.

7

The Administrative State,

1930S–2010S

As the nineteenth century progressed, the need for a law-making body that could bring expertise to particular areas of economic, social, or governmental activity became increasingly apparent. Starting in the 1880s with the Interstate Commerce Commission, which mainly dealt with railroads, administrative law developed fitfully until the 1930s, when the pace of development increased, the need for order was recognized, and order was implemented.

Today there is a large, well-developed body of both federal and state administrative law. Administrative law includes the law that governs governmental administrative agencies and the law created by those agencies. The powers of agencies are limited by the Constitution and by the grant of power, usually by the legislative body, to an agency. There are many administrative agencies, and these agencies can make law and adjudicate disputes. Most administrative agencies reside in the executive branch but are children of the legislative branch. The legislature creates an agency or devolves power to an agency and allows it to make law in certain limited areas. The executive also has some constitutional ability to make law. Since administrative law research is much the same whether the power to make law comes from the legislature or from the executive's inherent constitutional power, we will treat them in the same fashion here. However, when considering whether an action of an agency exceeds the scope of its authority, a researcher must take into account the source of the authority. In that case, the source addressed will differ.

There are four types of administrative materials: (1) materials created by administrative agencies or executive departments other than the president before the mid-1930s, (2) presidential materials, (3) materials created by administrative agencies or executive departments other than the president after the mid-1930s, and (4) some miscellaneous materials.

Regulations

Since 1936, the *Federal Register* has published the rules and regulations created by administrative agencies, including administrative notices and proposed and final rules and regulations. The *Federal Register* has been published every business day since March 14, 1936, and is available, from 1994, for free online at the GPO's Federal Digital System website, or, from 1936, through HeinOnline, Lexis, and Bloomberg Law. Westlaw's coverage extends back to 1980. Annual and semiannual indexes also accompany the *Federal Register*.

Very quickly, Congress realized that the chronologically arranged *Federal Register* would not be conducive to research, so in 1938 it passed the Code of Federal Regulations (CFR) Act. The CFR, published annually in four parts, organizes the regulations in force by topic and within each topic by agency. The

CFR is organized into fifty titles, although CFR titles do not necessarily match U.S. Code titles. It can be browsed, entered via index, and searched by full text.

When working with federal regulations, a researcher will often want to know two pieces of information: the enabling legislation, that is, the congressional act that gave the agency the right to make the regulations; and the *Federal Register* citation to the initial publication of the regulations. When first published, a regulation is accompanied by a discussion of the rationale for it as well as the history of its proposal and adoption. Each chapter of the CFR will include the citation to the regulation's enabling legislation and its appearance in the *Federal Register*. If any of the sections within a chapter rely on different enabling legislation or were added or amended by a later regulation, a citation to the correct information will appear with the section.

Regulations change frequently, so finding a regulation as of a particular date is both important and somewhat complex. Examining the annually published CFR for the year in question will give researchers the regulation as it was for that date. Since the CFR is updated in four parts, the "current through" date depends on the CFR title under consideration. The first quarter of the CFR is published with material updated as of January 1 of the year published, the second quarter has material updated as of April 1, the third quarter as of July 1, and the fourth as of October 1. The research can get a little tricky when researchers are interested in the regulations as of a date between annual releases—for example, if they want to find out about the state of a regulation in Title 7 as of July 1, when Title 7 is current only through January 1.

The first step is to see whether there was a change during the year; to do this, researchers should examine the CFR for the following year. If the sections are the same and they find no reference to a *Federal Register* from the prior year that might have changed the regulation and then reverted, researchers can be sure that the regulations are the same. If there has been a change, the newer version of the CFR will refer to the *Federal Register* page on which the change was made.

The process becomes more complicated when updating a very recent version of the CFR, one for which the next year's version has not been published. This issue falls outside the scope of this book, although many legal research texts explain the process fully.

Researchers interested in a "regulatory history" will begin with the *Federal Register* issue that contains the final regulation. When an agency proposes a regulation, the process for adoption generally requires publication in the *Federal Register;* an opportunity for citizen comment; and, accompanying the publication of the final regulation, responses to the classes of comments, including how the agency took the comments into consideration and what changes the comments may have engendered. The publication of the final regulation in the *Federal Register* includes prefatory material that describes the issue to be solved, the regulation proposed and a description of how it would solve the identified problems, the comments received and responses to the comments received, and the text of the regulation. Although this is not a complete regulatory history, it is perhaps the most important and easiest to locate rationale for any regulation.

Presidential Materials

Congress and the courts are not the only branches of government to produce law and to create materials of interest to attorneys, historians, and others. The executive branch also produces a large volume of materials. In addition to the law that the president can make based on the powers granted in the Constitution, a great deal of other documents come from the executive that can shed light on the process and development of law and government.

The president has the power to issue several types of documents that create legal obligations; the two most important are executive orders and proclamations. Executive orders are legally binding orders directing governmental departments or agencies to do something. These orders can have a wide effect on society. For example, the armed forces were integrated in July 1948 by Executive Order 9981. Other types of documents that go by a variety of names have the same legal effect as an executive order. A good discussion of these can be found in "Presidential Directives: Background and Overview" by Harold C. Relyea (CRS Report 98–611GOV). Proclamations are generally not as important as executive orders (other than those like the Emancipation Proclamation) and are generally issued to recognize a person or a group.

The first executive order was promulgated by President George Washington, but executive orders were not widely published or even noted until the end of the nineteenth century. Regular publication did not start until the 1930s, and even today, not all executive orders are published, including some entire categories, such as secret national security directives.

Finding executive orders issued since 1935 is relatively straightforward. They are first published in the *Federal Register*, then they are placed in Title 3 of the CFR. While most of the CFR is organized topically, Title 3 is different. It contains presidential material from the prior year. The GPO occasionally publishes a codification of the executive orders. The most recent covers from 1943 to 1989.

For executive orders published before the mid-1930s, the Congressional Information Service has an excellent *Index to Presidential Executive Orders and Proclamations* covering from George Washington forward. Clifford L. Lord's *List and Index of Presidential Executive Orders* is also an excellent finding tool. Other resources that bring together earlier executive orders include James D. Richardson's *A Compilation of the Messages and Papers of the Presidents, 1789–1921* and Clifford L. Lord's *Presidential Executive Orders: Numbered Series (1862–1938)*. Richardson's collection is also available at HeinOnline. The American Presidency Project of the University of California, Santa Barbara (http://www.presidency.ucsb.edu/), also offers a good collection.

Proclamations can easily be found in the *Statutes at Large,* and they are also printed in Title 3 of the CFR. Proclamations furthermore are available from the American Presidency Project from 1789.

Presidential administrations create many more public documents than executive orders and proclamations. Since the 1920s, these documents have been systematically collected and published in the *Public Papers of the President,* which cover administrations from Herbert Hoover to the present. All of these are available at many libraries and online through Hein-Online, the Federal Digital System, and the American Presidency Project.

The one post–Hoover administration not included in the *Public Papers of the President* is a big one: Franklin D. Roosevelt. However, the *Public Papers and Addresses of Franklin D. Roosevelt* have been published and are available at many libraries and online through HeinOnline and the American Presidency Project.

It takes several years for the *Public Papers* to be published. A much more timely resource for presidential material is the

Weekly Compilation of Presidential Documents (1965–2009), continued by the *Daily Compilation of Presidential Documents* (2009–). These are available at the GPO's Federal Digital System website.

Papers from presidents before Hoover can be found in a variety of sources, though none is as complete as the *Public Papers* sets. Richardson's previously mentioned *Compilation of the Messages and Papers of the Presidents, 1789–1921* is a good resource. There are a variety of additional resources, including collections of the addresses of the presidents—for example, *The State of the Union Messages of the Presidents, 1790–1966*—and the collection of inaugural addresses online at Yale Law School's Avalon Project (http://avalon.law.yale.edu/subject_menus/inaug.asp).

Administrative Decisions

Congress grants agencies the right to make regulations and the right to adjudicate disputes arising under those regulations. The resulting administrative decisions make up a huge body of law. Administrative decisions differ from court decisions in several important ways. First, while an agency will attempt to be consistent from one decision to another, the rules of authority and stare decisis are much weaker in administrative law. Second, process and procedure are often much less formal in administrative adjudications. Finally, and most important for researchers, locating administrative decisions is far more complex and difficult than locating court decisions.

The Administrative Procedure Act governs broad adjudicatory and other procedural outlines that agencies must follow. Within each agency, the rules of procedure are usually laid out in the regulations promulgated by the agency. When dealing with an administrative agency, a researcher will want to examine how it is organized, what its adjudicatory system looks like, and what publications come from the agency. Of the several good guides to the organization of administrative agencies, many have a long publishing history and can be used to see how the agency was organized historically. One of the most useful is the official *United States Government Manual.*

Rules and regulations of administrative agencies are fairly coherently published; the adjudicatory decisions of administrative agencies are not. Each agency has its own adjudicatory system, and each differs from the other agencies. Agencies also have different methods of publishing their decisions: some are published by the government, some are commercially published, and some are not published at all. Several resources can help a researcher discover the published decisions. Looseleaf services tend to be published in areas that have a lot of administrative actions. They bring together all materials related to a subject, often including administrative decisions. A guide to research within an administrative area, such as Gail Levin Richmond's *Federal Tax Research: Guide to Materials and Techniques,* or a guide to several areas of administrative law, such as *Specialized Legal Research* by Penny A. Hazelton, can offer useful information about adjudication within a particular agency. Major treatises that deal with topics that contain a great deal of administrative law will also provide guidance to the researcher new to a topic and agency.

Many other documents created by agencies besides those associated with adjudicatory matters may be of interest to a researcher. Some of these are readily available, and others are more difficult to locate. Today, agency websites are very useful for finding these materials. Farther back in time, the materials not published in the *Federal Register* or CFR or as administrative decisions may be published by the GPO and indexed in its catalog. If material is not available from any of those resources, it may be available in the U.S. National Archives (discussed in chapter 8) or by contacting an agency directly. To acquire material from an agency, a researcher may need to file a Freedom of Information Act request (see chapter 11).

State Administrative Law

Federal regulations are initially published in the chronologically arranged *Federal Register* and then compiled into the topically arranged CFR. The same model holds true in many states. State agencies granted the power to make law promulgate regulations that are often printed in a regular "register," although at times the regulations will instead be collected into a topical code. The creation and publication of regulations vary by state, and a researcher will often do well to start with a state legal research guide.

States also publish governmental documents. Many early records, up to 1900, are included in a microform collection titled *Records of the States of the United States of America,* published in the middle of the twentieth century. This set, put together by the Library of Congress and the University of North Carolina, is indexed by a print volume by W. S. Jenkins, *A Guide to the Microfilm Collection of Early State Records.* The Law Library Microform Consortium is currently publishing *Early State Records,* which is a digitization of the *Records of the States.* The first phase will include the records of fifteen Atlantic Coast states and Native American tribes. Other resources for identifying state records include the *Monthly Checklist of State Publications, Records of the States of the United States of America,* and *Documents Illustrative of the Formation of the Union of the American*

States. Each of these indexes will inform a researcher that a document exists but will lead to further research into the records of the state. Some states collected and published sets of their legislative and other governmental records from colonial times (see chapter 3), with some continued coverage into the nineteenth century. The records available for each state vary widely, and a research guide into the state of interest will provide further information about availability. The state library and state archives are other resources worth investigating.

Bibliographies

A list of some excellent bibliographies of materials published by administrative agencies appears at the end of this chapter. A good catalog search to locate materials like these will include requirements that "government publications" and "bibliographies" appear as subjects in the bibliographic record.

Government Documents

From its earliest times, the federal government has produced documents of public interest. In the early nineteenth century the important documents were collected and published in *American State Papers,* which includes material released or created between 1789 and 1838. In 1817, Congress, which was at the time the largest producer of government material, began publishing the *United States Congressional Serial Set.* While *American State Papers* and the *Serial Set* mainly include legislative materials, they also publish many documents from a variety of departments and agencies from 1789 to date. The *Serial Set* also includes a great deal of material that Congress received from other departments. In 1861, the GPO was founded, and the importance of the *Serial Set* as a publisher of noncongressional material began to decline. Researchers can often find documents dating from the nineteenth century, and even the twentieth, such as annual reports from executive departments and agencies, within the *Serial Set.*

In 1903, the superintendent of documents created a classification system for government publications. The system, which is based on the governmental unit that created the document, is used to organize U.S. governmental documents in federal depository libraries and in the online collections of government documents. A great introduction to government documents is Joe Morehead's *Introduction to United States Government Information Sources.* This text, although published in 1999, thoroughly introduces the types of resources that the government has produced and the best methods for using them.

The tools for locating federal government documents can be separated into three time periods. The first covers the early Republic, the second covers the bulk of the nineteenth century, and the third continues through the twentieth and into the twenty-first centuries. One of the most important resources for identifying material from the early years is J. H. Powell's *The Books of a New Nation: United States Government Publications, 1774–1814;* another is the *American State Papers.*

For most of the nineteenth century, Benjamin Perley Poore's *A Descriptive Catalogue of the Government Publications of the United States* is the most important resource. It includes a brief chronological listing of government publications published from 1774 through 1881, as well as a brief index by name and subject. It also includes many congressional documents and documents from various departments such as the Department of the Interior, the Library of Congress, and the Department of Justice.

Another important resource is the *Checklist of United States Public Documents, 1789–1909.* Intended as a multivolume index of government documents, only volume 1, *Lists of Congressional and Departmental Publications,* was actually published. The *Checklist* introduces the superintendent of documents numbering system, or SuDoc number, which is the GPO's structure for organizing federal publications. Documents are organized under the issuing department, indicated by a one- or two-letter designation. For example, congressional material is located under the letter Y, materials from the Justice Department can be found under J, and Civil Service Commission materials bear the designation CS. Materials are then further organized. For example, the annual reports of the attorney general are filed under J1.1, the Official Opinions of the Attorneys General under J1.5, and the annual reports of the Assistant Attorney General for Indian Depredation Claims under J3.

Another important tool for researching nineteenth-century government documents is a microform collection of executive branch documents prepared by the CIS. The microform set by CIS is accompanied by the *CIS Index to U.S. Executive Branch Documents, 1789–1909.* Although the index and accompanying microforms are available at many large libraries, most researchers will want to use the related ProQuest *Executive Branch Documents* database. Since ProQuest purchased CIS, this microform set played an important roll in the development of the database.

ProQuest's *Executive Branch Documents, 1789–1932,* follows the structure and models its contents on the *Checklist of United States Public Documents.* The *Checklist,* like Poore's, is an excellent guide to the types of publications and the organization of the publications, but it does not provide more than the bibliographic information that describes the material. *Executive Branch Documents* includes the full text of all of the document types listed in the *Checklist* in searchable PDF format with indexing. At many libraries this is available as an add-on to ProQuest Congressional.

Several other guides to government documents cover parts of the nineteenth century. These are far more detailed than either Poore's or the *Checklist*; however, they cover only a small number of years. The *Comprehensive Index to the Publications of the United States Government, 1881–1893* by John G. Ames is a detailed two-volume index to the publications. A slightly longer coverage window with slightly less detail is provided by the *Catalogue of the Public Documents of the 53rd Congress, 2d Session—76th Congress, 1st Session, March 4, 1893–December 31, 1940 and of All Departments of the Governments of the United States*. The latter becomes less important when it covers the early twentieth century because better indexes appear.

Starting in 1895, the federal government began issuing the *Monthly Catalog of United States Government Publications*, an index that is still being published. Researchers can find and consult it in print in depository and other libraries, though it is most often held in the microform version. Two electronic versions have made this an even more useful tool. The first is a for-fee database from ProQuest simply titled *Monthly Catalog of United States Government Publications, 1895–1976*, which can be browsed chronologically or searched by a variety of means, such as keyword, title, author, date, and SuDoc number, though not by full text. The other database picks up in 1976 and takes researchers into the present. This is a free index available at the GPO website (https://catalog.gpo.gov).

Several collections of governmental documents gather around particular topics. *American Archives* was planned as a documentary history of the American colonies up to the ratification of the U.S. Constitution in six multivolume series, but only nine volumes were published, covering 1774–1776. Researchers can find them in many academic and law libraries and online from Northern Illinois University (http://amarch. lib.niu.edu/). The *Documentary History of the Constitution of the United States, 1786–1870,* a terrific resource for investigating how the Constitution was seen early in its history, includes materials created between 1786 and 1870 relating to the development of the Constitution.

This brief discussion of governmental materials touches only the surface of all possible documents that researchers may want to use. Inventive researchers will also use tools such as the *United States Government Manual* to fully understand an administrative agency or department and locate areas within the department that may house materials of interest. They can also investigate materials published elsewhere by using library catalogs and Google Books or by contacting archives and investigating materials collected there. Researchers may need to submit a Freedom of Information Act request to obtain materials not widely disseminated (see chapter 11). The Justice Department's Office of Information and Privacy publishes an excellent annual *Freedom of Information Act Guide.*

The Current Era

Research has not remained static since the 1930s. In fact, the past twenty-five to thirty years have seen the most dramatic changes in research tools and methods than any previous era. Today, researchers can accomplish research tasks and develop research projects that would have been possible to imagine but practically impossible to undertake even twenty-five years ago. New tools allow them to find materials that would have been unfindable until very recently. Researchers can comb through and manipulate data in ways and to an extent that until recently was the province of science fiction.

One can think of the early twentieth century as the era in which structure was imposed on the law, but the current era is one in which researchers are freed from the constraints of structure. It is important to note that freedom from the constraints of structure is not the same as rejecting structure or even moving beyond structure. Rather, researchers today can use tools that impose structure when desired and eschew structure when needed.

In the late nineteenth and early twentieth centuries, legislation, judicial opinions, and regulations were all broken apart and placed into a preexisting theoretical structure. This was the era of structure. While the idea of and human desire for classification has ancient roots, the late nineteenth and early twentieth centuries was a time of sweeping dramatic classification. The zoological taxonomies were developed and regulated, and the Dewey Decimal System, a system for organizing libraries that attempts to describe all knowledge, was established.

These taxonomies, best described as precoordinate indexing, in that a structure exists before items are placed within it, should be compared with postcoordinate indexing, in which a structure follows a collection. The Dewey Decimal System is a precoordinate system, and the Library of Congress Classification System, the system used in many academic libraries, is a postcoordinate system. The existence of references in a postcoordinate system means that what is referred to actually exists in what is being described. Nothing is included in the description unless it appears in the collection. Although precoordinate schemes can be modified when it is found that they are too far from representing reality, such modification is a tremendous undertaking.

In the law, a major classification scheme is the West Key Number system, which has undergone some significant changes over time. By merely expanding the outline, or looking at the spines of a print digest, one can easily see that digest topics vary in size and complexity. Sometimes, especially as the law is changing and developing, a piece of a case may not fit into the structure very well. Because changing the classification scheme is so difficult, some ill-fitting topical assignments can persist for years.

In the mid- to late twentieth century, full-text searching became a reality. With full-text searching, every word, or as in most databases, almost every word, became searchable. One of the first full-text databases available in the United States was LexisNexis. Beginning in the 1970s, Lexis began to make law accessible in new ways. One of the advantages of the taxonomic system in which laws are categorized was that one could identify a preexisting topic and find the law surrounding the topic. Categorization had another effect as well: it created the belief that the law has a structure, that the categories defined relationships of ideas and that the categories described the range of thinkable thoughts about the law. But the law is messy. In many cases, ideas that are separated in the West scheme can occur in close temporal or theoretical proximity in the world. Some relations in the law are not described by the West system or by any other system of categorization. Full-text searching allows researchers to break free of the constraints imposed by categories so they are able to think new thoughts and combine new ideas.

At first, researchers had to learn an arcane system of logic and symbols in order to use these collections. After learning how to use these, practiced researchers were able to make new logical connections and find previously unfindable material. As freeing as this new paradigm was, it came with some freight. First, researchers had to learn the system of logic and symbols, and in order to conduct useful searches, they needed to be experienced. Attorneys already knew how to use indexes and print digests; would they think it worthwhile to spend the time and effort to learn a new system? Would the benefits outweigh the costs?

At about this time a new problem with full-text searching became apparent: simple full-text Boolean searches do not work very well. In 1985 David C. Blair and M. E. Maron published their study "An Evaluation of Retrieval Effectiveness for a Full-Text Document Retrieval System" (*Communications of the ACM* 28, no. 3, 280–99), which showed that particular kinds of full-text searches return roughly 20 percent of relevant items. This study has generated a valuable discussion, and the facts it elucidated have led to the development of algorithmic or natural language searching and the inclusion of more structure in some databases. Search algorithms have their own limitations for legal research. At this point the benefits of full-text searching appeared to carry with them some significant problems. The major legal database providers responded in two ways. West, which had started its online venture by making only its head-notes available online, continued with the rollout of the full text of cases; but West made clear online the underlying structure to the case law. The structure that West had imposed on the cases became a search element and not just a landing place. Lexis also began to add structure to its collection of cases.

Natural language searching, that is, using a search algorithm to determine what the searcher is looking for and returning what the algorithm thinks the researcher wants, is ubiquitous today, but its takeover in the law has not been universal. As we will see, the most powerful search tools today allow elements of both Boolean searching and natural language searching. One of the truths about natural language searching is that it can be improved. With a Boolean search, researchers construct a logic statement, and everything that matches that statement is returned. The only way to improve such a search is to improve the skills of users and, perhaps, provide some firm, controlled references on which they can rely. A natural language search can be improved from both ends. Users can learn to pose better queries, and over time some have learned about querying databases in this way. But much more important is that vendors, or the algorithms themselves, can improve their search algorithms. They need not rely on users becoming better searchers; owners of the databases can try to make the systems better able to tease out the meaning of the search and better able to pinpoint relevant material. As we have moved into the twenty-first century, the main legal database providers offer systems with well-developed natural interfaces and algorithms that also support the aspects of Boolean searching that are most useful.

As all of this was being developed to make cases and law review articles findable, issues with the other structured data, codes, in the databases began to become apparent. Experts had known that the type of language used in codes—both prospective and general, nonspecific—is difficult to search. For example, efforts to construct searches for finding legislative material on a particular topic for all states almost always end unsatisfactorily. Searches in annotated codes tend to return far too many results since the language that tends to appear in the headnotes and other annotations generates a lot of the results. On the other hand, searches in unannotated codes or searches that omit the annotations tend to return far fewer results and miss many relevant code sections since the language of the code can be inconsistent from state to state and can be difficult to conceive.

The databases first made the structure of the underlying data more apparent. The codes became browsable. One could approach the entire code and drill in. One could select an area of the code and search only within that area. Or one could work from an identified section and move back and forth or step back and look at the area around the identified section. These improved the usability of codes online, but finding relevant code-based law remained difficult. To remedy this problem, the databases returned to an old technology: the index. Westlaw has made many of its codes, encyclopedias, and other indexes available online. By pulling an old technology into the twenty-first century, West is merging the best of the old with the best of the new.

Thus far, much of what is new is a repackaging of an existing print resource into an online version. With some types of materials, the switch has been logical and seamless. Citators make much more sense online than they do in print. Indeed, Frank Shepard did the best that he could to mimic a computer in an economically advantageous way. Other kinds of materials, such as looseleaf services, which are topically arranged and are updated by having new information interfiled in the correct logical location, make a lot of sense as online products. With many other types of material, however, what we see today is merely a placing of the material online without really taking advantage of what being online provides.

Of course, merely placing material online and making it searchable does add significant value. Being able to search through millions of books has tremendous value, but one is still searching through "books." Most of the databases that we have seen contain a collection of items that are recognizable as books, articles, or index entries. Value has been added in that they may now be full-text searched or they have a structure imposed on them or have a controlled vocabulary describing them, but a nineteenth-century lawyer still would instantly recognize them.

In earlier chapters, we have looked at the books, serials, treatises, encyclopedias, citators, finding tools, and other materials that are used in conducting legal research. Many are widely available to a modern researcher in print, in the original printing or as a reprint, or online. When we get to the mid-twentieth century, the landscape changes. Fewer items from the 1920s on are available online.

Cases, codes, and other legal materials are all available for a fee from Lexis and Westlaw and other databases. And the availability of other cases online is growing. Google Scholar contains the vast majority of appellate cases from the 1950s forward, and Ravel Law has teamed with the Harvard Law Library to scan and make freely available all reported cases. The current U.S. Code is available for free online, but older versions are generally behind pay walls—and this is the case with federal government material, that is, material for which no copyright is claimed. When we get to state materials, where a copyright may be claimed, and to privately created and published materials, where copyright is often claimed, it can be difficult or impossible for researchers to find online versions.

Research Example

Let's assume an interest in the regulations relating to educational television facilities during the 1970s. Using some of the government resources mentioned in the introduction as well as in this chapter, we need to look into whether any government reports exist and then locate the regulations in place between 1965 and 1980. To find government reports published from the 1960s, after the first wave of educational television had settled, and the 1970s, when the government provided grants for educational television under the Federal Communications Commission (FCC) and the Department of Health, Education, and Welfare (HEW), we start with the *Monthly Catalog of Government Documents.* Since the dates that interest us run through the 1970s, we also need to use the GPO's online Monthly Catalog search tool. We should further look into any legislation and congressional reports, documents, or hearings.

A very broad search in the Monthly Catalog database for the terms "education" and "television" anywhere in the record gets us twenty-two items from January 1, 1965, through December 31, 1975. Note that we are interested in material published through 1980, but this database ends in 1975. We can look through the list to gain an idea of the agencies and organizations involved and see the types of subjects covered. We can also sort the material by date and determine whether we can discern any topical trends. In looking through the records, we note that Congress was interested in public television, and there were several studies by HEW: some about the finances of educational television organizations along with a very interesting guide for public schools.

We must remember to search the Monthly Catalog broadly because the only material being searched is the brief Monthly Catalog record; an initial broad search can open the research to alternative ways of seeing the issue. After we have identified materials in the Monthly Catalog, we still need to obtain them. Government documents can be found at depository libraries, but to avoid an unnecessary trip, we can contact a library, even the ones that are "complete depositories," before visiting to make certain the materials are available there. Frequently, libraries are unable or unwilling to lend unique government documents, although it is frequently possible to acquire a scan of a shorter item.

Since our Monthly Catalog search covered only from 1966 to 1975, we must search the GPO-provided online *Catalog of U.S. Government Publications* to find material from 1976 to 1980 (available at www.gpo.gov/fdsys). When we search for publications from January 1, 1976, to December 31, 1980, we find twenty-eight very interesting documents, including a 1978 report titled "Television, the Book, and the Classroom: A Seminar."

We should now look at the regulations in place in 1975. Initially, we considered the FCC as the most important agency, but now we can see that, depending on our research interests, perhaps we should start with HEW. The free online version of the CFR made available on the Federal Digital System website goes back only to the mid-1990s, so we can find either a print or microform archive of the CFR or use HeinOnline's archival version.

We can find the relevant regulations through a search using the CFR indexes or a search of the full text of the CFR. Let's start with a full-text search for 1975 to see whether we can get a handle on where within the CFR relevant regulations might be generally located. At this point, missing a relevant document is not a matter of extreme concern because we hope to be directed to an area of the CFR. Since the CFR is organized topically, we need only one hit within the relevant section. Again, we should conduct a fairly broad search: "education," truncated after the "n" to allow other variants, and "television," limiting the search to 1975. We find 218 sections of the CFR; by scanning these results we see that Title 45 (Public Welfare), Part 153 (Educational Broadcasting Facilities Program) looks promising. Looking at the part, we note the authority that the agency cited for creating the regulations: P.L. 87–447, 76 Stat. 64–67, as amended. We also note that the regulations were indeed put in place in 1975 at 40 F.R. 11243, March 10, 1975. By turning to that date in the *Federal Register,* we find the original regulations and, starting a couple of pages before the final regulations, the agency's rationale, the types of comments that it received, and its responses to the comments.

Now we should look to see whether there were any amendments to the regulations during the rest of the 1970s. The easiest way to do this is to look at the sections of interest in the 1980 edition of the CFR and check the date the sections were added or amended. If the date given is March 10, 1975, then we have already seen the version of the regulations that was in force for the end of the 1970s; if the sections have been amended, we will see the date of amendment. When we turn to Title 45, Part 153, in the 1980 edition of the CFR, we see that the entire part was revised on November 1, 1977, at 42 F.R. 57286. Next, we can turn to the November 1, 1977, issue of the *Federal Register,* and, by looking at the rationale, we may be able to gain some insight into why the changes were made.

Further Reading

Ackerman, Bruce A. *We the People.* Cambridge, MA: Belknap, 2014.

Armstrong, Robert D. "'The Matter of Printing': Public Printing in the Western Territories of the United States." *Journal of Government Information* 21, no. 1 (1994): 37–47.

Berring, Robert C. "Collapse of the Structure of the Legal Research Universe: The Imperative of Digital Information." *Washington Law Review* 69 (January 1994): 9–34.

Cohen, Morris L. "Researching Legal History in the Digital Age." *Law Library Journal* 99 (2007): 377–93.

Danner, Richard A. "Legal Information and the Development of American Law: Writings on the Form and Structure of the Published Law." *Law Library Journal* 99, no. 2 (2007): 193–227.

Feinberg, Lotte E. "Mr. Justice Brandeis and the Creation of the Federal Register." *Public Administration Review* 61, no. 3 (2001): 359–70.

Gellman, Robert. "Who Should Publish the Law?" *Journal of Government Information* 23, no. 3 (1996): 253–63.

Katsh, Ethan. "Law in a Digital World: Computer Networks and Cyberspace." *Villanova Law Review* 38 (1993): 403–85.

Mart, Susan Nevelow. "Let the People Know the Facts: Can Government Information Removed from the Internet Be Reclaimed." *Law Library Journal* 98 (2006): 7–31.

Martin, Peter W. "The Internet: 'Full and Unfettered Access' to Law— Some Implications." *Northern Kentucky Law Review* 26, no. 2 (1999): 181–209.

———. "Reconfiguring Law Reports and the Concept of Precedent for a Digital Age." *Villanova Law Review* 53 (2008): 1–45.

Schmeckebier, Laurence Frederick, Roy B. Eastin, and Brookings Institution. "Catalogs and Indexes." In *Government Publications and Their Use,* 6–13. Washington, DC: Brookings Institution, 1969.

———. "Congressional Publications." In *Government Publications and Their Use,* 134–93. Washington, DC: Brookings Institution, 1969.

Sears, Jean L., and Marilyn K. Moody. "Historical Searches." In *Using Government Information Sources: Electronic and Print,* 482–95. Phoenix: Oryx, 2001.

Stubbs, Walter. "Finding Congressional Journals in the U.S. Serial Set." *Journal of Government Information* 24, no. 1 (1997): 39–45.

Zink, Steven D. "Clio's Blindspot: Historians' Underutilization of United States Government Publications in Historical Research." *Government Publications Review* 13, no. 1 (1986): 67–78.

Important Sources Mentioned in This Chapter

American State Papers: Documents, Legislative and Executive, of the Congress of the United States. Washington: Gales and Seaton, 1832.

Ames, John G. *Comprehensive Index to the Publications of the United States Government, 1881–1893.* Washington, DC: GPO, 1905.

Congressional Information Service. *CIS Index to Presidential Executive Orders and Proclamations.* Washington, DC: Congressional Information Service, 1987–.

————. *CIS Index to U.S. Executive Branch Documents, 1789–1909*. Bethesda, MD: CIS, 1990–.

————. *CIS Index to U.S. Executive Branch Documents, 1910–1932: Guide to Documents Not Printed in the U.S. Serial Set*. Bethesda, MD: Congressional Information Service, 1996–.

Hazelton, Penny A., ed. *Specialized Legal Research*. Boston: Little, Brown, 2014–.

Morehead, Joe. *Introduction to United States Government Information Sources*. Englewood, NJ: Libraries Unlimited, 1999.

Poore, Benjamin Perley. *A Descriptive Catalogue of the Government Publications of the United States, September 5, 1774–March 4, 1881*. Washington, DC: GPO, 1885.

Powell, J. H. *The Books of a New Nation: United States Government Publications, 1774–1814*. Philadelphia: University of Pennsylvania Press, 1957.

Richmond, Gail Levin. *Federal Tax Research: Guide to Materials and Techniques*. Westbury, NY: Foundation Press, 1990.

United States. *United States Congressional Serial Set*. Washington, DC: GPO, 1817–.

United States and Bureau of Rolls and Library. *Documentary History of the Constitution of the United States of America, 1786–1870*. Washington, DC: Department of State, 1901.

United States Department of Justice. *Freedom of Information Act Guide & Privacy Act Overview*. Washington, DC: Office of Information and Privacy, Office of Policy and Communications, 1992.

United States Department of State, Library Division. *Documentary History of the Constitution of the United States of America, 1787–1870. Derived from the Records, Manuscripts and Rolls Deposited in the Bureau of Rolls and Library of the Department of State*. Washington, DC: Department of State, 1894.

United States National Archives and Records Administration and Office of the Federal Register. *Weekly Compilation of Presidential Documents*. Washington, DC: GPO, 1965–2009.

United States Office of the Federal Register. *The Code of Federal Regulations of the United States of America*. Washington, DC: Office of the Federal Register, 1938–.

————. *The United States Government Manual*. Washington, DC: GPO, 1974–.

United States Office of the Federal Register, U.S. National Archives and Records Service, and National Archives and Records Administration. *Federal Register*. Washington, DC: GPO, 1936–.

United States President, U.S. Federal Register Division, and U.S. Office of the Federal Register. *Public Papers of the Presidents of the United States.* Washington, DC: National Archives, 1958–.

United States Superintendent of Documents. *Catalogue of the Public Documents of the 53rd Congress, 2d Session—76th Congress, 1st Session, March 4, 1893–December 31, 1940 and of All Departments of the Governments of the United States.* Washington, DC: GPO, 1896.

———. *Monthly Catalog of United States Government Publications.* Washington, DC: GPO, 1895–.

United States Superintendent of Documents and Mary Ann Hartwell. *Checklist of United States Public Documents, 1789–1909, Congressional: To Close of Sixtieth Congress; Departmental: To End of Calendar Year 1909.* Washington, DC: GPO, 1911.

Databases

Northern Illinois University. *American Archives.* http://amarch.lib.niu.edu/.

ProQuest. *Monthly Catalog of U.S. Government Publications, 1895–1976.* http://monthlycatalog.chadwyck.com/home.do.

———. *ProQuest Executive Branch Documents, 1789–1932.* https://www.proquest.com/products-services/ProQuest-Executive-Branch-Documents–1789–1932.html.

United States Government Printing Office. *Monthly Catalog of United States Government Publications.* http://purl.access.gpo.gov/GPO/LPS844.

United States Office of the Federal Register and U.S. Government Printing Office. *Daily Compilation of Presidential Documents.* Washington, DC: GPO, 2009–. http://purl.access.gpo.gov/GPO/LPS107897.

Selected Bibliographies of the Work of Government Agencies

Burns, Richard Dean, and the Society for Historians of American Foreign Relations. *Guide to American Foreign Relations Since 1700.* Santa Barbara, CA: ABC-Clio, 1983.

Dubester, Henry J. *Catalog of United States Census Publications, 1790–1945.* Washington, DC: GPO, 1950.

Hasse, Adelaide Rosalie. *Index to United States Documents Relating to Foreign Affairs: 1828–1861; in Three Parts.* Washington, DC: Carnegie Institute, 1919.

Smithsonian Institution. *List and Index of the Publications of the United States National Museum (1875–1946)*. Washington, DC: GPO, 1947.

Smithsonian Institution and Bureau of American Ethnology. *List of Publications of the Bureau of American Ethnology: With Index to Authors and Titles*. Washington, DC: GPO, 1971.

Stemple, Ruth M. *Author-Subject Index to Articles in Smithsonian Annual Reports 1849–1961*. Washington, DC: Smithsonian Institution, 1963.

United States Bureau of Labor Statistics. *Bureau of Labor Statistics Publications, 1886–1971: Numerical Listings, Annotations, Subject Index*. Washington, DC: GPO, 1972.

———. *Subject Index of the Publications of the United States Bureau of Labor Statistics up to May 1, 1915*. Washington, DC: GPO, 1915.

United States Department of Commerce Library. *Publications Catalog and Index, 1790–1950*. Washington, DC: GPO, 1952.

United States Geological Survey. *Publications of the Geological Survey, 1879–1961*. Washington, DC: GPO, 1964.

United States Office of Education. *Bibliography of Publications: 1867–1959*. Totowa, NJ: Rowman & Littlefield, 1971.

8

Archives and Practice Materials

The savvy legal history researcher is constantly aware that much of the material that lends insight into the law is unpublished. While official documents that make law and some background materials are published, much background material is not. For instance, many appellate decisions beginning in the nineteenth century have been published, but most briefs and other documents that provide the researcher with a fuller understanding of the circumstances have not. Occasionally, participants will publish their recollections, or law-making bodies and individuals may leave a trove of documents, letters, and other papers. Archives and special collections have obtained some of these papers and make them available. Archival research is where the most exciting and rewarding items are often found, offering new insights into the past.

Archival Research

Archival collections are diverse, ranging in size, scope, creator, and format. Some collections contain only a few items; others are mammoth. Some relate to all activities of a particular person or organization; others focus narrowly on a topic. Some contain the records of an organization, for example, the American Civil Liberties Union or the U.S. Justice Department; while others may contain the records of a family or an individual, as in the Kent Family Papers or the papers of Justice Harry Blackmun. A researcher may find it more difficult to identify relevant materials in archival research than in other types of historical research.

The integrity of archival collections is extremely important to archivists and affects how archival research is conducted. Archivists try to respect the donor and the collection. For example, archivists endeavor to retain the arrangement of materials and will keep materials from different sources separate: "original order" and "provenance" are watchwords for archivists. A researcher interested in learning about a specific person may need to consult a great many archives. Relevant material might reside in collections of the subject's personal papers or organizations with whom that person corresponded. The researcher may also consult collections that contain materials about the subject or collections created by an employer or other organization or person with whom the subject interacted.

Many archival collections have finding aids, and a finding aid is the first thing that researchers should look for. Finding aids vary in their completeness and detail, but they are the best windows into a collection. A finding aid should provide an overview of the collection, including the provenance and information about access; perhaps a brief biography and/or description of the collection; and a list of the contents of the collection that describes the contents as specifically as the name of each box or folder. It should also provide a list of the people, other than the creator of the collection, who play a significant role in the content as a correspondent or subject. Researchers will try to locate finding aids at whatever archive might hold the material they are interested in. An example of a database of finding aids is the Yale Finding Aid Database of the Yale Library Manuscripts and Archives, available online at the Yale University Library's website.

There are two parts to an archival research project: (1) determine which archive holds the needed materials, and (2) determine, as much as possible, where in a collection relevant materials might be found. Several widely available resources can help a researcher determine which archives to consult. WorldCat is the resource most reliably available and includes many archival collections. These records will provide the name of the collection, perhaps a brief general description, and the names of the most important correspondents, but they will offer little other detail. A search for the research topic as a subject combined with the word "papers" as the title will often reveal the location of a relevant collection of papers.

Although WorldCat includes numerous collections of papers, other more specialized databases can also help a researcher find archival collections. The most important are ArchiveGrid and Archive Finder.

ArchiveGrid is from the Online Computer Library Center (OCLC), the same organization that provides WorldCat. ArchiveGrid covers more than three million collections in more than one thousand archives, most in the United States and a preponderance in the English-speaking world. Searches cover the detailed descriptions of collections as well as the expected names and subjects, making ArchiveGrid very useful for finding materials within collections that might not be obvious. The "summary view" lists the archives that contain material responsive to the search collected by the creator of the collection, whether an individual or group; the subject of the collection; and the location of the archive or the name of the archive itself.

The latter are useful because archival work often requires that the researcher visit a collection in person.

Archive Finder pulls together two lists of archives: *ArchivesUSA* and the *National Inventory of Documentary Sources in the United Kingdom and Ireland* (NIDS UK/Ireland). Researchers can search in the list of repositories or in the description of the collections or in both simultaneously. The descriptions in Archive Finder tend to be less in-depth that those in ArchiveGrid, but Archive Finder is useful for locating collections that might be worth examining, and it provides good practical information about repositories. Fairly broad searches using a subject's name will often yield a list of the collections and/or repositories in which the name appears. By clicking on the collection name, researchers can examine further information: details about the location of the repository, the type of materials included in the archive, the extent of the materials included, and a description of the materials. They may also find notes and subject headings. The best searches start broadly to identify a person of interest, who may then be found as a subject heading, prompting a further search for any collection that includes substantial material about the person.

As an example, a researcher may conduct an initial search for James Kent in Archive Finder. This search will return more than 150 collections. Looking through that list he or she can locate the Kent Family Papers. From the description of the papers, the researcher learns that "Kent, James, 1763–1847" is included as an index term. Clicking on this yields ten collections that contain papers by, to, or related to Chancellor Kent. The results include the George Jacob Abbott Papers at Yale University, the Goodhue Family Papers at the New York Society Library, the Jones Family Papers at the New York Public Library, a collection of microfilms of James Kent's papers at the Library of Congress, the Kent Family Papers at Columbia, and more.

The Library of Congress offers a description of its collection on James Kent, including biographical information on him, some of the major types of papers included in the collections, and some of his correspondents. The index terms list correspondents and other important people mentioned in Kent's papers, such as John Quincy Adams, Henry Clay, Francis Lieber, and Daniel Webster. In addition, the collection has been assigned subjects such as "law practice New York," "New York legal affairs," and others. Searching in the Library of Congress manuscript collection for other collections related to "law practice New York" returns Kent's papers as well as others.

A search for "James Kent" using ArchiveGrid, available without a subscription from OCLC Research, returns more than three thousand collections. Narrowing the search to "James" within four words of "Kent" ("James Kent"~4) reduces the list to about three hundred collections. Interestingly, the list includes many single items related to Kent. For example, one collection contains two letters from James Kent to one of his successors as chancellor of New York. One is related to a particular case, and the other requests the admission of a colleague from South Carolina as counsel before the New York Court of Chancery. ArchiveGrid also returns a page titled "Results Overview," which allows the researcher to narrow the results by a variety of means, including a person related to the collection and listed as a subject of the collection, the topic assigned to the archival collection, the general geographical location of the archive, and the particular geographical location of the archive.

Archives Made Easy (AME) is a different kind of resource. Rather than function as a finding tool for materials within an archive, this site collects archives and provides a short discussion

of how to use each one. For example, when a researcher choos-
es the United States on Archives Made Easy, he or she gets a list
of around twenty archives located in the United States. For each
archive, AME provides a link to its website as well as signed and
dated "easy archive tips" that provide information about how
to use it. While not many archives are included, the information
provided by AME can make using archives easier.

Another extremely important resource is the National
Union Catalog of Manuscript Collections (NUCMC), whose
mission is to describe archival and manuscript collections at
eligible U.S. repositories. The NUCMC project began in 1959
and continues today. The early records, from 1959 through 1993,
were published as print catalogs and can be found at the largest
academic and public libraries. The records from 1986 forward
are included in WorldCat.

Once researchers have identified and located a collection,
they will want to learn whether there are any restrictions on its
use. Donors often place restrictions on their papers, or there
may be limits for a particular time or for a particular use. Certain records, such as student records, might be restricted because
of privacy concerns. Information regarding limits may be available in the collection's description. If not, researchers may have
to contact the archive.

By using WorldCat, Archive Finder, and ArchiveGrid researchers can begin to get an idea of where they might find the
papers of a particular individual or organization. Next, they
must find particular materials within the papers. Because archivists hold it as an article of faith that an archival collection
should not be rearranged, each collection will be organized
differently. Archivists know that an archive's organization can
give insight into the person who created and organized it.
Therefore, researchers will want to begin by locating the guide

to the collection, understanding that the quality of and detail in such guides vary widely. Some provide only a box-level general description; others offer folder-level descriptions. Item-level descriptions are rare. However, in a well-organized collection, a folder-level description should guide researchers to the correct folders, or at least boxes, to examine.

Sometimes an archive will copy materials and deliver them to researchers, but only if they know enough details to choose specific items. Often, they will have to visit an archive to examine the materials themselves. It is important to plan ahead for any trip to an archive. Most archives have web pages or other publications that describe their rules and offer other information that visitors should know. Or researchers may want to contact an archivist for practical information regarding a visit to an archive, such as whether the archive allows digital photography, and if so, whether there is sufficient light to take legible pictures. Researchers might also want to know whether an archive will make copies of materials, and if so, how much they cost and how long they will take. Some archives allow only notes to be taken.

Before planning a trip to an archive, researchers should determine whether the materials they seek might have been deemed valuable enough to be published in print or on microform, making them available more locally. For example, James Madison's papers have been published in print several times and are available for free on the web. Chancellor Kent's papers have been published on microform, as have Felix Frankfurter's and Oliver Wendell Holmes's. Records of some courts have been published on microform, as have the records of some federal administrative agencies.

The National Archives is the most important archive for researchers interested in federal law. Archival material is organized into record groups. Material from each branch of government is treated differently. Congressional material is housed at the National Archives but is under the control of Congress and is administered by the Center for Legislative Archives. The center should be contacted with any questions about access. Most judicial material is housed at regional archives, and executive material is generally housed at the nearest archival branch, with material from the central office in the District of Columbia or Maryland and regional material at the closest regional location. Some material has been microfilmed by the National Archives and is available for purchase. Researchers may gain access to other material by making a request to or visiting the archives. The National Archives website (www.archives.gov) has several finding aids, information about archival locations, information about obtaining materials that have been microfilmed, obtaining other materials, and visiting.

Practice Materials

Practice books or manuals are one of the most long-lived type of legal material. They were designed to help attorneys and laypeople work with the law. Other than sensational trial accounts, it was the legal publication most designed for wide distribution beyond the practicing bar. The genre began with John Rastell's *The Boke of the Justyce of Peas,* published in the last half of the 1520s. The most popular practice book in America, *Conductor Generalis,* originated in London in the middle of the seventeenth century; the American version was published in New York as early as 1711. *Conductor Generalis* remained in print, with various publishers and authors, until 1819. However, 1819 did not signal the end of practice materials. The field remains an important type of legal publishing today.

While early practice materials were designed for anyone
who needed to work with the law, from the nineteenth century,
they can be considered in two classes: those meant for the
public and those meant for lawyers. Manuals designed for
nonlawyers were especially important in the early United States
as many officials and others who worked with the law or came
in contact with it had no legal education. The *Conductor Generalis* and its descendants served the needs of these people,
whether officials, such as constables or justices of the peace, or
business leaders. The manuals also provide great insight into
the ideas about law that laypeople held at particular times and
the type of legal problems that were most often raised. Other
than some excellent bibliographies, there are no easy searches
that can lead a researcher to practice materials. The best possibility is to conduct a subject search for "practice of law" or a
topical search in a catalog, then browse through the results.
Manuals designed for laypeople were often not published by
established law publishers, making searching more difficult.
However, once a researcher identifies a publisher or series, finding additional manuals either earlier or later than the one at
hand becomes easier.

Attorneys also often use practice materials, but these can
differ from those aimed at the layperson. Practice materials
designed for lawyers are more detailed, provide related references and more information, and are more voluminous. Dis-
tinguishing among legal encyclopedias, legal treatises, and legal
practice materials is, in many respects, a meaningless exercise.
Practice materials will look like treatises and encyclopedias, but
their purpose is different. The early twentieth century was the
high-water mark for the publication of large practice materials
collections. The major legal publishers each had their own collections and endeavored to keep researchers within materials

that they published. These tools described a transaction or a lawsuit step by step and provided checklists, tips, references to statutes, regulations, and interpretive cases. Many are available today through the large legal databases, and many are still in print.

One class of practice materials aimed at attorneys is the deskbook. These are published privately and sometimes by the state. They may contain rules of practice and procedure. Some of the privately published state-specific versions contain brief synopses of the major areas of law.

Some practice materials contain legal forms; one type is designed to ensure that a standard set of information is collected. These forms are sometimes published by the state, but more often they are required by the state—for example, one form is required to file a lien, another to apply for workers' compensation. A second type of form is not required by the government but designed to ease the way for an attorney. The great legal realist Karl Llewellyn explained that the doctrine of precedent perhaps made legal forms popular because of "laziness as to the reworking of a problem once solved; the time and energy saved by routine, especially under the pressure of business; the values of routine as a curb on arbitrariness and as a prop of weakness, inexperience and instability; the social values of predictability; the power of whatever exists to produce expectations and the power of expectations to become normative" (K. N. Llewellyn, "Case Law," in Edwin R. A. Seligman and Alvin Johnson, eds., *Encyclopedia of the Social Sciences* [New York: Macmillan, 1937], 249). Of these, expectation and predictability are, one hopes, the driving force behind most decisions to work with a legal form.

There are two classes of legal forms: procedural forms and those meant for transactional work. The procedural forms are often set by statute, and the basic forms are available within the statutory sets. For-profit legal publishers also produce procedural forms, adding value through annotations and other practice tips.

Many legal forms were initially created and distributed by stationers' shops. These early forms can be difficult to locate and are rarely found in bound or published collections. A sort of ephemera, they are found in some archival collections, in the libraries of practicing lawyers, and even as blank note pages inserted by printers in other books. In the nineteenth century, legal publishers began to collect the forms and publish them in topical and jurisdictional sets to include in some of their publications geared toward the practicing bar, though the stationers' forms never did completely disappear. Today, forms might be printed by the government, but individual forms can still be purchased as one-offs or in bulk. To locate legal forms, a researcher can add the term "forms" to a catalog search in the subject field.

Court rules encompass the final class of practice materials. Over time a great many rules about the practice of law have grown up. In the twentieth century a movement to rationalize the practice of law led to the elimination of the court of equity and the combination of the equitable and legal practice into the court of law. As a part of the movement, rules of procedure in civil and criminal actions were adopted at the federal level and, eventually, by all states. Various jurisdictions also developed and adopted rules of evidence and rules of practice before particular courts. In a civil suit, the rules of civil procedure dictate how the suit is initiated and how it will proceed; however, the major rules remain silent on a number of issues. In those instances local court rules step in. How many copies must be served? What does the cover look like? Is there a particular size of paper or color of cover to be used? Local rules govern all of these issues. For the past seventy years, such material has been fairly easy to locate within various publications of jurisdiction-specific court rules or sets of collected court rules; today, they are also invariably available on a court's website. Finding this information from before the 1930s poses more of a challenge. The researcher's best option is to look for practice manuals with a jurisdictional focus.

Research Example

Let us assume that we are interested in the dissent by the first Justice John Marshall Harlan in *Plessy v. Ferguson* and want to look at his papers. We can turn to several sources in order to locate them. Perhaps surprisingly, a good place to start our research is Wikipedia, where we see reference to his papers held at the University of Louisville, the Manuscript Division at the Library of Congress, and other locations. When we try to verify the information at the cited website, the history pages at the Sixth Circuit Court of Appeals, a "Page Not Found" message appears. When we go to the Sixth Circuit page and try to find the material there, we come to another dead end. The foray to Wikipedia was not a waste of time, however, because we have picked up some information for free and can now turn to other resources.

We can next try another free resource, WorldCat. When we search for the subject "Harlan John Marshall" and the title "papers," we get sixty-five results, many of them very interesting. The first two, by relevance, are of microform copies of his papers at the Library of Congress and the University of Louisville. Also in the top ten are a description of his papers at both of those places and an article from the *American*

Journal of Legal History discussing his papers at the University of Louisville.

The WorldCat search has refocused our efforts. We have learned that there are good guides to the papers that we can obtain so that we can be better informed when we speak with archivists or visit the archives in Louisville or D.C. and our trip to the archive can be more productive. We now know to look more closely at the scholarship since it appears that Justice Harlan's papers have been well examined. Our next step is to obtain the guides and to read any articles or books that a subject search for Justice Harlan gives us that appear to describe or rely on his papers. WorldCat also returned some materials that relied on his papers, as well as published collections of his letters and collections of other people's papers.

We might also examine a number of additional sources to determine whether other archives hold relevant information. Archive Finder contains the records available in *ArchivesUSA* and NIDS UK/Ireland. We can search Archive Finder by a number of variables. Most of the records contain a description of the highlight of the collection. Also, most of the collections will have index terms or subject headings assigned to them. Unfortunately, the record may use index terms from NUCMC or NIDS UK/Ireland or both or neither. At Archive Finder, we can search for a repository, a collection, or both. It is usually advisable to start with a broad search and include both types of collections and not limit by index terms. If we search for "Harlan John Marshall," we get two repositories and fifty-seven collections. A search for "John Marshall Harlan" returns the same results. The repositories are at Princeton and the University of Louisville. We are familiar with Louisville, but Princeton is new. One wrinkle with our search, of course, is that there have been two Justice John Marshall Harlans. Since the second

Justice Harlan attended Princeton, we can assume that the papers there are his, but we should give the Princeton collection a closer look to be certain.

As we examine the collections uncovered by Archive Finder, we encounter a difficulty resulting from the fact that the two justices have the same name. We can, of course, look for a collection that contains a NUCMC or NIDS index term for the correct Justice Harlan, or we can limit the display by clicking on the heading. But with only fifty-seven collections to examine, we would be hesitant to do so because the subjects can be overly limiting; a common heading in NUCMC is "Harlan, John Marshall, as correspondent." If we find Justice Harlan in the NIDS index terms, we will miss archives in the United States.

Once we select a record in Archive Finder, we get a brief description of the collection and information about the archive as well as a link to the archive's website. The page describing the archive will provide a great deal of useful information, including hours, phone numbers, addresses, and more.

ArchiveGrid includes the bibliographic records of archives from WorldCat as well as finding aids and other archival descriptions that it harvests from the web. ArchiveGrid isn't limited to the United States, but it is strongly focused on the United States. At ArchiveGrid, we can browse by geographical location to find an archive or to conduct a search in a single Google-style box. A search for "John Marshall Harlan" yields 582 records as well as tabs that provide an overview of the results. The result list can be overwhelming; for example, the first is for a one-page statement held by Cornell University that accompanied a petition Harlan wrote during the Civil War. When we turn to the overview, the system becomes much more useful, as it breaks the results down by people, groups, places, archives, locations of archives, and subjects. At the top of the list of people are "Harlan, John Marshall, 1833–1911," with forty collections; next is "Harlan, John Marshall, 1833–1911, correspondence," with twelve collections; and third is "Harlan, John M. (Marshall), 1899–1971." Not only does this easily limit the list of resources to examine, it also contains a great deal of interesting information. For example, Felix Frankfurter is tied for fourth with Abraham Lincoln, Franklin Roosevelt, and Adlai Stevenson on the list of people with eight collections.

Once we have identified the archives that hold material we wish to examine, our next step is to look for a good description of the collection. We may get lucky and locate a description in our WorldCat search, but more likely we'll need to visit the archive's website. In this case, we go to the Library of Congress's site to look for a description of its Harlan holdings. At the Manuscript Division site we can select "Finding Aids for Collections." When we click through, we can browse by name and select "Harlan," where we discover that the entire Harlan family from 1810 to 1971 is included in the collection. The guide gives us box-by-box and folder-by-folder or reel-by-reel descriptions. It also includes subject headings and the ability to search. The library also offers information about using the collection and obtaining copies of documents as well as information about reference services.

Further Reading

Beck, Karen S. "A Working Lawyer's Life: The Letter Book of John Henry Senter." *Law Library Journal* 99, no. 3 (2007): 471–523.

Callier, Michael, and Achim Reeb. "The Industrial Age of Law: Operationalizing Legal Practice Through Process Improvement." *Oregon Law Review* 93, no. 4 (2015): 853–79.

Finnane, Mark. "Law as an Intellectual Vocation." *Melbourne University Law Review* 38, no. 3 (2014): 1060–79.

Fordham University School of Law. *Symposium: The Legal Profession: Looking Backward. Fordham Law Review* 71, no. 4. New York: Fordham Law School, 2003.

Kruse, Katherine R. "Legal Education and Professional Skills: Myths and Misconceptions About Theory and Practice." *McGeorge Law Review* 45, no. 1 (2013): 7–49.

Lambert, Mark W. "More Than You Imagined: Sources of History in the Records and Papers of the Federal Courts of Texas." *UMKC Law Review* 75, no. 1 (2006): 81–101.

Lepore, Jill. "On Evidence: Proving Frye as a Matter of Law, Science, and History." *Yale Law Journal* 124, no. 4 (2015): 1092–1158.

Parrillo, Nicholas R. "Leviathan and Interpretive Revolution: The Administrative State, the Judiciary, and the Rise of Legislative History, 1890–1950." *Yale Law Journal* 123, no. 2 (2013): 266–411.

Shilling, Patrick. "Attorney Papers, History and Confidentiality: A Proposed Amendment to Model Rule 1.6." *Fordham Law Review* 69, no. 6 (2001): 2741–81.

Sugarman, David. "From Legal Biography to Legal Life Writing: Broadening Conceptions of Legal History and Socio-Legal Scholarship." *Journal of Law and Society* 42, no. 1 (2015): 7–33.

Westbrook, Jay Lawrence. "Empirical Research in Consumer Bankruptcy." *Texas Law Review* 80, no. 7 (2002): 2123–60.

Important Sources Mentioned in This Chapter

Franklin, Benjamin, David Hall, and James Parker. *Conductor Generalis: or, the office, duty and authority of Justices of the Peace, . . .* Philadelphia, 1750.

Great Britain Foreign Office. *National Inventory of Documentary Sources in the United Kingdom and Ireland: The Public Record Office Registers and Indexes.* Cambridge: Chadwyck-Healey, 1988.

Library of Congress. *National Union Catalog of Manuscript Collections.* Washington, DC: Library of Congress, 1961.

Databases

OCLC. ArchiveGrid. https://beta.worldcat.org/archivegrid/about/.

ProQuest. Archive Finder. http://archives.chadwyck.com/infoCentre/about.jsp.

9

International and Civil Law in the United States

There are several different sources of international law, and the extent to which the United States is bound by the law depends on the source of the law and the formality with which the United States has recognized it. While international law may obligate the federal government, the Supreme Court has held that the states are not necessarily bound. The issue of standing, whether the person bringing suit to enforce the law has suffered a recognized injury that the judicial system can remedy, can often bar suit. Finally, the question of whether a treaty creates an obligation within the nation, an obligation to anyone other than the signatory states, may depend on whether subsequent legislation has made the laws of the treaty the law of the United States as well.

The term "international law" is most often used to refer to public international law, which regulates behavior among nation-states. Private international law refers to the law that regulates conduct among or between private actors who happen to be from different nation-states. A government can be subject to private international law when it acts as a private actor. For instance, if the Commonwealth of Massachusetts contracted with a Canadian company to purchase subway cars, the relationship would, in some aspects, be governed by private international law. If the United States contracted with a German farmer to supply vegetables to a U.S. air base in Germany, the relationship may be governed, in part, by private international law.

In addition to public and private international law, foreign law can arise in American life and American litigation. In some areas of law, the parties can designate the law to be applied; in other issues, choice of law concepts may dictate use of the law of the site where the action occurred. The former often arises in contract issues and the latter in family and matrimonial disputes. Finally, the concepts of comparative law can play a role in historical and legal research. Researchers might approach comparative law from two directions. First they can approach from the nation by directly comparing the law of one nation on a particular topic with the law of another nation, or nations, on the same topic. Second, they might start from the legal concept and explore any discernable trends.

International law will most often arise in treaties. As the Supremacy Clause of the U.S. Constitution states:

> This Constitution, and the Laws of the United States which shall be made in Pursuance thereof; *and all Treaties made,* or *which shall be made, under the Authority of the United States,* shall be the supreme Law of the Land; and the Judges in every State shall be bound thereby, any Thing in the Constitution or Laws of any State to the Contrary notwithstanding. (art. VI, sec. 2; italics added)

The Supreme Court, in *The Paquete Habana* (175 U.S. 677, 700 [1900]), noted, "International law is part of our law, and must be ascertained and administered by the courts of justice of appropriate jurisdiction as often as questions of right depending upon it are duly presented for their determination."

Finally, the unofficial, but important, *Restatement (third) of the Foreign Relations Law of the United States* (sec. 111[1], 1987) states:

> (1) International law and international agreements of the United States are law of the United States and supreme over the law of the several States.
>
> (2) Cases arising under international law or international agreements of the United States are within the Judicial Power of the United States and, subject to Constitutional and statutory limitations and requirements of justiciability, are within the jurisdiction of the federal courts.

Prepared by members of the Society for Historians of American Foreign Relations, *American Foreign Relations Since 1600: A Guide to the Literature* has been described as "magisterial" and is an extremely important resource that should be among the first stops in any research project touching on this topic. It is a seminal multivolume reference guide that covers materials related to U.S. foreign relations. The set is available at many research libraries and as an updated database that can be browsed and searched. It provides bibliographic references to various subjects of law in a subject/chronological arrangement and is one of the first topical sources that should be considered. A general encyclopedic look at foreign relations, in, for example, the *Encyclopedia of United States Foreign Relations,* is often a valuable place to start a research project that involves international law.

International Law at the Founding

Researchers should recognize that the founders were very knowledgeable about the law of nations. They read widely and deeply on the subject and understood it as a part of their intellectual framework. Examining the libraries of the founders reveals that many owned a large number of what would now be considered the classic writings of international scholars. The founders not only owned the material, but they also used it, citing it in ratification documents and elsewhere.

What are the classic writings of international law? Many methods can be used to define the body of work; one of the better and most convenient is through a collection that the Carnegie Endowment published in 1911 and Hein reprinted in 1995. Among the classic texts are those by Hugo Grotius, Samuel von Pufendorf, Emer de Vattel, and others. Researchers can find these in many libraries as well as at HeinOnline. Many of the titles and many volumes of the Classics of International Law series can also be found online through Google Books, HathiTrust, and the Internet Archive.

Sources of International Law

In beginning to look at U.S. practice in international law, a researcher needs to consider the sources of the law. The most important sources that may impose requirements or restrictions are treaties, which are agreements entered into between states. In one view, they can be seen as a sort of contract. Other sources of international law are less obvious and more open to interpretation. The Statute of the International Court of Justice lists four sources of law, including treaties or, in its formulation, international conventions as the most important:

a. international conventions, whether general or particular, establishing rules expressly recognized by the contesting states;
b. international custom, as evidence of a general practice accepted as law;
c. the general principles of law recognized by civilized nations; [and]
d. ... judicial decisions and the teachings of the most highly qualified publicists of the various nations, as subsidiary means for the determination of rules of law. (art. 36[1], Statute, International Court of Justice, 59 Stat. 1031)

Treaties and Treatylike Legislation

Black's Law Dictionary defines a treaty as "an agreement formally signed, ratified, or adhered to between two nations or sovereigns; an international agreement concluded between two or more states in written form and governed by international law" (Thomson Reuters, 2014, p. 1732). The Constitution makes it clear that a treaty is part of the laws of the land. The Constitution requires that to be effective, a treaty must be negotiated by the executive branch, signed, given the advice and consent of two-thirds of the Senate, and proclaimed. Two other types of international agreement with somewhat different requirements have been developed over the past two hundred years: international executive agreements and congressional-executive agreements. The methods by which they are made differ from each other and from treaties. Aside from the "legislative history" aspect of their development, research into these documents proceeds exactly as with treaties.

When the president undertakes an international executive agreement alone, he is generally relying on the powers granted by the Constitution to conduct foreign policy, as the commander in chief, or when an act of Congress or an earlier treaty grants him the power. These are generally of limited import or duration because a president is less likely to act to bind a future president unless Congress is involved. Congressional-executive agreements look a great deal like treaties, but they are made into law with the assent of both houses of Congress. In a congressional-executive agreement, the executive will negotiate an international agreement, usually with a great deal of input from the legislative branch. The agreement will then be submitted to each house of Congress as a regular bill. If the agreement passes both houses and is signed, it will become the law. The North American Free Trade Agreement is a notable recent agreement of this sort. A congressional-executive agreement has the advantage of requiring only a majority in both the Senate and the House, whereas a treaty needs a two-thirds supermajority to be ratified.

In *Missouri v. Holland* (252 U.S. 416 [1920]) the Supreme Court held that treaties can authorize Congress to deal with matters that it otherwise could not. However, executive agreements and congressional-executive agreements are limited by the Tenth Amendment. Other important considerations about treaties and other agreements include who the treaty limits and when it begins to affect various players. Internationally, the United States is clearly bound by a treaty when the treaty is proclaimed, thus completing the ratification, and by publication in the case of executive agreements or signature in the case of congressional-executive agreements.

Another problem is raised by the question of when a treaty begins to affect internal U.S. law. An international agreement will make U.S. law when it is either published or signed. For treaties that require ratification, in order to make domestic law, the treaty must either be "self-executing" or a statute must have been passed making the treaty law in the United States. In domestic law, the Supreme Court held in *Medellin v. Texas* (522 U.S. 491 [2008]) that a treaty is not self-executing unless the treaty conveys the intention that it is self-executing.

It is less clear that the other sources of international law have a legally recognizable effect on domestic law. Foreign law and international norms, or the "law of nations," have a long history in U.S. courts and in the deliberations of Congress. However, at most, the authority of this material would be persuasive, not mandatory. The United States might be required to adhere to a treaty's agreement, but if it is not a self-executing agreement and no separate law has been passed implementing the agreement, the subsidiary governments in the United States will not be held to the agreement.

Finding Treaties

When approaching treaty research, researchers must consider three major steps. First, they must identify and locate the treaty; second, they must determine whether the treaty is "in force" and against whom; and third, they must consider how the terms of the treaty will be interpreted.

Treaties and other international agreements were published in the *Statutes at Large* from 1845 to 1949. The agreements made with foreign nations from 1778 to 1845 were included in volume 8, and agreements with Native American tribes made between 1778 and 1842 were included in volume 7. Agreements with both classes made between 1846/3 and 1949 were included in the *Statutes at Large* volume for the year in which they were proclaimed.

Since the 1940s, agreements have first appeared in the Treaties and International Agreements Series (TIAS). TIAS is a series of "slip" treaties, with each published as a separate pamphlet, which many libraries have collected and bound. The TIAS pamphlets, including more recent pamphlets, are available at HeinOnline. After a period of time, the TIAS pamphlets were collected and published in the United States Treaty series (UST). UST is available in print and at HeinOnline, but researchers should note that it was recently officially discontinued and includes treaties only to 1984. TIAS, available at the Department of State's website, is current within days (https://www.state.gov/s/l/treaty/tias/).

Statutes at Large, UST, and TIAS are the official and often best sources for the texts of treaties to which the United States is a party. The most important older, unofficial, but still government-published sources of treaty texts are the Executive Agreement Series (E.A.S.), 1928–1945, and the Treaty Series (TS), 1795–1945. Before 1928, executive agreements were included in the TS. In addition, several unofficial, privately published treaty sources may be useful to researchers. The official publications and many of the unofficial ones are available at HeinOnline. The unofficial series available include Charles Bevans's *Treaties and Other International Agreements of the United States of America, 1776–1949;* David Hunter Miller's *Treaties and Other International Acts of the United States of America, 1776–1863;* and William M. Malloy's *Treaties, Conventions, International Acts, Protocols, and Agreements, 1776–1937.* Miller and

Malloy have been superseded by Bevans but still contain several useful tables not found in Bevans. Miller, for example, includes a bibliography of U.S. treaty collections, a chronological list of documents, a list by contracting country, a list of documents included in the TS, a list of documents included in the Executive Agreement Series, a chronological and a classified list of proclamations affecting foreign relations, a bibliography of materials related to treaties, and a subject list of agreements. Malloy includes a chronological list of agreements by country and within them by chronology. Bevans has a general index to the entire set of agreements and then divides the agreements into "multilateral" and "bilateral" and prints the multilateral in chronological order; the bilateral agreements are first organized by country and then printed chronologically.

Some international agreements, for whatever reason, are not assigned a number or published in the tools described above. The annual *Guide to the United States Treaties in Force* and *Current Treaty Index,* published since 1982, both include references to unnumbered agreements. In 1990 the editors, Igor Kavass and Adolf Sprudzs, began to number the unnumbered agreements, first dividing the documents into a pre-1950 group and a post-1950 group. They assigned each document in the pre-1950 group an AD (additional documents) number and each document in the post-1950 group a KAV (short for Kavass) number. Many of these agreements later had a TIAS number assigned, so both the *Guide* and the *Index* contain conversion tables. For a while in the 1990s and 2000s, there was a significant lag between the proclamation of a treaty and its publication in TIAS. To address this, HeinOnline publishes the agreements with KAV numbers, giving researchers a place to find treaties and other agreements that are in force but not yet published in TIAS. Another way to find such treaties is through the most current version of the Senate Treaty Document. Each treaty submitted to the Senate for ratification is assigned a Senate Treaty Document number; a researcher can use that number to find the most "official" version of the text of a treaty before it is published in TIAS.

Two additional classes of treaties have generated their own publications. *Indian Affairs: Laws and Treaties*, compiled by C. J. Kappler, contains laws relating to Indian affairs from the *Revised Statutes* to 1979 and treaties, in volume 2, from 1778 to 1883. It is probably the best collection of treaties between the United States and the Native American nations. *Unperfected Treaties of the United States of America, 1776–1976*, edited by C. L. Wiktor, contains information about treaties that never became effective, including the proposed text of each agreement, any legislative history, and an analysis.

Several of the unofficial treaty sources mentioned, most notably Bevans, include excellent tools that enable researchers to identify treaties by a variety of criteria, including date, party, and subject. However, most researchers will choose one of the treaty index/finding tools to identify a treaty.

Several indexes to treaties to which the United States is a party exist, including the annual *Treaties in Force* published by the Department of State since 1929, which lists all of the treaties and other international agreements to which the United States is a party and that the department believes are in force as of January 1 of the title year. Each volume is divided into two parts: the first lists bilateral treaties, and the second, multilateral treaties and other agreements. In the bilateral section the lists are organized by party and then by subject, and in the multilateral section the list is organized by subject. For each treaty or agreement, *Treaties in Force* includes the title, the dates signed and entered into force, and citations to U.S. and some major international treaty sources. Any amendments are also listed. The multilateral section adds a list of the parties to the treaty.

The annual *Guide to United States Treaties in Force* is also an extremely useful tool. It contains much the same information as *Treaties in Force* and the organization is similar, but it includes several additional means of organization, including original publication source, a chronological list of treaties, and a subject list of bilateral treaties that includes all treaties under a particular subject, not just a subject list under the country. Another index is I. L. Kavass and M. A. Michael's *U.S. Treaties and Other International Agreements Cumulative Index, 1776–*. Finally, the *Current Treaty Index* is the most up-to-date of the indexes. All of these publications are available at HeinOnline.

Treaties: Legislative History and Interpretation

After determining whether a treaty is in force and locating the text of the treaty, a researcher will often consider three questions: What is the legislative history of the treaty? When the treaty passed the Senate, were any reservations, understandings, or declarations attached? How has the treaty been interpreted?

Much of the general legislative history research covered in chapter 6 is also true for treaties, with a few differences. One is that a true treaty requires only Senate approval, and the Senate Committee on Foreign Relations is responsible for its consideration. A congressional-executive agreement must pass both houses of Congress, but its path through them is similar to the one taken by other bills. A second major difference is that a treaty does not "die" with the end of a congressional session. When a Congress ends, all bills that have been proposed but not passed will die. Any law on the same subject must be resubmitted to be considered in the next Congress. But a treaty can wait for consideration at the Foreign Relations Committee for years or even decades. A researcher therefore must consult tools that cut across many Congresses, or, when using tools limited to a single Congress, use several editions.

After a treaty has been negotiated and signed, it is sent to the Senate for advice and consent. The Senate forwards the treaty to the Foreign Relations Committee. Since 1981 treaties are sent to the committee as Senate Treaty Documents; before 1981 treaties were labeled Senate Executive Documents, which could cause confusion, as other documents are also called Senate Executive Documents. A Treaty Document contains the text of a treaty and, perhaps, a message from the president and/or the secretary of state. Treaty Documents are numbered sequentially, starting a new sequence with each Congress. A treaty will maintain its Treaty Document number even as it works its way through subsequent Congresses. If the Treaty Document is treated as confidential, as often occurs, it will not appear in the *Monthly Catalog of United States Government Publications* or other indexes until the confidentiality is lifted, at which time the document becomes available and is indexed under its original number.

As the committee considers a treaty, additional documents may be created, reflecting hearings or other committee events or requests. These documents do not differ from the hearing and congressional documents discussed in chapter 6.

After the Foreign Relations Committee has considered a treaty, it will go to the full Senate with a recommendation for or against ratification. A Senate Executive Report will accompany the treaty. This report is the most useful element of a treaty's legislative history. It provides the researcher not only with the committee's rationale and concerns, but also with any reservations, understandings, or declarations that the committee recommends.

Reservations are specific limitations or qualifications that limit the effect of the treaty but don't change the treaty language; understandings are statements that clarify or elaborate how the nation interprets specific provisions of the treaty; and declarations are more general policy statements related to the subject of the treaty.

While the Foreign Relations Committee's Senate Executive Reports concerning treaties are among the most important, it should be noted that other committees can, and do, publish Senate Executive Reports. These reports usually deal with issues such as judicial and ambassadorial nominations. All of the Senate Executive Reports are numbered and published as one set, regardless of issuing committee or subject.

Choosing the best tools for tracking a treaty through the various Congresses depends on when the Senate considered the treaty. Any treaty that has been submitted to the Senate since 1975/1976 or was pending in 1975 is indexed in the online legislative information system at Congress.gov. There, the treaty's link at the bottom of the page leads to a page that allows for a variety of search tools, including the Congress during which the document sought was created, the committee, treaty status, or treaty topic. The bibliographic record created for each document can be searched from the Treaty Documents page. Once the treaty is identified, the site provides information such as the treaty number; any older treaty numbers; the date the treaty was transmitted to the Senate; the type of treaty; if bilateral, the partner country; if multilateral, the other signatories; the formal title; reference to the Senate Executive Report (or Treaty Report); and related documents. All committee and floor actions are also listed, with links provided to floor amendments if the *Congressional Record* is available through the Federal Digital System website. Finally, the text of the resolution in which the Senate gave its advice and consent is reprinted. If advice and consent to the treaty has not been given, then the information included will reflect committee and floor actions to that date.

The Foreign Relations Committee's website (https://www. foreign.senate.gov/) has a treaties section that contains information about all treaties still before the committee. The site provides PDF access to treaty documents and treaty reports, as well as brief listings about the status of all treaties.

The *CCH Congressional Index* is another tool that makes tracking a treaty from Congress to Congress a little easier. Unfortunately, it is available only from 1953. The *Congressional Index* is a print looseleaf service that is updated regularly, though the archival volumes will most interest the historical researcher. The index contains a table that tracks the status of a treaty. Another useful resource for tracking the status and committee actions of a treaty is the Legislative Calendar of the Senate Foreign Relations Committee, which is usually published as a Committee Print. A researcher will also find useful other resources that help track the doings of Congress, such as the *Congressional Quarterly* publications and the *Congressional Record* indexes. Finally, the *CIS Index to U.S. Senate Executive Documents and Reports* published by the Congressional Information Service lists all such documents that were not included in the *Serial Set* and were published between 1817 and 1969.

Treaty interpretation can be gathered by examining the practice of the government in the conduct of foreign affairs (the tools are described below) and by examining court decisions. The case-finding tools described in chapter 6 can be used to find cases that relate to a treaty. In addition, the USCS, the annotated version of the United States Code published by Lexis, includes a little over forty treaties. The annotations in the

Code contain references to some interpretive court decisions. This is one of the easiest print tools to use to find cases interpreting treaties and is often a very good place to start hunting for material interpreting aspects of treaties.

Customary Law

In addition to treaties, the main sources of international law included in the Statute of the International Court of Justice are customary law, general principles of law, judicial decisions, and the writings of scholars or other publicists. While a treaty may possibly rise to the level of mandatory authority, none of these other sources of law can dictate an outcome. However, all of them can provide great insight into the behavior of actors and their beliefs about what the law is. The sources that a researcher will consult to determine what customary law is, to discover what constitutes general principles of law, or to find judicial decisions or the writings of legal scholars are, in large part, the same.

International law can be considered much the way the common law once was: there is an existing edifice of law, and the job of the court or lawyer or actor is not to make the law but to discover it. We can see this strand of thought in international law by the reliance on custom and principles, and on cases and writings. These all describe how issues were treated or should have been treated. The process used to determine what customary international law is, working through materials that describe state action, is similar to the process that lawyers use to determine the state of common or statutory law by reading and rationalizing the interpreting cases.

There are three aspects to customary international law: state practice, *opinio juris,* and *jus cogens.* All can be derived from an examination of the resources below, where the aspects of law that differ are mainly in the mind of the actor and therefore in their force. State practice is, simply, what a state has actually done. *Opinio juris* is state practice with the added benefit that the state was doing (or not doing) an action because it believed that the law required (or prohibited) the action. Finally, *jus cogens* is a norm that is widely considered so fundamental that one would expect a nation to never violate it. Genocide is an example of something typically considered banned by *jus cogens*. The power of *jus cogens* is such that one cannot avoid it even by agreement or treaty.

Principles of law and *jus cogens* are often difficult to distinguish, and general principles are often described as being relatively unimportant in international law. However, there is a difference. *Jus cogens* is a peremptory norm of law; it is considered so compelling or fundamental that it overrides every other law. General principles of law are concepts like estoppel or equity—concepts that are a part of many systems and that allow a system to function and represent basic fairness.

Of course, international law is powerless without an enforcement mechanism, usually state power and state influence. The historical researcher should recall that the status of the United States as a superpower is a relatively recent phenomenon. For a significant portion of its history, the United States could assert strong international rights but could not really back them up.

The critical sources for finding out what the U.S. government thought it was obliged to do (or refrain from doing) given international law are the various digests of U.S. practice in international law published originally in print by the government but now widely available online, including at HeinOnline:

- J. L. Cadwalader, Digest of the Published Opinions of the Attorneys-General and of the Leading Decisions of the Federal Courts: With Reference to International Law, Treaties, and Kindred Subjects (1877).
- F. Wharton, A Digest of the International Law of the United States: Taken from Documents Issued by Presidents and Secretaries of State, and from Decisions of Federal Courts and Opinions of Attorneys-General (1887)
- J. B. Moore and F. Wharton, A Digest of International Law: As Embodied in Diplomatic Discussions, Treaties, and other International Agreements, International Awards, the Decisions of Municipal Courts, and the Writings of Jurists (this covers developments from 1776 to 1906, superseding Cadwalader and Wharton) (1906)
- G. H. Hackworth, Digest of International Law (covers 1906–1939; published 1940–1944)
- Marjorie M. Whiteman and G. H. Hackworth, Digest of International Law (covers 1940–1960; published 1963–1973)
- Digest of United States Practice in International Law (covers 1973–present; published 1989–present)
- Cumulative Digest of United States Practice in International Law (covers 1981–1988; published 1993)

Another source, Francis Wharton's *Revolutionary Diplomatic Correspondence of the United States,* provides wonderful insight into the conduct of the Revolutionary War. It is also a House document, available in the *Serial Set.*

Another critical resource, *Foreign Relations of the United States,* contains the official documentary record of the U.S. government's actions when conducting foreign policy. The digests listed above provide information about what the United States *says* is customary law, but *Foreign Relations* provides information about what the actions of the United States *show* is customary law. *Foreign Relations* has been published since 1863 and contains reprints of the actual documents that were the tools of international law, including cables, memos, letters, and so on. Because of the sensitive nature of much of the material, a significant amount of time passes before the material is made public. Currently, the set is about thirty to thirty-five years in the past. *Foreign Relations* is available in print at many large research libraries, and the most recent volumes are available at the Department of State's website. The University of Wisconsin–Madison libraries has placed the volumes covering from 1861 to 1960 online at its Digital Collections website (http://uwdc.library.wisc.edu/collections/FRUS). An extremely valuable new addition to the literature is a study by the State Department's Office of the Historian; *Toward "Thorough, Accurate, and Reliable": A History of the Foreign Relations Series* provides an in-depth history of this important resource.

Another type of information a researcher will want to consult is mainly found within judicial decisions or scholarly discourse. Most of the case-finding tools and methods described in chapters 5 and 6 are useful for finding cases that interpret various aspects of international law; however, a few sources might make the research a little easier. *American International Law Cases* (1st series, 31 vols., 1783–1979; 2nd series, 10 vols., 1980–1989), a collection of case opinions that deal with international law, is useful in that it brings the material together; however, a researcher should understand that all of the cases that appear here can be found in the other case reporters discussed elsewhere.

The highly regarded Restatements of the Law were developed through a long negotiation by members of the American Law Institute, all attorneys and legal scholars with expertise in the area of law to be restated. The *Restatement of Law (Third) Foreign Relations of the United States* is an excellent and highly regarded statement of what U.S. legal scholars believe international law requires. Like other restatements, it is not law unless expressly adopted, but it is considered a thoughtful statement of the law and is frequently followed by U.S. judges. The *Restatement (Second), Conflict of Laws* is also often important to researchers involved in international and foreign law research.

For finding American scholarship on aspects of international law, researchers should use the same tools and methods for research as for finding American scholarship on any aspect of law: library catalogs, periodical indexes, and full-text periodical databases. Researchers who want to see how a particular issue of international law has been treated by international scholars can consult one of several resources that reach beyond the United States. WorldCat, for example, includes library catalogs from many libraries worldwide, making it a good place to start to find treatise scholarship from outside the United States. National library catalogs, even if their records are included in WorldCat, may be worth a search. Several other bibliographic sources can be fruitful. National versions of Amazon.com will return items concerning the nation selected. A virtual catalog available online through the Karlsruhe Institute of Technology (kvk.bibliothek.kit.edu) allows searches across a large number of European bibliographic resources.

The basic American legal periodical indexes cover some journals from outside the United States that contain articles considering the law of many nations as well as international issues from many perspectives. Researchers can find authors from around the world who publish in journals covered by the indexes. While most of the journals are American, some have an international focus; several journals are from outside the United States, though mainly from English-speaking jurisdictions. These indexes are discussed more fully in chapter 6. Another periodical index fairly widely available to U.S. researchers covers more international journals and non-English-language journals. The *Index to Foreign Legal Periodicals*, published since the 1960s, indexes a somewhat idiosyncratic list of journals from around the world. Available in print and at HeinOnline, it uses English-language subject headings. Researchers who want to search farther afield will find that many indexes or full-text databases of journals or other scholarly writing are becoming available to subscribers. Beck-Online from Germany or PKULaw from China, or others, may be available, but often, English translations of the material are not found in these systems.

Many excellent international law portals are available, including a guide to electronic research sources from the American Society of International Law (Electronic Resource Guide [ERG], https://www.asil.org/resources/electronic-resource-guide-erg). A print version is available at many libraries. Another is a portal created by librarian-members of the society, the Electronic Information System for International Law (EISIL).

Foreign Law

While research within the laws of other nations is beyond the scope of this book, an American researcher looking for historical foreign law resources might consult a guide to the research and legal history of the nation under consideration. Bibliographic resources and collections of national legal research guides are available online. A guide to foreign law sources at the Yale Law Library's website pulls together many of these, organized by country. The *Foreign Law Guide: Current Sources of Codes and Basic Legislation in Jurisdictions of the World* by Thomas H. Reynolds and Arturo A. Flores, or the online version, the *Foreign Law Guide* compiled by Marci Hoffman, should get special mention. This print and online resource available by subscription and held by many U.S. and other libraries includes sections on most countries. For each country, it provides a brief background on the legal system and legal history and bibliographic references to the main official legal publications, often extending back to the nineteenth century. It also includes a list of the most useful websites for researching the law of the nation of interest and concludes with a list of subjects, with reference to the major law(s) implicated in those topics.

Native American Law

Researching the relations between the U.S. government and Native Americans is often exceedingly complex. In some instances, laws governing the relations strongly resemble international law and in others, domestic law. Before 1871, the United States often treated Native American tribes as foreign sovereign nations, and the relationship was governed by treaty. These treaties were considered and followed the same ratification process as other treaties. After 1871, the relationship changed. When researching relations with Native Americans before 1871, and insofar as the United States still treats Native American tribes as sovereign nations, both international law

resources and some aspects of foreign law research are implicated. The foreign law resources described above do not include
Native Americans; therefore, a researcher must look for research
guides devoted to Native American legal research generally or
to the law of a particular tribe. Only recently has a fairly large
amount of legal material from Native Americans become available to most researchers. Previously, researchers could easily
locate the U.S. government's position and materials, but materials from the other side of the relationship were nonexistent
or extremely difficult to find.

Today, there are published versions of the codes of many
Native American tribes, and the recent decisions of some Native
American courts are available in print and online at many law
libraries. The Law Library Microform Consortium's *Early State
Records* includes a great deal of early Native American tribal
materials. However, for in-depth research in older Native
American materials, a serious researcher will want to start with
the National Indian Law Library in Boulder, Colorado.

Volume 7 of *Statutes at Large* includes early treaties between the United States and Native Americans, and the annual
Statutes at Large volumes add later ones. Other resources include
Indian Affairs: Laws and Treaties by Charles J. Kappler, which
is freely available on the web as part of the Oklahoma State
University Library digital collection (http://digital.library.ok-
state.edu/Kappler/), at HeinOnline, and in print. Early Recognized Treaties with American Indian Nations is a free website
hosted by the University of Nebraska (http://treatiesportal.unl.
edu/earlytreaties/) that includes nine treaties created between
1722 and 1805 not published in the *Statutes at Large* or Kappler.
LexisNexis's database *Native American People Treaties Ratified
and Unratified* has ratified and unratified treaties created between 1787 and 1883. *Documents of American Indian Diplomacy:*

Treaties, Agreements, and Conventions, 1775–1979 (2 vols.; 1999) by Vine Deloria Jr. and Raymond J. DeMallie is available in print. Finally, Felix Cohen's *Handbook of Federal Indian Law* (1942, rpt. 1982, 1986) is an extremely useful resource for historical work.

Civil Law

The place of foreign and international law in U.S. legal history leads to at least two related inquiries: the first considers citations to foreign law by early American courts and references to foreign law by early American legal scholars; the second considers the place civil law had in the historical development of American law. Many states determined that English law as of some date would be considered part of their law. And because of the lack of American precedent, many early courts found it necessary to look outside of the United States for guidance. The historical use of foreign law has been widely discussed in the scholarly legal literature (see chapter 6), but one study deserves special mention.

In 1991, R. H. Helmholz in "Use of the Civil Law in Post-Revolutionary America" published the results of an investigation of how civil law was used in state courts up to 1825. He surveyed decisions from the reports of fourteen states and the federal courts, including the U.S. Supreme Court, from 1790 to 1825. He found that lawyers and judges in all of the states, including Kentucky and Tennessee, used civil law, including Roman law texts and continental law treatises by authors such as Hugo Grotius, Samuel von Pufendorf, Jean Domat, Jean-Jacques Burlamaqui, and Emer de Vattel, plus Roman law institutes and Justinian's *Corpus Juris Civilis*. Proponents of natural law were cited as well as writers on the law of nations.

In addition, writers on particular subjects were also often consulted, including Robert Pothier on commercial law, Cesare Beccaria on criminal law, and Ulrich Huber on conflicts of law. In cases involving last wills and testaments, the English civilian scholars Henry Swinburne and John Godolphin were regularly cited. Civil law was most frequently used in cases involving maritime and commercial law, as well as the law of civil and criminal procedure and, generally, as a resource for demonstrating principles of justice. It was used where English law was nonexistent, inconclusive, or deemed to be wrong. Interestingly, civil law was also used where civil and common law were identical but where English law seemed to need buttressing from outside sources. Civil law was not used when the issues involved real property or the rules of pleading or in cases regarding slavery.

Other signs point to the importance of civil and other foreign law in early America. Some examples are the success of Thomas Cooper's *Institutes of Justinian with Notes* published in 1812 and republished in 1841 and 1852, which related American case law to civil law; and Jean Domat's *The Civil Law in Its Natural Order,* from 1850. James Kent, one of early America's greatest jurists, was interested in the civil law and in codes. He participated in the development of New York's code and made frequent use of civil law sources in his writing. Civil law and other foreign law was not afforded the precedential authority that a state case or even an English case would have, but it was frequently respected as useful and could inform the law.

Civil law also played a role in the law reform, simplification, and codification movements of the early nineteenth century. The codification movement in Europe strongly influenced the codification efforts led by Edward Livingston's draft Louisiana code and David Dudley Field's slightly later efforts in New York law. While Livingston's codes were adopted, their popularity in Europe shows how much of the codification movement of the early nineteenth century moved back and forth across the Atlantic. Jeremy Bentham, in a letter to President James Madison, offered his assistance in developing a code for the United States. There is no evidence that Bentham received a reply. He also sent a circular letter to all governors offering to help codify state laws. Although he received no takers, early America was fully participating in the global legal conversation.

Law reformers of the time questioned the utility of the common law. William Sampson, who argued that the common law cemented inequality, called for codification to meet the promise that "all men are created equal." While Jesse Higgins didn't specifically call for codification, his critique of the common law drew on the same criticisms as the codifiers, and his proposals look a great deal like codification. See the chapter "Legal Profession" in volume 2 of Michael Grossberg and Christopher L. Tomlins, eds., *Cambridge History of Law in America* (Cambridge: Cambridge University Press, 2008), for more information.

As the United States expanded, it took on jurisdictions with civil law history and systems, such as Florida, Louisiana, Texas, and California, to mention only a few states carved from the former civil territories of the Louisiana Purchase, the Florida acquisition, and the territory acquired in the Mexican War.

American codes are not the same as continental codes; they rely heavily on court interpretation to add substance. However, they offer a far more specific, clear, and widely available statement of the law than the common law. The American common law system sits somewhere between the civil law code-based system and the traditional common law system in place in the United Kingdom and parts of the British Commonwealth. The United States took guidance from both its historic common law and the benefits that some observers saw in the civil law systems, which became apparent as familiarity with civil law developed through the addition of territories with civil law in place, through movements toward a code in New York and elsewhere, and as the civil law itself appeared revitalized by the Napoleonic Code.

Research Example

Let us take a look at the relationship between the United States and Iraq through the lens of extradition. Wikipedia tells us that the United States and Iraq signed an extradition treaty on June 7, 1934; that it went into effect on April 23, 1936; and that it was published at 49 Stat. 3380. Since this information is from Wikipedia, it should be verified. To ensure that we have the most up-to-date information, we turn to the 2016 edition of *Treaties in Force*. Had we been interested in the law as of some earlier date, we could examine an earlier edition of *Treaties in Force*. By looking for "Iraq" in the bilateral treaties section and then for "law enforcement," we find that Wikipedia is correct. The 1936 treaty is the current extradition treaty. *Treaties in Force* provides three additional citations for the treaty: the Treaty Series, Bevans, and the League of Nations Treaty Series. But since *Statutes at Large* is the official source for treaties before 1949, the Wikipedia-provided citation is sufficient.

We can examine the treaty as it was being ratified and can find whether any discussion occurred. Turning to ProQuest Congressional and searching for the terms "Iraq" and "extradition" in the Seventy-Third and Seventy-Fourth Congresses, we find no documents from the Seventy-Third Congress and three documents from the Seventy-Fourth. The first is the Message from the President delivering the treaty to the Senate on January 17, 1935. The second is the favorable report from the Senate Foreign Relations Committee, reported on February 4, 1935, in volume 79, page 1426, of the *Congressional Record.* The Iraq extradition treaty was offered, along with extradition treaties with Bulgaria, Estonia, Switzerland, Latvia, and San Marino. Clearly, the Iraq treaty was not considered especially important. The third document is from the February 6, 1935, *Congressional Record.* On pages 1573 and 1574, the treaty is printed along with the motion for ratification and its passage.

We can check whether the treaty was of concern to the President or the State Department. A search of *Foreign Relations of the United States* at HeinOnline for the terms "Iraq" and "extradition" appearing within fifty words of each other yields four items. Two precede the treaty, one from the administration of Calvin Coolidge and the other from the administration of Herbert Hoover. The documents from the Coolidge and Hoover administrations demonstrate a concern for the necessity of an extradition treaty with Iraq as Great Britain's position was changing. A document from the Roosevelt administration contains the text of the treaty itself. That leaves the fourth document: a telegram from the U.S. Embassy in Iraq to the State Department expressing mild concern about whether Iraq might invoke the extradition treaty and ask the United States to return to Iraq Mustafa Barzani, the Kurdish leader exiled in Iran. Interestingly, the telegram, dated August 30, 1976, expressed the opinion that Barzani was a "spent force" and might potentially cause a problem only in "the almost unthinkable situation in which Iran and Iraq were at war." Of course, after a change in the Iranian regime in 1979, the Iran-Iraq War began almost exactly four years later.

There are a few more sources to examine. A search of the *Public Papers of Franklin D. Roosevelt* (available at Hein-Online and for free at the Presidency Project at the University of California at Santa Barbara) for the terms "Iraq" and "extradition" within fifty words of each other yields no documents. The same search in the *Public Papers of the Presidents* from Hoover to George W. Bush, excluding Roosevelt, yields two documents. Both, one from 1987 and the other from 1997, appear only by happenstance. Two documents are in proximity, one from the Venice Economic Summit Conference's discussion of terrorism in which an annex expressed commitment to the Bonn Declaration of 1977. It was agreed that, if a country refused to extradite or prosecute an airplane hijacker, flights to the country would be suspended. The document was the conference's statement on the Iran-Iraq War. On July 31, 1997, President Bill Clinton's message to Congress reporting on the national emergency with respect to Iraq was immediately followed by the transmittal of an extradition treaty with Barbados.

Further Reading

Abebe, Daniel, and Eric A. Posner. "The Flaws of Foreign Affairs Legalism." *Virginia Journal of International Law* 51, no. 3 (2011): 507–48.

Babusiaux, Ulrike. "The Future of Legal History: Roman Law." *American Journal of Legal History* 56, no. 1 (2016): 6–11.

Bodansky, Daniel. "The Use of International Sources in Constitutional Opinion." *Georgia Journal of International and Comparative Law* 32, no. 2 (2004): 421–28.

Cleveland, Sarah H. "Embedded International Law and the Constitution Abroad." *Columbia Law Review* 110, no. 2 (2010): 225–87.

Falstrom, Dana Zartner. "Thought Versus Action: The Influence of Legal Tradition on French and American Approaches to International Law." *Maine Law Review* 58 (2006): 338–76.

Farber, Daniel A. "The Supreme Court, the Law of Nations, and Citations of Foreign Law: The Lessons of History." *California Law Review* 95 (2007): 1335–65.

Glensy, Rex D. "Constitutional Interpretation Through a Global Lens." *Missouri Law Review* 75, no. 4 (2010): 1171–1241.

Golove, David M., and Daniel J. Hulsebosch. "A Civilized Nation: The Early American Constitution, the Law of Nations, and the Pursuit of International Recognition." *New York University Law Review* 85, no. 4 (2010): 932–1066.

Jay, Stewart. "The Status of the Law of Nations in Early American Law." *Vanderbilt Law Review* 42 (1989): 819–49.

Kearley, Timothy G. "From Rome to the Restatement: S. P. Scott, Fred Blume, Clyde Pharr, and Roman Law in Early Twentieth-Century America." *Law Library Journal* 108, no. 1 (2016): 55–76.

Kent, J. Andrew. "Congress's Under-Appreciated Power to Define and Punish Offenses Against the Law of Nations." *Texas Law Review* 85, no. 4 (2007): 843–946.

Martinez, Jenny S. "International Courts and the U.S. Constitution: Reexamining the History." *University of Pennsylvania Law Review* 159, no. 4 (2011): 1069–1140.

"Review of *Review of Code Civil, . . .*" *North American Review* 20, no. 47 (1825): 393–417.

Shelton, Dinah. "Challenging History: The Role of International Law in the U.S. Legal System." *Denver Journal of International Law and Policy* 40, no. 1–3 (2011): 1–21.

Vagts, Detlev F. "The Treaty-Making Process: A Guide for Outsiders." *ILSA Journal of International and Comparative Law* 17, no. 1 (2010): 127–46.

Wedgwood, Ruth. "The Revolutionary Martyrdom of Jonathan Robbins." *Yale Law Journal* 100 (1990): 229–68.

White, G. Edward. "The Marshall Court and International Law: The Piracy Cases." *American Journal of International Law* 83 (1989): 727–35.

Young, Ernest A. "Treaties as Part of Our Law." *Texas Law Review* 88, no. 1 (2009): 91–141.

Important Sources Mentioned in This Chapter

Beisner, Robert L. *American Foreign Relations Since 1600: A Guide to the Literature.* Santa Barbara, CA: ABC-CLIO, 2003.

Bevans, Charles I. *Treaties and Other International Agreements of the United States of America, 1776–1949.* Washington, DC: GPO, 1968.

Kappler, Charles Joseph, ed. *Indian Affairs: Laws and Treaties*. 2nd ed. Washington, DC: GPO, 1904–.

Kavass, Igor I., and Adolf Sprudzs. *A Guide to the United States Treaties in Force*. Buffalo, NY: William S. Hein, 1982–.

McAllister, William B., Joshua Botts, Peter Cozzens, and Aaron W. Marrs. *Toward "Thorough, Accurate, and Reliable": A History of the Foreign Relations of the United States Series*. Washington, DC: U.S. Department of State, Office of the Historian, Bureau of Public Affairs, 2015.

Malloy, William M. *Treaties, Conventions, International Acts, Protocols and Agreements between the United States of America and Other Powers*. Washington, DC: GPO, 1910–1938.

Miller, David Hunter. *Treaties and Other International Acts of the United States of America*. Washington, DC: GPO, 1931.

Moore, John Bassett, and Francis Wharton. *A Digest of International Law: As Embodied in Diplomatic Discussions, Treaties and Other International Agreements, International Awards, the Decisions of Municipal Courts, and the Writings of Jurists . . .* Washington, DC: U.S. Department of State, 1906.

Peters, Richard Peters, George Minot, George P. Sanger, U.S. Department of State, and U.S. Federal Register Division. *United States Statutes at Large, Containing the Laws and Concurrent Resolutions . . . and Reorganization Plan, Amendment to the Constitution, and Proclamations*. Washington, DC: GPO, 1845.

United States. *Treaty Series*. Washington, DC: U.S. Department of State, 1926–1935.

United States Department of State. *Foreign Relations of the United States*. Washington, DC: GPO, 1861–.

———. *United States Treaties and Other International Agreements*. Washington, DC: GPO, 1950–.

United States Department of State, Office of the Legal Adviser. *Cumulative Digest of United States Practice in International Law*. Washington, DC: GPO, 1993–1995

———. *Digest of United States Practice in International Law*. Washington, DC: GPO, 1974–1986 and 2001–.

United States Department of State, Treaty Affairs Staff, and Office of the Legal Adviser. *Treaties in Force: A List of Treaties and Other International Acts of the United States in Force on . . .* Washington, DC: GPO, 1941.

Wharton, Francis. *A Digest of the International Law of the United States: Taken from Documents Issued by Presidents and Secretaries of State, and from Decisions of Federal Courts and Opinions of Attorneys-General.* Washington, DC: GPO, 1886.

Wharton, Francis, and John Bassett Moore. *The Revolutionary Diplomatic Correspondence of the United States.* Washington, DC: GPO, 1889.

Whiteman, Marjorie M., and Green Haywood Hackworth. *Digest of International Law.* Washington, DC: GPO, 1963–1973.

Wiktor, Christian L. *Unperfected Treaties of the United States of America, 1776–1976.* Dobbs Ferry, NY: Oceana, 1976.

Databases

Hoffman, Marci, ed. *Foreign Law Guide.* BrillOnline Reference Works. http://referenceworks.brillonline.com/browse/foreign-law-guide.

10
Language and Biography

More than almost any other human endeavor, the law is concerned with language. Because a dispute may turn on the meaning of a single word, legislatures will often define words within legislation. In the common law, cases from the Middle Ages, unless revised, can still be in effect, so understanding what a word meant in the past can be critically important to the present. Consider the plight of the law student today in every common law jurisdiction who must master the Rule in Shelley's Case, a rule of law related to future interests in real property that was first applied in the *Provost of Beverley's Case* in 1366 (Y.B. 40 Ed. 3, f9, 18). While it has been abrogated during the past century in most of the United States, it remains in effect in most of common law Canada today! The U.S. Supreme Court often seeks to determine the meaning of the Constitution at the time of its passage. When interpreting a statute, a court must often do the same. To understand the law in a historical context, researchers face the same dilemma.

Almost more than words, the law is about people. People make the law; it shapes and constrains people and society; it regulates human affairs. Very often the answers to "why" come through reference to the individuals involved in shaping the law. Especially in America, lawyers have shaped the government, as many of the founders and legislators throughout American history have been lawyers. Biographical studies of individuals can lend insight into the law-making process. Prosopography, the study of the common characteristics of a group, can be especially enlightening in understanding why the law favors or disfavors who it does.

Dictionaries of English

When trying to determine what a law means, researchers must understand what the terminology meant at the time the law was crafted. Researchers working with historical materials and interested in determining how a term was used or what a word meant at a particular time have three avenues to attack the problem. First, they can find dictionaries published at the time under consideration. Second, they can use a modern dictionary that provides guidance to a word's historical use. Finally, they can find the word in documents from the time of interest and try to work out the meaning from context. The first two options are preferred. Since the law is a specialized field, terms may be used in a way that a general dictionary might not offer; therefore, specialized legal dictionaries should be consulted when possible.

The first modern English dictionary, Samuel Johnson's *Dictionary of the English Language,* was published in 1755, and the first modern American dictionary, Noah Webster's *American Dictionary of the English Language,* was published in 1828. A researcher wishing to determine the general usage and meaning of words contemporary to the Revolution might start with Johnson's dictionary. There are no real English dictionaries before Johnson's, but there are several word lists and some specialized glossaries that, while not always clearly defining a word, can offer some sense of the meaning of a word—for example, Edward Phillips's *The New World of Words: or, a general English dictionary*, from 1658.

Johnson's dictionary is available for free online at the Internet Archive, and another project is developing a searchable copy (http://johnsonsdictionaryonline.com/). Many of its early editions are also available at Eighteenth Century Collections Online.

After the Revolution, American society was determined to diverge from British society. A sign of this divergence was Webster's *American Dictionary of the English Language*. Webster, himself educated in the law at the Litchfield Law School in Litchfield, Connecticut, wanted not only to create a good dictionary, but also to demonstrate how different America was from Britain.

Whether or not Webster demonstrated American difference or superiority, he did demonstrate the demand for a dictionary of American English. His first volume was priced low and sold very well. Webster published a second edition in 1841, which was reprinted by others in 1844 and 1845. The Merriam brothers then purchased the rights to the dictionary and hired Chauncey A. Goodrich to revise it. In 1847, the "New and Revised" edition was published. In 1864 they published a newly revised and enlarged version, the first Webster's to be called unabridged. Through the rest of the nineteenth century, *Webster's Unabridged Dictionary* of 1864 was supplemented and has retained its place as one of the most important dictionaries of the English language.

In 1890 Merriam published *Webster's International Dictionary of the English Language*, the new title recognizing the worldwide impact that *Webster's Unabridged Dictionary* had. This was supplemented in 1900 and revised; the word "New" was added to the title in 1909. A second edition was published in 1934 and a very controversial third edition in 1961. Herbert C. Morton's *The Story of Webster's Third: Philip Gove's Controversial Dictionary and Its Critics* (1995) offers a good history of Webster's, though it mainly concentrates on the controversies surrounding the third edition.

Webster's was not the only American dictionary. Webster claimed that Joseph E. Worcester's *Comprehensive Pronouncing and Explanatory Dictionary of the English Language* (1830) was plagiarized. In 1883, an American edition of the *Imperial Dictionary of the English Language* was published. An expanded version, the *Century Dictionary,* came out between 1889 and 1891. In 1894, Funk and Wagnall's *Standard Dictionary,* a one-volume competitor to Webster's, was published to great success and was expanded in 1913.

Webster's 1828 and 1913 editions, the *Century Dictionary,* and others are available online through the Internet Archive, and several other editions can be found through HathiTrust or by using a Google search.

Legal Dictionaries

Law has its own vocabulary and language. In the Middle Ages, the language of English law was Latin and "law-French." From 1066 to 1362, proceedings were held in Norman French, and statutes, writs, and records were in Latin. In 1362, the Pleading in English Act required proceedings to be held in English, although records were still kept in Latin. Law-French continued to be used in some documents and areas until the seventeenth century, although it became less and less "French." Resources written in English and designed to help lawyers and others deal with specialized legal language first appeared in the sixteenth century. The original guide to legal language, John Rastell's *Exposiciones terminorum legum anglorum,* also known as *Termes de la ley,* was published in 1523. It was so popular that it appeared in twenty-nine editions up to 1819.

The seventeenth century saw many more guides to legal language, including the following:

- John Cowell, *The Interpreter, or Booke Containing the Signification of Words* (1607)
- William Sheppard, *An Epitome of All the Common & Statute Laws of This Nation Now in Force: Wherein More Than Fifteen Hundred of the Hardest Words or Terms of the Law Are Explained* (1656)
- Edward Leigh, *A Philologicall Commentary, or an Illustration of the Most Obvious and Useful Words in the Law* (1658)
- Henry Spelman, *Glossarium archaiologicum: continens latino-barbara, peregrina, obsoleta, & novatae significationis vocabula* (1664)
- Thomas Blount, *Nomo-Lexicon: A Law Dictionary* (1670)

In 1729, *A New Law Dictionary* by Giles Jacob was published. Because it delved more deeply than its predecessors, Jacob's dictionary became one of the more important and influential eighteenth-century legal publications. *A New Law Dictionary* contained elements of a dictionary and an abridgment of law; it went through eleven editions in the eighteenth century. Though not nearly as important as Jacob's dictionary, two additional eighteenth-century English law dictionaries deserve mention: Timothy Cunningham's *A New and Complete Law-Dictionary, or, General Abridgement of the Law* (1764) and Richard Burn's *A New Law Dictionary, Intended for General Use as Well as for Gentlemen of the Profession* (1792).

Although by the eighteenth century law-French had fallen into disuse and was mainly of antiquarian interest, it had been an important language of the law for many years, and eighteenth-century lawyers needed a guide: Robert Kelham's *A Dictionary of the Norman or Old French Language* (1779) is a good, relatively contemporary guide. An excellent modern guide to law-French is J. H. Baker's *Manual of Law French* (2016).

The first American legal dictionary was John Bouvier's *A Law Dictionary* (1839). It was so important that fifteen editions were published before 1885. A century edition appeared in 1926 as well as many student editions from the 1930s. Bouvier's *Law Dictionary* is still published today; the early versions are available for free online through the Internet Archive, and the fifteenth edition is available in the *Making of American Law: Primary Sources, 1620–1926*. The *Making of Modern Law* and HeinOnline have the 1897 "new edition." Among the most interesting editions of Bouvier is the 1914 version, *A Law Dictionary and Concise Encyclopedia*. This version, while not published in subsequent editions, became a part of the legal encyclopedia building movement in the early twentieth century.

In 1891 Henry Campbell Black published *Black's Law Dictionary*, which became the dominant law dictionary in the United States during the twentieth century. The tenth edition was published in 2014, with previous editions in 1891, 1910, 1933, 1951, 1979, 1990, 1999, 2004, and 2009. The current version of Black's is available online through Westlaw. The second edition is available for free online at The Law Dictionary (http://thelaw-dictionary.org/) and through the Internet Archive.

Modern Dictionaries

One of the great lexicographic achievements, *The Oxford English Dictionary* (OED), is also useful for researchers in legal history. The OED attempts to track each shift in a word's meaning through references contemporary to the shift. With the help of the OED, a researcher can approximate the meaning of a term at a particular point in time with relative confidence. If possible, a researcher should consult the online version, which is updated regularly, rather than the print version. It is a subscription database, and most universities, some library consortia, and some larger public libraries subscribe. Not only is the OED easier to search and work with online, but the editors constantly search out references to words that demonstrate or illustrate differences in meaning or older uses of a particular meaning. It may take years or even decades before new information appears in the print version.

Biographical Materials

There are three types of biographical sources: book-length biographies, directory-type resources that provide brief biographical data, and (perhaps the most useful starting point) encyclopedic biographical sets. The most prominent of these are national in scope and provide researchers with a brief biographical sketch written by an expert. Accompanying the biographical sketch is a brief bibliography that will help researchers delve more deeply into their subject.

The two critical encyclopedic sets covering Americans are the *American National Biography* and *Dictionary of American Biography*. They provide both brief biographies of important individuals and also a bibliography of more in-depth biographies of individuals. Published in 1999 by Oxford University Press, *American National Biography* is in many ways a more modern version of the *Dictionary of American Biography* (both were published under the auspices of the American Council of Learned Societies), which was published in the 1920s and 1930s. The *Dictionary of American Biography* was updated by several supplements into the 1980s. Researchers should be aware that to be eligible for inclusion in the *Dictionary of American Biography,* subjects have to be dead. In addition, the *Dictionary of American Biography* has been criticized for excluding some notable women and people of color. Both of these resources are available in print at most larger libraries; *American National Biography* is also available online through a subscription database.

Researchers should also be aware of the *Dictionary of National Biography,* which was published in the 1880s. This resource is critically important not just because of its quality and completeness, but because it set the standard for biographical dictionaries and brief biographical sketches. It covered British citizens and citizens of Britain's present and former colonies. Since it also required that the subject be deceased, it soon became apparent that it needed supplementation. The *Dictionary of National Biography* was supplemented at various times to 1996 and is available in print. In 2004, the *Oxford Dictionary of National Biography* was published, succeeding the *Dictionary of National Biography.* This book took a broad view of British history when determining whom to include, but it makes no attempt to be comprehensive. American colonists were eligible for inclusion, as were citizens of other former and present colonies if they were a part of British culture. The *Oxford Dictionary of National Biography* is available in print and online.

Before beginning a search for an individual, a researcher should note the person's characteristics because they will often govern the kind of material available and will do much to shape the nature of the research. Things to consider include the person's gender, birth and/or death dates, country or state of origin and/or death, century and decades of activity, nationality, and religion. The person's profession will also play a dramatic part in discovering available information. Was he or she a lawyer, judge, educator, politician? a member of Congress, of state government, or of the military? a diplomat? a writer? a criminal (if so, what crime)? Occupational directories exist for many professions. Was the person involved in litigation, and if so, as the plaintiff or defendant? What was the nature of the litigation? How famous or notorious was this interaction with the law? If the person was a criminal defendant, what was the crime and in what court was the case heard? If the person attended college or law school, additional resources may be available. How well known was this person?

In addition to biographical information, prosopography, the investigation of similarities among a group of people, can serve as an important means of investigation. What are the characteristics of graduates of a particular law school in the 1880s? What was the background of the federal judiciary in 1910? How much does gender or race affect sentencing?

Biographical and prosopographical research can be an end in itself. Such research can enlighten and help answer many questions as well as add depth and spice to research that generally uses other kinds of resources to examine issues.

A great number of biographical resources are available. Perhaps the most obvious is the biography or autobiography, which can be located through library catalogs. A search using the person's name as the subject will return materials about the

person, including biographies. The same search may also identify the individual's papers or the papers of others that substantially refer to the subject.

While information about people who were well known
during their lifetimes is easily available, searching for those who
were not well known can prove difficult or nearly impossible.
In such cases, a researcher can turn to prosopography or descriptions of people similarly situated as the best tools to get a
handle on ordinary people.

The U.S. Census Bureau has collected a great deal of information over the past two hundred years. Most of this material can be accessed through Ancestry.com, a for-fee database
especially popular among people interested in genealogy. Researchers can conduct searches by name, address, occupation,
and so on. Once they have located relevant items, they can view
the actual census pages. Information about neighbors, their
occupations, the number of people residing in a house, and
more can be gleaned from this data. For example, if a researcher has the address of a defendant obtained in a case file or
other document, he or she can search the address and get a good
idea about the socioeconomic background of the defendant's
neighborhood.

The Church of Jesus Christ of Latter-Day Saints (Mor-
mons) has collected a large volume of genealogical data. Their
website, familysearch.org, contains a number of tools that help
researchers learn about and conduct genealogical research.

Newspapers can be a tremendous biographical resource
for both famous and not-so-famous people (see more in chapter 11). For famous, infamous, and otherwise important people,
obituaries can provide a wealth of biographical information.
For people who were not so well known, death notices often
include information about date and place of birth and death,

education, profession, and family. Wedding announcements are also informative, often containing information about the people getting married and their families. Newspaper articles discussing particular crimes, or public meetings, or anything else of note can contain information about subjects and their views.

Several online tools aggregate other biographical articles— resources such as EBSCO's *Biography Reference Bank,* Gale's *Biography and Genealogy Master Index,* and Gale's *Biography in Context* provide access to some biographical resources as well as reference biographical materials that appear elsewhere. *Biography in Context* contains *Marquis Who's Who,* a collection of small biographical sketches of important people. The most important version of *Who's Who* for the researcher in U.S. legal history is *Who's Who in American Law.* All are available online and allow searching by a number of criteria. These tools skew greatly toward Americans. If the subject is not an American and unlikely to appear in American resources, the *World Biographical Information System* is worth examining.

Biographical sketches can appear in other places as well. If the subject was a renowned scholar, a researcher may discover festschrifts or other memorials in law reviews and other scholarly periodicals. The resources that allow searching for law reviews, such as the legal periodical indexes, HeinOnline, Lexis, and Westlaw can locate these. JSTOR and the indexes to the periodical literature of other disciplines may also unearth useful information. In addition, the transcripts of some memorial ceremonies for federal judges appear in West's federal reporters. These are indexed in an article by Barbara L. Fritschel, "An Index to Special Court Sessions in West's Federal Reporters" (*Law Library Journal* 93, no. 1 [2001]: 109–71).

A researcher may find books by or about figures of interest in some of the full-text treatise databases such as *Early American Imprints* and the *Making of Modern Law.*

A specialized database, *Notable American Women,* provides biographical information about women of note in U.S. history and can help a researcher find information about women who played an important role in the development of the law. Another database, ProQuest's *Heritage Quest Online,* brings together a great deal of information from census records, Freedman's Bank records, family histories, and Revolutionary War pensions. *Appleton's Cyclopedia of American Biography,* an older biographical directory and encyclopedia, provides biographical information about people who were once notable in America and may have become forgotten.

Tombstones and other gravesite information can also provide important biographical details. Two websites collect information about graves and cemeteries. The Political Graveyard (http://politicalgraveyard.com) provides information about and locations of politicians' gravesites. This searchable database can be very useful for finding birth and death dates. Another searchable database is Cemetery Records Online (http://www.interment.net).

To find information about current and former members of Congress, the *Biographical Directory of the U.S. Congress* is an important resource. This database and print resource is freely available online and can be searched in a variety of ways. A good resource for finding information about members of the legal profession is Morris Cohen's *Bibliography of Early American Law* (BEAL). It covers information up to 1861 and contains an author index, parties index, and subject index.

For finding information about lawyers and judges, researchers will find a terrific resource in legal directories. Two large and important directories especially deserve mention. The first is *Livingston's Law Register,* published through the mid-nineteenth century and held by many libraries. Many volumes are available for free through the Internet Archive, Google Books, or HathiTrust. The other, *Martindale-Hubbell Law Directory,* has been published continuously since 1868. As more people rely on the Internet for directory information, however, it has become a less important resource. For much of its history, *Martindale-Hubbell* consisted of two parts. One listed most members of the bar with an indication of where they went to college and law school and their graduation dates. The second, and the bulk of *Martindale-Hubbell,* was a paid directory service that listed, for its subscribers, more detailed information about every attorney in particular firms. Since *Martindale-Hubbell* is an annual, a researcher can track lawyers and firms from year to year. Current *Martindale-Hubbell* data is available online (https://www.martindale.com/), and many law libraries hold older directories.

There are several very good resources for finding information about judges. Bernan's *Biographical Directory of the Federal Judiciary, 1789–2000,* one of the most complete, provides biographical sketches of all federal judges. A free online version at the Federal Judicial Center breaks the listing into type of judge and covers from 1789 to the present. An older directory, *Biographical Notes of the Federal Judges prior to 1894,* provides information similar to that in the *Biographical Directory of the Federal Judiciary.* The *Supreme Court Compendium* is a tremendous resource that, as we will see in chapter 11, provides statistical information about the Court. However, it also contains a great deal of biographical information about the justices. Other important early books are Henry Flanders's *Lives and Times of the Chief Justices of the Supreme Court of the United*

States (1855–1858) and George Van Santvoord's *Sketches of the Lives and Judicial Services of the Chief-Justices of the Supreme Court of the United States* (1854 and 1882). Both of these books delve in some depth into the first several Supreme Courts chief justices. The *Almanac of the Federal Judiciary* (1984–present and updated regularly) is a more recent resource. It provides biographical sketches of current and recently retired federal judges and also delivers a great deal of biographical data and lists of important opinions, as well as the perceptions of the local bar about each judge.

Other directories also can provide basic biographical information, such as details about particular levels of government, agencies, judges, or other categories of people. These tools offer birth dates and often include educational information about each subject. To find these types of directories, conduct a subject search for "directory" and another term of interest.

Organizations can provide information about legal figures from the past. For example, the Federal Judicial History Office, the Supreme Court Historical Society, and the Women's Legal History Biography Project give information about federal judges, the U.S. Supreme Court, and women in the law, respectively.

Researchers can find additional biographical information in a variety of places. For example, regional bench and bar periodicals, many of which are available online through the *Making of Modern Law,* provide information about former judges and lawyers. Biographical sketches and obituaries often appear in the same journals. One tool that often offers great insight into how attorneys worked is their library catalogs, many of which can be found in estate inventories and as separately published guides to their collections. Finally, over the past decades many people have begun collecting oral histories, which can be investigated for important information about interviewees and their contemporaries.

Often, researchers can find directories based around particular law schools, such as *Biographies of Graduates of the Yale Law School, 1824–1899*. Samuel H. Fisher's *Litchfield Law School, 1774–1833: A Biographical Catalogue of Students* gives information about the many important people who attended that school. Marianne McKenna's biography of the founder of the Litchfield Law School, *Tapping Reeve and the Litchfield Law School,* provides information about the school and biographical sketches of both Tapping Reeve and some of the illustrious students who attended the school.

If the person under investigation was a part of the government, a researcher might try the *Biographical Directory of the United States Congress,* which provides information about members of the Continental Congress in 1774 to Congress today. The *Biographic Register of the Department of State* includes basic biographical information of major State Department officials, and the *Biographical Directory of the Governors of the United States, 1789–1978* offers information about state-level politicians; occasional supplements have brought this forward to the mid-1990s. The *Biographical Annals of the Civil Government of the United States During Its First Century* profiles people at various levels of government throughout the nineteenth century, and the *Biographical Directory of the United States Executive Branch, 1774–1989* includes biographical information about high-level individuals who served in the U.S. executive branch.

These directories, organized by profession, provide basic biographical information, but scholarly legal publications may provide more, as might bar journals, newspapers, and even case reporters. When hunting for biographical information about a person, researchers will find that almost any resource may provide the key. Histories of various organizations, papers of the person of interest or those with whom he or she may have interacted, biographies of the subject's contemporaries—all can provide insight into a person.

In the nineteenth and early twentieth centuries, several directories offered information about important attorneys who worked in various regions of the United States:

- William Davis, *The New England States, Their Constitutional, Judicial, Educational, Commercial, Professional, and Industrial History* (1897)
- Herbert Parker, *Courts and Lawyers of New England* (1931)
- Conrad Reno, *Memoirs of the Judiciary and the Bar of New England for the Nineteenth Century* (1901)
- Henry Foote, *The Bench and Bar of the South and Southwest* (1876)
- Charles Taylor, *Eminent Judges and Lawyers of the Northwest, 1843–1955* (1954)
- InterOcean Newspaper Company, *Notable Lawyers of the West* (1902)
- Dorothy Thomas, *Women Lawyers in the United States* (1957)

Many states have published their own histories of the bar. These and directories provide information about the important lawyers in any particular location over a particular time. Some examples include

- *The Bench and Bar of Georgia: Memoirs and Sketches* (1858)

- *The Bench and Bar of Chicago Including Biographical Sketches* (1883)
- *The Bench and Bar of Southern California* (1909)
- *History of the Bench and Bar of California* (1912)
- *The Reference Biography of Louisiana Bench and Bar* (1922)

Many similar books appeared in the nineteenth and twentieth centuries covering almost every state. A catalog search for items that contain the name of a state or region in the title and "bench" or "lawyers" or "judges" or "bar" in the title and the subject term "directory" will point researchers to these resources.

Research Example

Let us consider the use of the term "appeal" in the law. We will see how we can use dictionaries to understand at least two very different definitions of the word. *Webster's Third International Dictionary* provides six definitions for the noun form:

1. "A legal proceeding by which a case is brought from a lower to a higher court for rehearing"
2. "A formal accusation of a felony or heinous crime made against a person by another who demands punishment for the private injury rather than for the public offense"
3. A demand to defend oneself against a charge (considered obsolete)
4. Relating to an application to a recognized authority for corroboration, vindication, or decision
5. An earnest plea or request

6. "The power or property of arousing a sympathetic response"

Webster's further tells us that the word is a Middle English word
from the Old French, *apel.* Since the third definition is considered obsolete, the fourth appears to be derived from the first
two meanings, and the fifth is further removed from the law,
we will concentrate on the first two.

Webster's definition of the transitive verb form has four
meanings:

1. "To institute a private criminal prosecution against
   for a felony or heinous crime"
2. To take steps to remove a case from a lower to a
   higher court
3. To challenge (archaic)
4. To call to witness

The intransitive verb meanings are

1. "To apply for the removal of a case from a lower
   to a higher court for rehearing"
2. "To call upon or refer to another as a recognized
   authority for corroboration, vindication, or decision"
3. To make an earnest request
4. To arouse a sympathetic response

Interestingly, the noun form and the transitive verb form start
off with the idea of appealing from one court to another, while
the first definition for the transitive verb form is to institute a
private prosecution.

By turning to the *Oxford English Dictionary*, we can gain some history behind the meanings and see their roots. The OED provides roughly the same etymology, though with more detail, but when we look at the definitions, things become interesting. The first two appear to be the most relevant to our inquiry.

1. "A calling to account before a legal tribunal; in *Law:* A criminal charge or accusation, made by one who undertook under penalty to prove it"
2. The challenge idea
3. An appeal to a higher court
4. The call to a higher authority, not necessarily legal, for a decision
5. A call for help of any kind
6. Language specifically addressed to invoke sympathy
7. A summons by bell ringing

In the OED the transitive verb definitions are as follows:

1. To call one before a tribunal
2. The challenge idea
3 and 4. To invoke or claim as a judge and to invoke or call a witness (both obscure and rare).

In the OED, the intransitive verb definitions continue the numbering, so we will as well:

5. An appeal to a higher court
6. To call upon a recognized authority
7. To call to a witness for corroboration
8. To call for a favor

9. To attempt to be attractive or pleasing to another
10. A transitive verb with the thing as an object: to appeal to a higher tribunal

The OED definitions and examples date from 1885 and have not been updated yet, but let's look at the dates that it has found for some of the meanings. Starting with the noun form, the first citation for the private cause of action is from *Piers Plowman* in 1377. The first use of "appeal" for the idea of moving a case to a higher tribunal comes from 1297 from the chronicle of Robert of Gloucester: "To the bissop fram ercedekne [h]is apel [he] solde make." The second example is from John Gower's *Confessio Amantis*: "Fro thy wrath . . . To thy pite stant min appele."

For the verb form, the OED supplies *Mandeville's Travels* from 1366: "Straungeres . . . schulle thus appelen us & holden us for wykked Lyveres"; and for the appeal to a higher court, it supplies Robert Mannyng's *Chronicle* from 1330: "S. Anselm þerfor appeld vnto þe courte of Rome."

For both meanings, the OED provides citations from the fourteenth century, although one citation is from the very end of the thirteenth. As we look more closely at the definitions, though, it appears that the idea of appealing to a higher court might come from the ecclesiastical law world. Robert of Gloucester specifically refers to a bishop, and Robert Mannyng refers to Saint Anselm appealing to Rome; even Gower uses "wrath" and "pity," and an appeal from one to the other certainly feels biblical. Is this, perhaps, a common law/civil law distinction? We can look at law abridgments and dictionaries that might pin the meanings down a little.

The earliest version of John Rastell's *Termes de la ley* available in Early English Books Online is from 1624, although it was written a century earlier. In it, "appeal" is defined as the private cause of action against one who has committed a murder, robbery, or mayhem. He does not mention any alternative definition. In *The Interpreter* (1607), John Cowell provides a long explanation of "appeal" as "a lawful declaration of another man's crime before a competent judge," with a citation to Henry de Bracton, *De legibus et consuetudinibus Angliae* (1275). He next provides definitions of two types of appeal: an "appeal of mayhem" and an "appeal of false imprisonment." Finally, he mentions that at "diverse times" the term is used in the common law as it is used in the civil law to mean removal of a cause from an inferior judge to a superior, "as appeale to Rome." By the 1684 version, by which time Cowell had been dead for seventy-three years, the definitions are almost identical. The language is somewhat modernized, but the only significant change from our perspective is that the second definition of "appeal," an appeal to a higher tribunal, is now "many times used in the common law as it is in the Civil Law."

Even as late as 1756, Giles Jacob, in *A New Law Dictionary*, stresses the appeal as a private cause of action by a victim or a victim's heirs or by an accomplice against one who commits a felony. Jacob does state in the first definition that an appeal is the "removal of a cause from an inferior" to a superior court. However, in the next clause, he says that an appeal is "more commonly for an accusation of a murderer by a party who had interest in the person killed."

In the second edition of *A Dictionary of the English Language* (1755), Samuel Johnson provides four definitions for the verb form of the word: the first is "the transfer of a cause from one to another"; the second, "to refer to another as judge"; the third, "to call another as witness"; and the fourth, "to charge with a crime; accuse." In the noun form, Johnson also provides four definitions: first, "a provocation from an inferior to a superior judge"; second, "in the common law, an accusation; which is a lawful accusation of another man's crime before a competent judge"; third, "a summons to answer a charge"; and fourth, "a call upon any as a witness."

Further Reading

Eskridge, William N., Jr. "All About Words: Early Understandings of the Judicial Power in Statutory Interpretation, 1776–1806." *Columbia Law Review* 101 (2001): 990–1106.

Fenster, Mark. "The Folklore of Legal Biography." *Michigan Law Review* 105 (2006): 1265–82.

Holborn, Guy. *Sources of Biographical Information on Past Lawyers*. Warwick: British and Irish Association of Law Librarians, 1999.

McEldowney, John. "Challenges in Legal Bibliography: The Role of Biography in Legal History." *Irish Jurist* 39 (2004): 215–42.

Mellinkoff, David. "The Myth of Precision and the Law Dictionary." *UCLA Law Review* 31 (1983): 423–42.

Post, Robert C. "Judging Lives." *New York University Law Review* 70 (1995): 548–55.

Scalia, Antonin. *A Matter of Interpretation: Federal Courts and the Law*. Edited by Amy Gutmann. Princeton, NJ: Princeton University Press, 1997.

Thumma, Samuel A., and Jeffrey I. Kirchmeier. "The Lexicon Has Become a Fortress: The United States Supreme Court's Use of Dictionaries." *Buffalo Law Review*. 47, no. 1 (1999): 227–561.

Important Sources Mentioned in This Chapter

American Council of Learned Societies. *Dictionary of American Biography*. New York: Scribner, 1928.

Black, Henry Campbell. *A Dictionary of Law Containing Definitions of the Terms and Phrases of American and English Jurisprudence, Ancient and Modern: Including the Principal Terms of International, Constitutional, and Commercial Law: With a Collection of Legal Maxims and*

Numerous Select Titles from the Civil Law and Other Foreign Systems.
St. Paul, MN: West, 1891.

Blount, Thomas. *Nomo-Lexikon = A Law-Dictionary.* London, 1670.

Bouvier, John, and Robert Kelham. *A Law Dictionary, Adapted to the Constitution and Laws of the United States of America, and of the Several States of the American Union with References to the Civil and Other Systems of Foreign Law.* Philadelphia: T. and J. W. Johnson, 1839.

Bouvier, John, and Francis Rawle. *Bouvier's Law Dictionary and Concise Encyclopedia.* Kansas City, MO: Vernon Law; St. Paul, MN: West, 1914.

Burn, Richard, and John Burn. *A New Law Dictionary . . . Continued to the Present Time by John Burn.* London: T. Cadell, 1792.

Cowell, John. *The Interpreter: Or Booke Containing the Signification of Words: Wherein Is Set Foorth the True Meaning of All . . . Words and Termes, as Are Mentioned in the Lawe Writers, or Statutes of This . . . Kingdome.* Cambridge, 1607.

Cunningham, Timothy. *A New and Complete Law-Dictionary, Or, General Abridgment of the Law: On a More Extensive Plan than Any Law-Dictionary Hitherto Published, Containing Not Only the Explanation of the Terms, but Also the Law Itself, Both with Regard to Theory and Practice. Very Useful to Barristers, Justices of the Peace, Attornies, Solicitors, &c.* London, 1674.

Garraty, John A., and Mark C. Carnes, and American Council of Learned Societies. *American National Biography.* 24 vols. New York: Oxford University Press, 1999.

Jacob, Giles. *A New Law-Dictionary Containing, the Interpretation and Definition of Words and Terms Used in the Law; and Also the Whole Law, and the Practice Thereof . . . By Giles Jacob, Gent.* London, 1729.

Johnson, Samuel. *A Dictionary of the English Language.* London, 1756.

Kelham, Robert, and David Wilkins. *A dictionary of the Norman or Old French language; collected from such acts of Parliament, Parliament rolls, journals, acts of state, records, law books, antient historians, and manuscripts as related to this nation. To which are added the laws of William, the Conqueror, with notes and references.* London: E. Brooke, 1779.

Leigh, Edward. *A Philologicall Commentary, Or, an Illustration of the Most Obvious and Usefull Words in the Law . . . By E. L[eigh], Gentleman, Etc.* London, 1658.

Martindale, James B., and Hubbell, John Henry. *Martindale-Hubbell Law Directory.* New York: Martindale-Hubbell Law Directory, 1868–.

Matthew, H. C. G., and Brian Howard Harrison. *Oxford Dictionary of National Biography: In Association with the British Academy: From* the Earliest Times to the Year 2000. Oxford: Oxford University Press, 2004.

Murray, James A. H., and R. W. Burchfield. *The Oxford English Dictionary; Being a Corrected Re-Issue with an Introduction, Supplement, and Bibliography of a New English Dictionary on Historical Principles.* Oxford: Clarendon, 1933.

Murray, James A. H., William A. Craigie, and C. T. Onions. *A New English dictionary on historical principles; founded mainly on the materials collected by the Philological Society.* Oxford: Clarendon, 1888.

Porter, Noah. *Webster's International Dictionary of the English Language, Being the Authentic Edition of Webster's Unabridged Dictionary, Comprising the Issues of 1864, 1879, and 1884.* Springfield, MA: G. & C. Merriam, 1890.

Rastell, John. *Exposicio[n]es T[er]mi[n]or[um] Legu[m] Anglor[um]: Et Natura Breuiu[m] Cu[m] Diversib[us] Casub[us] Regulis et Fundame[n]tis Legum Tam de Libris Magistri Litteltoni Qua[m] de Aliis Legum Libris Collectis [et] Breuit[er] Compilatis p[er] Iuuinib[us] Valde Necessariis = The Exposicions of Ye Termys of Ye Law of England [and] the Nature of the Writts with Diuers Rulys [and] Principalles of the Law as Well out of the Bokis of Mayster Littelton as of Other Bokis of the Law Gaderyd and Breuely Compylyd for Yong Men Very Necessarye.* London, 1523.

Sheppard, William. *An Epitome of All the Common & Statute Laws of This Nation Now in Force: Wherein More than Fifteen Hundred of the Hardest Words or Terms of the Law Are Explained; and All of the Most Useful and Profitable Heads or Titles of the Law by Way of Common Place, Largely, Plainly, and Methodically Handled . . .* London, 1656.

Spelmann, Henry, and Alice Warren. *Glossarium archaiologicum: continens Latino-Barbara, peregrina, obsoleta, & novatae significationis vocabula; . . . Scholiis & commentariis illustrata; in quibus prisci ritus quamplurimi, magistratus, dignitates, . . . & consuetudines enarrantur. Authore Henrico Spelmanno equite, Anglo-Britanno.* London, 1664.

Stephen, Leslie, and Sidney Lee. *Dictionary of National Biography.* London: Smith, Elder, & Co., 1885.

United States Congress, Bruce A. Ragsdale, and Kathryn Allamong Jacob. *Biographical Directory of the United States Congress, 1774–1989: The Continental Congress, September 5, 1774, to October 21, 1788, and the Congress of the United States, from the First Through the One Hundredth Congresses, March 4, 1789, to January 3, 1989, Inclusive.* Washington, DC: GPO, 1989.

Webster, Noah. *An American Dictionary of the English Language: Intended to Exhibit, I. The Origin, Affinities and Primary Signification of English Words, as Far as They Have Been Ascertained. II. The Genuine Orthography and Pronunciation of Words, according to General Usage, or to Just Principles of Analogy. III. Accurate and Discriminating Definition, with Numerous Authorities and Illustrations. To Which Are Prefixed, an Introductory Dissertation on the Origin, History and Connection of the Languages of Western Asia and of Europe, and a Concise Grammar of the English Language.* New York: S. Converse, 1828.

Webster, Noah, Chauncey A Goodrich, and Noah Porter. *An American Dictionary of the English Language: Containing the Whole Vocabulary of the First Edition in Two Volumes Quarto, the Entire Corrections and Improvements of the Second Edition in Two Volumes Royal Octavo: To Which Is Prefixed an Introductory Dissertation on the Origin, History, and Connection, of the Languages of Western Asia and Europe, with an Explanation of the Principles on Which Languages Are Formed.* Springfield, MA: George and Charles Merriam, 1864.

Wilson, James Grant, and John Fiske. *Appleton's Cyclopedia of American Biography.* New York: D. Appleton, 1889.

Databases

EBSCO. *Biography Reference Bank.* https://www.ebsco.com/products/research-databases/biography-reference-bank.

Gale. *Biography and Genealogy Master Index.* http://www.gale.com/c/biography-and-genealogy-master-index.

———. *Biography in Context.* http://www.gale.com/c/biography-in-context.

Federal Judicial Center. *Biographical Directory of Article III Federal Judges, 1789–Present.* https://www.fjc.gov/history/judges.

———. *History of the Federal Judiciary.* https://www.fjc.gov/history/home.nsf.

Oxford University Press. *OED: Oxford English Dictionary.* http://www.oed.com.

ProQuest. *Ancestry Library Edition.* https://www.proquest.com/products-services/ale.html.

———. *HeritageQuest Online.* https://www.proquest.com/products-services/HeritageQuest-Online.html.

11

Nonlaw Research

Since the law defines the relationships that people have with the state and, frequently, with each other, it is intimately related to many other areas of scholarship and inquiry. Legal researchers will often have to expand their research beyond the law and delve into politics, sociology, economics, psychology, current or historical events, and many other areas. This chapter looks at several types of nonlaw resources. The list is not exhaustive but includes the most important and frequently used sources: newspapers; periodical literature, monographs (also discussed in chapter 1) and dissertations; statistical resources; and public records. There are many guides to research in each of these areas.

As researchers move beyond this introduction, they should search for guides to research in the areas of their interests. Many academic libraries provide topical research guides for free on their websites. For more in-depth guidance, researchers should use library catalogs. Searches for their subject followed by methodology or by research can be useful subjects. For example, a search for "economics research" limited to 2016 returns the *Handbook of Research Methods and Applications in Heterodox*

Economics published by Edward Elgar. A subject search for materials published since 2013 containing the terms "sociology" and "research" returns, among others, Marcelo Bucheli and R. Daniel Wadhwani, *Organizations in Time: History, Theory, Methods* published by Oxford University Press. It is important to notice that for the latter search the terms were required to appear in the subject field, but their order, relationship, and the existence of additional terms were unspecified. The broader search allowed the subject "organizational sociology research methods," the subject assigned to the Bucheli book, to be included.

Newspapers

Newspapers can aid researchers in understanding what was publicly known and what was considered important as particular events unfolded, through both the information included and that omitted in news accounts. Newspaper reporting can also expose the prejudices and assumptions of various groups of people at the time an event occurred. Newspapers are often geared toward particular audiences; not only do they report what their readers want to hear about, but they can also reflect readers' prejudices. By reading several newspapers on a topic, researchers can often learn a great deal about the tenor of the time and the environment within which a legal event occurred.

Of course, researchers will want to ensure that they have equipped themselves with a basic understanding of the development of the press in the United States as well as how and why stories were gathered and reported. A critically important introduction to early American newspapers is Clarence Brigham's *History and Bibliography of American Newspapers, 1690–1820*

(1961). A useful companion, Winifred Gregory Gerould's *American Newspapers, 1821–1936: A Union List of Files Available in the United States and Canada* (1937), will allow researchers to understand the corpus of early American news. Other valuable introductions to the history of the press in the United States are Leonard Levy's *Emergence of a Free Press* (1985), Richard L. Kaplan's *Politics and the American Press: The Rise of Objectivity, 1865–1920* (2002), and Christopher B. Daly's *Covering America: A Narrative History of a Nation's Journalism* (2012).

Before the development of online databases, newspaper research was a time-intensive undertaking. Major research libraries had microform back files of important newspapers, but gaining access to smaller newspapers often required searching local libraries or historical society collections or going through a newspaper's own "morgue." Even when a newspaper was located, finding relevant articles was difficult. Articles in most newspapers were not indexed in periodical indexes, and the *New York Times* was one of the few that published its own index. Researchers could easily find materials about an event as long as the materials appeared in a relatively close temporal proximity to the event. Stories that long preceded an event, which may have placed the event in a larger context, were unavailable except to those researchers with the time and budget to read beyond the time of their topic.

Today, many newspapers are available for full-text online searching. Several databases aggregate newspapers, and other newspapers are available as stand-alone digital resources. Some newspapers have not been digitized, but resources are available that can help a researcher locate a microform version of a newspaper. *America's Historical Newspapers* from Readex includes the full text of more than one thousand newspapers published between 1690 and 1922. Researchers can conduct complex Boolean searches that return article and page images of the newspaper. ProQuest has several products that supply researchers with access to fully searchable newspapers with page and article images. ProQuest's list of titles is smaller than Readex's, but ProQuest supplies national newspapers like the *Chicago Tribune, Los Angeles Times, New York Times, Wall Street Journal,* and *Washington Post* available in their Historical Newspapers databases. Heritage Archive's database Access Newspaper Archive is another full-text-searchable collection of newspapers with article and page images. What sets it apart is that it includes newspapers from smaller towns and cities. Coverage can be spotty, but when the database's coverage and an important local event converge, the material can be invaluable. More recent material from newspapers, wire services, and other sources is available from LexisNexis, Westlaw, and Factiva. Coverage in these databases frequently goes back to the 1980s, and page images are often not available, but the title lists are extensive. Most of these databases are available at academic libraries, and some may be available through public library consortia.

In addition to the general collections of newspapers described above, several collections limited by topic or date can also be useful. For example, researchers can find collections of African-American newspapers, Jewish newspapers, Hispanic-American newspapers, newspapers from the entertainment industry, military newspapers, the alternative press, and the music press. In addition to these smaller collections, several important newspapers are available as stand-alone resources. Examples of the latter include the Northern New York Historical Newspapers and the *Brooklyn Eagle,* the former a project of the NY3Rs Association and the latter a project from the Brooklyn Public Library.

Several additional collections of full-text newspapers and periodicals are important. Accessible Archives is a database that contains many nineteenth-century newspapers, journals, and monographs. Its collection is especially strong on Civil War and African-American history. The Library of Congress's Chronicling America website is digitizing many newspapers. In 2017, it had twelve million pages available for full-text searching covering from 1789 to 1924. Gale's database *17th and 18th Century Burney Newspapers Collection* includes the full text of newspapers from around the world covering from 1604 to 1804. Gale's database of British newspapers provides full-text access from 1600 to 1950. There are many additional newspaper resources; the best resource to use to identify them is the print *Guide to Reference Books,* by Robert Balay (11th ed., 1996), which is available at most libraries. Unfortunately, this is the last edition of this title. There are few guides to or lists of newspaper databases. Researchers might use several strategies to identify and locate a database. The major database providers can be checked; many academic libraries post guides to research in an area and will list databases that they have access to; World-Cat can be searched; and Wikipedia has a nice page that includes many individual newspaper's archives, many of which are free (https://en.wikipedia.org/wiki/Wikipedia:List_of_online _newspaper_archives). If researchers know about databases that exist but that are not available through libraries they frequent, they may be able to help guide the library's acquisitions decisions.

Many newspapers that are not available in a digital format are available to researchers in print or microform. WorldCat is a good resource for locating libraries that hold print or microform copies of newspapers. Once a newspaper is located, the next step is to find relevant material within the newspaper.

Browsing through a newspaper surrounding a date is one common method, but indexes can often help researchers. The *New York Times Index* is a print index that has been published since 1913 and is available at many libraries. Legal researchers might also consider the legal periodical index LegalTrac, which also includes several legal newspapers. The *New York Law Journal,* a legal newspaper, has been published every business day since 1888. It is now available online to subscribers at Law. com. The *New York Law Journal Digest-Annotator* and its predecessor *Clark's Digest-Annotator* index the cases reported in the newspaper.

When all of the databases are taken into account, most important newspapers in the United States and some small newspapers are available for much of the country's history. The newspapers included in the databases can be easily searched; those that are not available online are more difficult to use, but the material is often available. As more newspapers are digitized by commercial and nonprofit organizations, finding relevant articles covering events from a variety of perspectives will become even easier.

Periodicals, Dissertations, and Monographs

Periodicals, monographs, conference proceedings, and other less regular publications are important means of scholarly communication in legal scholarship and many other disciplines. It is critical for researchers to work with these materials to understand the scholarly debates in context. In chapter 1 we discussed finding monographs and in chapter 6 journal articles related to legal scholarship. Here, we consider resources that researchers can use to find materials that cover other areas of scholarship.

When searching for scholarly materials outside of the law, researchers will find that the resources they use work much the same as law-related resources. For example, finding monographs in areas of scholarship other than law is much the same as searching for law-related monographs. The catalogs are the same and the search strategies are much same. What differs is the terminology. Researchers new to an area can use several strategies to identify important terminology. Most obviously, they can read any books, articles, encyclopedias, or other material that they already know about to begin to develop a foundation and vocabulary. They can search in a catalog for known items or conduct searches with terms that they are already familiar with, examine the found items and identify the most relevant, note the subjects or other descriptions added to the item, and conduct new searches using the newly identified terms. They can also speak with experts in the area or experts in conducting research in the area.

As researchers develop familiarity with a subject, they will move from more general works, such as encyclopedias and introductory texts and treatises, to more specialized ones. Then as they develop familiarity with the concepts and terminology of the subject, they will also begin to track authors and to notice citations. Together, the concepts, terminology, authors, and citations are the blocks on which further searching is based. As new concepts and terminology are identified, the resources that have already been examined should be reexamined in light of the new data.

As we have seen with the law, encyclopedias dedicated to specific topics can be useful for researchers new to a field and are often good places for neophytes to start their research. Once a field is familiar to researchers, they will find that the value of encyclopedias may diminish; however, an encyclopedia can be useful even to experts if the subtopic under investigation is unfamiliar.

As in the law, specialized periodicals and journals publish scholarship in almost every area of study and play an important part in scholarship. When conducting periodical research, researchers should identify three things: relevant articles, the most prestigious journals, and the most important articles in a particular area. To identify articles, researchers should examine either general scholarly full-text or index databases or specialized databases. Almost all of the databases work as described in chapters 1 and 6. As with any database, researchers new to one will want to see whether it supports a controlled vocabulary (many do) and how logical expressions should be represented.

In determining the databases to search, researchers should consider what databases exist that cover the field and, more importantly, which databases they can access. The best means for determining possible databases are the methods already mentioned, catalogs, lists of databases and subject guides at large specialized libraries, and, once the major publishers that cover the area are identified, the lists of databases provided by a publisher. Another method is to conduct searches in a free database such as Google Scholar, identify the most relevant articles, note the journals in which they appear, and then, using a resource like the subscription Ulrichsweb, determine which databases include the journal. Ulrichsweb provides information about more than three hundred thousand journals, including where they are indexed or abstracted.

Several databases include runs of important journals in a range of disciplines. The most important is JSTOR, which includes journals from many disciplines and coverage back to the beginning of each journal. Project MUSE is a similar collection. It contains full-text books and journals from more than

260 mainly academic publishers. Project MUSE is strongest in the humanities and social sciences, while JSTOR's collection also includes journals in the sciences. There are also large collections of full-text databases of journals in more limited topical areas. For example, Medline is limited to journals in the medical and allied fields. All of these are subscription databases, but they are often more widely available; for example, both JSTOR and Project MUSE have programs that allow academic institutions to pay a fee and for alumni access to the databases.

In addition to full-text databases, index databases are also available for many disciplines. As discussed in chapter 7, index searching differs from full-text searching. There are many topically oriented indexes, such as *EconLit*, *Sociological Abstracts*, and *Humanities Index*. Most academic libraries and some larger public libraries have access to a number of topical indexes. Several resources are available to help researchers determine whether there is an index that covers a topic; one of the most widely available is the print *Guide to Reference Books* and the online Guide to Reference.

In contrast to topical indexes, many indexes in some disciplines include journals. In truth, the distinction between an index and a full-text database is becoming less clear as many of the following "index" databases contain some full-text content or allow libraries to easily and seamlessly imbed links to full-text content within the search results. Among these are Academic Search, the Web of Science, Google Scholar, and the *Readers' Guide to Periodical Literature*. The *Readers' Guide* is skewed toward general-interest publications, while Academic Search covers both general-interest and scholarly publications. The Web of Science also includes journals in the social sciences. Google Scholar's coverage is a little more difficult to define, although it does include a large number of journals and does allow libraries with subscriptions to the underlying databases or journals to include links to the articles in the Google Scholar display.

In addition to the legal indexes and full-text sources already mentioned, historical legal researchers should remember the history indexes. *America: History and Life* covers scholarly research into U.S. history, and *Historical Abstracts* indexes the literature commonly available in the United States that deals with history in the rest of the world.

Two major periodical databases provided by ProQuest, *American Periodicals* and *British Periodicals Collection,* encompass the important periodical literature from the nineteenth century and into the twentieth and offer full texts of periodical materials. These databases include both general-interest and more scholarly publications. Researchers will find that in the nineteenth century, quite scholarly discussions on fairly esoteric topics, including legal topics, took place in certain general-interest periodicals. Finally, several long-standing periodicals have databases devoted solely to their literature; for example, the *New Yorker,* the *Economist, Frank Leslie's Weekly, Harper's,* the *Nation,* and the *National Review* each appear in their own database. As the market for complete runs of periodicals matures, many more titles will become available.

When investigating very specific events or issues, researchers may wish to examine dissertations and theses, in which authors delve deeply into an issue and generally conduct excellent research. Housed at the school granting the degree, dissertations are so valued that they have for years been distributed more widely. University Microfilms, Inc., has put many on microfiche, and they are available at many libraries. More recently, many have been added to the ProQuest database Dissertations and Theses.

Many of the documents are available in full text, and even more are indexed. Often, a dissertation or thesis identified through the index but not available in the database can be acquired through interlibrary loan. A few schools do not include their dissertations in the database or on microfilm. The best option for identifying such dissertations or theses is through the library catalog of the degree-granting institution.

More recently, preprint sites house scholarly papers before they are even published. The major players in this field, Social Science Research Network (SSRN) and Berkeley Electronic Press (BEPress), allow searching of, and access to, many papers. In addition, many institutions have repositories for the scholarship created by their faculty members. Examining these or searching Google Scholar may yield useful material.

Conference papers can also be very useful but difficult to locate. There are several guides to older materials, including Winifred Gregory Gerould's *International Congresses and Conferences, 1840–1937: A Union List of Their Publications Available in Libraries of the United States and Canada*, available at many libraries. Another great resource is *American Book Auction Catalogs, 1713–1934: A Union List*, by George J. McKay and Clarence Saunders Brigham.

Statistical Resources

Many organizations and governments collect a large amount of data. The most important collector of statistics in the United States is the U.S. Census Bureau. As the Constitution requires a census every decade, a great deal of information is thus available from the entirety of American history. There are several ways to gain access to census data. The U.S. Census website is often a good place to start, although it can be overwhelming. A better place to start may be the *Statistical Abstract of the United States*. This has been published since 1878 and is available for free through 2012 at the U.S. Census website. The census stopped publication of the *Statistical Abstract* in 2011, but the collection of data and publishing have been taken up by ProQuest. The *Statistical Abstract* provides tabular data covering the most important statistics. Often, a table may appear for many consecutive years, allowing for comparative research. Once researchers find the table in the *Statistical Abstract* that addresses the issue under consideration, they can identify the source of the statistics from the table. In addition to the annual *Statistical Abstract*, several special editions of information related to the census may be of interest. Collections have been published covering periods from 1790 to various ending dates. The most recent, published by Cambridge University Press, is the *Historical Statistics of the United States Millennial Edition*. As its name implies, it covers from roughly 1790 to about the year 2005.

For research, the most useful census material is likely the history page at the website of the U.S. Census Bureau (https:// www.census.gov/history/). The publications and catalog cover material that tends to be more recent, although the start dates for some of the data tables can go as far back as the mid-twentieth century. The history page contains links to information about every census since 1790. Among other items, it includes a list of the questions asked and images of the questionnaires for each census. Researchers should know that in order to maintain privacy, the Census Bureau uses a "rule of 72"; that is, the census will not release information that can identify people until seventy-two years after the data were gathered. For example, 1940 data were released through the National Archives on April 2, 2012, and the 1950 data will be released in April 2022. Researchers can seek census information through the National Archives; the main publications published by the Census Bureau related to each census since 1790 and through 2010 are also available online (https://www.census.gov/history/www/through_the_decades/ overview/). Each census can be selected for an overview of it and links to the publications related to it. Another easy Census Bureau tool is American FactFinder, which allows researchers to easily compile the most commonly sought type of statistics.

After the National Archives releases the data, individuals and organizations can collect the information and make it available to the public. Ancestry.com is the best-known and most useful of these vendors. Many libraries have subscriptions to Ancestry.com, as do many individuals.

In addition to the decennial census, the Census Bureau takes regular topical censuses, including the Economic Census that is taken every five years on the '2s and '7s (e.g., 2002 and 2007) since the 1935 Census of Business. Records from 1967 to 1997 are available online at Archive.org and from 1977 to the present at the Census Bureau site (https://www.census.gov/programs-surveys/ economic-census/year.html). Recall that the decennial census does include some economic data and that many other organizations and agencies also gather economic data.

Among those other governmental agencies that collect and publish a great deal of data are the Bureau of Justice Statistics, which publishes a great number of legal statistics; the Department of Commerce, which publishes commercial statistics, including historical statistics; and the Department of Labor, which publishes a number of statistical collections. Of course, the Census Bureau might be the most important producer of governmental statistics. Identifying the requisite agency and investigating the statistics it publishes, using the monthly catalog and other sources mentioned above, will usually reward a researcher. The *Statistical Abstract* contains and refers to a great deal of data published by these other governmental agencies. Again, it is often useful to use the *Statistical Abstract* as a guide to the data. In addition, many of the agencies that handle a lot of data have developed extremely sophisticated websites that allow researchers to find and manipulate data.

A great many agencies and departments collect statistics. Searching the website of an agency or department may yield helpful numbers. To find older statistics, turn to the publications of the agency or department. The *Monthly Catalog of Government Documents* is the best resource from 1895. Before 1895, the *Congressional Serial Set,* which also includes materials after 1895, is the first place to look, followed by the *Checklist of United States Public Documents.* The *Checklist* will not direct researchers to particular documents, but it will show whether an organ of the government regularly published such a report.

A great collection of information about Supreme Court opinions since 1946 is the Supreme Court Database through Washington University Law (supremecourtdatabase.org). This free resource, created by Professor Harold J. Spaeth and now supported by a team of academics, plans to take the data back to the first reported Supreme Court cases. It allows searching and sorting data by a variety of constraints, including the issues raised, the type of law considered (statute, etc.), the result at the Court, the author of the opinion, and many more. Another useful resource, the *Supreme Court Compendium: Data, Decisions, and Developments,* is a specialized resource, but it collects information about the Court and justices that is otherwise difficult to locate.

The Bureau of Justice Statistics and others produce the *Sourcebook of Criminal Justice Statistics,* available at many libraries and hosted online by one of the producers, the Michael J.

Hindelang Criminal Justice Research Center at the University of Albany (http://www.albany.edu/sourcebook/). Scholars continue to collect and create new data sets that allow for more and better analysis of the country in total. Many data sets are available to members of the Inter-University Consortium for Political and Social Research (ICPSR) (http://http://www.icpsr. umich.edu/icpsrweb/).

Several additional databases allow researchers to search across sets of statistics. One of the most important is ProQuest Statistical Insight. It covers research published since 1990, and the oldest research goes back to 1950. The best resource for finding government data sets, Data.gov (http://www.data.gov), contains more than 190,000 data sets from almost two hundred government organs. Data can be searched by tag, term appearing in the description, geography, agency, and other aspects. Data.gov contains data from a variety of sources, including federal and state governments and universities. While its focus is not historical, some of the data extend back to the early twentieth century.

Some new databases collect data from many sources. One concentrating on the law is Findout (https://findout.com/solution.html). Statistica (http://www.statistica.com) provides data and interpretive tools over a great many subjects. VoxGov provides access to a large number of government documents and reports. It allows users to create data visualization, timeline graphs, and multiyear comparisons. These are all expensive private databases, although some may be available at larger academic libraries or for-profit organizations.

Some resources allow researchers to post and share data sets that they have created. Academics and others, including governmental organs such as the Federal Judicial Center, supply data to resources like the ICPSR. The data are available for other researchers to use in their research.

Multinational organizations and other nongovernmental organizations also collect data that can be especially useful for comparative research over the past half century or so. Organizations such as the United Nations, the Organisation for Economic Co-operation and Development, and the World Bank hold very useful data, especially economic data.

Empirical legal research is a growing field, and more resources will continue to appear. A new guide, *An Introduction to Empirical Legal Research,* was published by Oxford University Press in 2014. Survey design and the use of sophisticated data and geographic data resources are beyond the scope of this book. However, legal and historical researchers should be aware that data tools exist and guides and experts are available that can begin to direct them in the use of empirical methods. A few additional titles—Peter Cane and Herbert M. Kritzer's *Oxford Handbook of Empirical Legal Research* (2010), Yun-chien Chang's *Empirical Legal Analysis: Assessing the Performance of Legal Institutions* (2014), and Frans L. Leeuw and Hans Schmeets's *Empirical Legal Research: A Guidance Book for Lawyers, Legislators and Regulators*—will help researchers get acclimated.

Public Records

Almost every interaction that a person has with the government is recorded in some fashion. Although the government withholds much of the data, especially during a person's lifetime, it is often possible to obtain it. We are in an interesting time with regard to data. Traditionally, some data have been completely public—for example, land records and records of liens filed. Many others, including most court records, are also public. Material gathered by the government that was not initially created to be a public record falls into another major class of records. Personal records of this type include a person's file with the Federal Bureau of Investigation. The third major type of public record is not specific to a particular person. These fall into two categories: the general operational records of departments and agencies, and other records. The processes used to identify and obtain many of these records are similar.

In the past, because of the difficulty of examining the necessarily public records, some level of privacy existed. A person may need to see whether a piece of property has a pre-existing lien before buying the property or whether a company has a lien before doing business with it, but the storage of property or business records, generally with a town clerk or the secretary of a state, ensured against frivolous examination. With the advent of computerized records, it became much easier for people to search records; however, since most governments rely on private companies to distribute their records and users must often pay to search them, some level of privacy has been retained at some cost to access. Because the money to be made in this field is generally with newer records, researchers must often use archival resources as described in chapter 8 to view older records of this type.

Chapter 5 covered finding case files, and that discussion holds true here as well. Researchers will find recent materials at a court clerk's office while older information may be at an archive or intentionally or unintentionally destroyed. Most courts and archives will organize their files by docket number, although they may have an index by main party name.

For research purposes, the material that the government creates or collects can be considered in two categories: material that is available for the asking, and material that requires a request through the Freedom of Information Act (FOIA).

Generally, the material a governmental organ generates in its day-to-day activities will eventually be stored at the National Archives. Most of this can be examined upon request and copies can be made. In this class, some of the most often requested or most important material may be published online or released on microform (see chapter 8 about archival research methods). If information has been previously published, researchers may obtain it fairly easily and inexpensively. But the more esoteric the information, the more difficult it may be to acquire.

The second class of information requires a FOIA request for access. The organ of government with control over the information will determine which information meets the criteria of the request and whether it can be released. The researcher wishing to make a request must first determine which agency has control of the information. It is usually the agency that created the information or its successor, although a certain amount of the material transferred to the National Archives is still under the protection of FOIA. In that case, the request should go to the FOIA officer at the National Archives, not the agency's FOIA officer. Most of the organs of government have web pages devoted to explaining the FOIA process. Once a researcher has filed a request, the agency will respond within thirty days. However, the response may simply state that it has received the request and is working on it. The length of time from filing a request to receiving documents can vary widely. One should not rely on a quick turnaround in this process.

Research Example

Let us look for some articles about the codification movement and the civil law. A search for contemporary newspapers and periodicals will provide us with a sense of how the subject was

perceived outside of the legislatures. A search in *America's Historical Newspapers* can be limited by time period; searching for
the terms "codification" and "civil law" in newspapers published
between 1790 and 1860 yields only thirty-six articles. The most
obvious initial thought is that we should expand the search;
however, before changing the search terms, we should examine
our results.

The first article, from the November 26, 1824, edition of
the *New York Spectator,* is a review, on page 3, of Georgia governor George Troup's message to the Georgia legislature. The
author reviewed the speech because "it forms altogether the
strangest medley of absurdity and vapouring bravado, that we
have ever seen." After several paragraphs, the author notes the
governor's "hostility to the common law" and his recommendation to have it "Jeremy-Benthamized into a codification." In a
letter to the editor published in the *Charleston (S.C.) Courier*
on September 1, 1826, a correspondent identified as "Amphicon"
wrote about the civilizing effect of the civil law and expressed
hope for the adoption of the civil law. Further articles appear
in papers from Salem, Massachusetts (1836); Albany, New York
(1839, 1846–1847, 1857); New York City (1847); Columbus, Ohio
(1850); Washington, D.C. (1859); and Baltimore, Maryland
(1860).

A search in the *American Periodicals* database, which includes the many periodicals from 1740 to 1940, for the phrase
"civil law" and the term "codification" in any articles published
through 1859 returns sixty-nine documents. The earliest, from
the *Atlantic* magazine, is from May 1824; and the latest is from
1859. The May 1824 *Atlantic* article is a response to an address
to the Historical Society of New York by William Sampson on
December 6, 1823. The next article, the August 1, 1824, issue of
the *Atlantic* also contains a long essay titled "On the Substitution

of a Written Code, in the Place of the Common Law." The third article listed is from the April 1825 issue of the *North American Review*, and it contains a book review of the Napoleonic Code. Throughout the period, regular articles about codification appear in journals of particularly legal interest such as *American Jurist* and *Law Magazine* and in general-interest periodicals such as the *North American Review* and the *New York Review*. The articles provide insight into the debates about the nature of law as the U.S. legal system was organizing.

Important Sources Mentioned in This Chapter

ABC-Clio Information Services, and American Bibliographical Center. *America: History and Life.* Santa Barbara, CA: ABC-Clio, 1989.

Brigham, Clarence S. *History and Bibliography of American Newspapers, 1690–1820.* Worcester, MA: American Antiquarian Society, 1947.

British Library and Gale Group. *British Newspapers, 1600–1900.* Gale Group, 2007.

Cane, Peter, and Herbert M. Kritzer. *The Oxford Handbook of Empirical Legal Research.* Oxford: Oxford University Press, 2010.

Carter, Susan B. *Historical Statistics of the United States.* Cambridge: Cambridge University Press, 2006.

Chang, Yun-chien. *Empirical Legal Analysis: Assessing the Performance of Legal Institutions.* London: Routledge, 2014.

Epstein, Lee, and Andrew D. Martin. *An Introduction to Empirical Legal Research.* Oxford: Oxford University Press, 2014.

Epstein, Lee, Jeffrey Allan Segal, Harold J. Spaeth, and Thomas G. Walker. *The Supreme Court Compendium: Data, Decisions and Developments.* 6th ed. Thousand Oaks, CA: CQ Press, 2015.

Gerould, Winifred Gregory. *American Newspapers, 1821–1936: A Union List of Files Available in the United States and Canada.* New York: H. W. Wilson, 1937.

———. *International Congresses and Conferences, 1840–1937: A Union List of Their Publications Available in Libraries of the United States and Canada.* New York: H. W. Wilson, 1938.

Hindelang, Michael J., U.S. Bureau of Justice Statistics, U.S. National Criminal Justice Information and Statistics Service, Criminal Justice Research

Center, and Michael J. Hindelang Criminal Justice Research Center. *Sourcebook of Criminal Justice Statistics.* Washington, DC: GPO, 1973.

Leeuw, Frans L., and Hans Schmeets. *Empirical Legal Research: A Guidance Book for Lawyers, Legislators and Regulators.* Northampton, MA: Edward Elgar, 2016.

Library of Congress, National Endowment for the Humanities, and National Digital Newspaper Program (U.S.). *Chronicling America: Historic American Newspapers.* Washington, DC: Library of Congress, 2006.

United States Department of the Treasury, Bureau of Statistics, U.S. Department of Commerce and Labor, Bureau of Statistics, United States, et al. *Statistical Abstract of the United States.* Washington, DC: GPO, 1878.

Databases

Accessible Archives. *Accessible Archives: Primary Source Material from 18th and 19th Century Periodicals.* http://www.accessible-archives.com/.

Heritage World Archives. Newspaper Archive. https://newspaperarchive.com.

Inter-university Consortium for Political and Social Research (ICPSR). https://www.icpsr.umich.edu/icpsrweb/.

ProQuest. *American Periodicals Series.* https://www.proquest.com/products-services/aps.html.

———. *ProQuest Historical Newspapers.* https://www.proquest.com/products-services/pq-hist-news.html.

Readex. *America's Historical Newspapers.* http://www.readex.com/content/americas-historical-newspapers.

Spaeth, Harold J., National Science Foundation, and Washington University, eds. *The Supreme Court Database.* http://scdb.wustl.edu/.

United States Census Bureau. American FactFinder. https://factfinder.census.gov/faces/nav/jsf/pages/index.xhtml.

———. Various resources at Census Bureau website. https://www.census.gov/.

Index